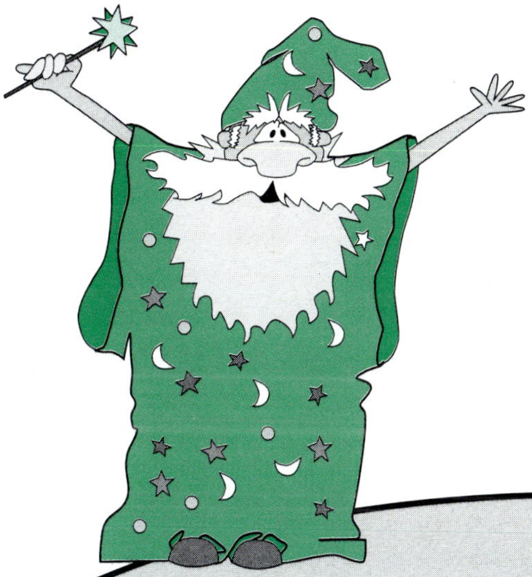

Instant Tools for Health Care Teams

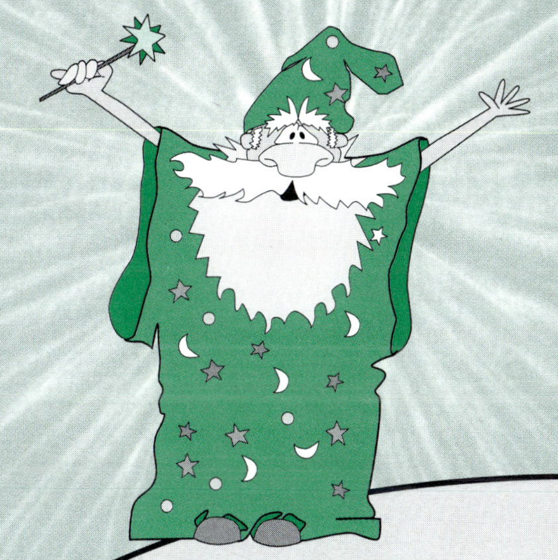

INSTANT TOOLS FOR HEALTH CARE TEAMS

Julia Balzer Riley, RN, MN

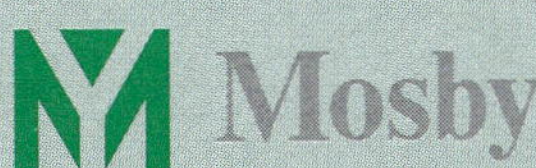

St. Louis Baltimore Boston Carlsbad Chicago Naples New York Philadelphia Portland
London Madrid Mexico City Singapore Sydney Tokyo Toronto Wiesbaden

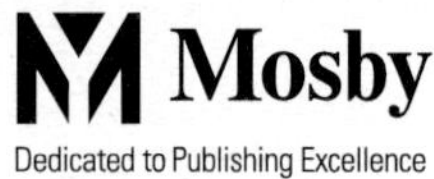

A Times Mirror
Company

Vice President and Publisher: Jacqueline Katz
Editor: Laurie Stahl
Developmental Editor: Barbara Watts
Editing, Production, and Design: Graphic World Publishing Services
Manufacturing Manager: Betty Richmond

Printed in the United States of America
Composition by Graphic World, Inc.
Lithography/color film by Graphic World, Inc.
Printing/binding by Mulligan Printing

Mosby–Year Book, Inc.
11830 Westline Industrial Drive
St. Louis, Missouri 63146

International Standard Book Number: 0-8151-5589-1

97 98 99 00 01 / 9 8 7 6 5 4 3 2 1

Julia Balzer Riley
RN, MN

Julia has worked in training and development, management development, and nursing education for more than twenty-five years. She received a diploma in nursing from Alexandria Hospital in Alexandria, Virginia; a bachelor of science degree in nursing from the University of Virginia in Charlottesville, Virginia; and a master's degree in psychiatric and mental health nursing from the University of Florida, in Gainesville, Florida. Julia has taught practical nursing students, diploma students, and baccalaureate and graduate nursing students. Julia has been a nurse entrepreneur for over twenty years as a consultant, workshop presenter, and writer. She writes home studies for nurses and other health care professionals through AKH Consultants, Inc., Jacksonville, Florida. She is a columnist writing for such publications as *Home Health Aide Digest, Florida Caregiver,* and the *North Georgia Star,* a local newspaper. Julia's first book, *Communications in Nursing,* was published by Mosby in 1996. Her book *Humor in the Workplace* was published by CSS in 1996. Julia has been listed in *Who's Who in Human Service Professionals, American Nursing,* and *Entrepreneurs.* Julia is president of Constant Source Seminars in Cumming, Georgia, and a member of the Adjunct Faculty at Brenau University in Gainesville, Georgia, where she teaches a management and leadership course to RN and BSN students.

Julia's mission is to engage people in the pursuit of commitment to survive, to thrive, and to grow in their professional and personal lives . . . and add humor and joy along the way.

Contributors

Enoch Albert, RN
Togus VAMC
Maine

Mila N. Baker, PhD
Director, Management Development and Organizational Development
Baptist Medical Center
Jacksonville, Florida

Kathy Beck, RN, MSN
Director of Case Management/Performance Improvement
St. Joseph Hospital
and Health Systems
Memphis, Tennessee

Deanna Berg
Co-founder
Innovation Strategies
Atlanta, Georgia

Camilla Bracewell, BS, MA
Director, Continuous Quality Improvement
Athens Regional Medical Center
Athens, Georgia

Frances Coltrane, RN, MSEd
Formerly Assistant Director for Clinical Programs
Northern Virginia Mental Health Institute
Falls Church, Virginia

Jaye Lynn Hall, RN
Director of Nursing Staff Development and Research
Children's Hospital of Oklahoma
Oklahoma City, Oklahoma

Cheri Kilian-Hoffer
Army Nurse
Kanohe, Hawaii

June Larrabee, PhD, RN
Assistant Professor
The University of Tennessee
QA/QI Manager
The University of Tennessee
Bowld Hospital
Memphis, Tennessee

Evelyn Lewis
Executive Secretary
Baptist Medical Center
Jacksonville, Florida

Duncan Moore
President and CEO
Tallahassee Memorial Regional Medical Center
Tallahassee, Florida

Joann Mulqueen
Chair, Department of
Cross-Disciplinary Studies
Iona College
Columbia School: Iona's College for Adults
New Rochelle, New York

Diane Raines, RN, MSN
Director of Corporate Development and Planning
Baptist Medical Center
Jacksonville, Florida

Peter Ramme, RN, CEN, CCRN
Owner
Idea Nurse
Santa Barbara, California

James T. Riley
Logistics and Transportation
U.S. Postal Service

Judy K. Scott, RN, MSN
Senior Assistant Administrator for Patient Services
St. Mary's Medical Center
Galesburg, Illinois

Contributors *continued*

Kathleen Shutrump, RNC, CNA
Woodside Hospital
Youngstown, Ohio

Judy Trawick, RN, BSN
Agency Operations Consultant
Simone Central, Inc.
Atlanta, Georgia

Julie Walters
Employee Relations Specialist
Columbus Regional
Columbus, Georgia

Beth Warner
Continuous Quality Improvement
Athens Regional Medical Center
Athens, Georgia

Reviewers

Camilla Bracewell, BS, MA
Director, Continuous Quality Improvement
Athens Regional Medical Center
Athens, Georgia

Michelle Deck, MEd, BSN, RN, ACCE-R
Senior Training Consultant
Creative Training Techniques International, Inc.
Edina, Minnesota;
Co-owner
Gimics and Mania Educate Staff (G.A.M.E.S.)
and
Tool Thyme for Trainers
Metairie, Louisiana

Rebecca Bouterie Harmon, RN, MN, CS
Instructor of Nursing
University of Virginia School of Nursing;
Clinical Nurse Specialist
Western State Hospital
Staunton, Virginia

Joyce Larson-Presswalla, RN, PhD
Assistant Professor
University of South Florida
College of Nursing
Tampa, Florida

Preface

BUILDING TEAMS TOGETHER

The Four M's

Teams can be Magical. Teams can be Mysterious. Teams can be Miserable. And if you are responsible for leading or facilitating teams, groups, meetings, or committees, they can be Mind-boggling. This book is written to give you strategies to move from misery to camaraderie, from mystery to an understanding of ways to help teams do their work, from a mind-boggling experience to the magic of injecting a little fun along the journey. Using the exercises in this book can help people in teams to relax, understand how teams work, do their best problem solving, and even look forward to team meetings.

The content we teach and the problems we have to solve change, but we are always working with people who long to be challenged, engaged, stimulated, and, yes, sometimes even entertained! Working in training and development and management development for thirteen years, I have had tremendous response to creative and humorous touches to meetings and educational offerings. Managers would request ideas to engage staff in problem-solving meetings, retreats, and celebrations.

My goal in writing this book is to offer a variety of easy-to-use activities that will help you add energy and fun to teamwork. Dare to be outrageous! Some people will be unsure of what you are trying to accomplish. For this reason, pay close attention to tips for debriefing activities. Evaluate how activities are received, and ask for feedback. Make notes so you can customize the exercises and modify them to suit your setting. Set the expectation that we can work together efficiently and yet still have fun. Use exercises on team dynamics to help team members understand the stages of teams and behaviors to expect. Encourage staff to add their own ideas for energizers, team celebrations, and funny or everyday examples to better understand quality improvement teams. I invite you to come out and play.

Acknowledgments

Thank you to Jackie Katz, Continuing Education, Mosby, who envisioned this book and invited me to write it, and to Laurie Stahl, whose description of the task intrigued me. To Barb Watts, Continuing Education, thank you for the delightful idea to use a magical theme, our great discussions about where to put the wizard, and all the detail work to make a finished product. Thank you to all the contributors who generously and with great enthusiasm shared their own work; it is a thrill to see your name and work in print. To the best of our knowledge, all these activities are original or the source is unknown.

To my husband, Jim, thank you for your enthusiasm and support of my work. To Sneakers and Dice, my very own feline alarm clocks, thanks for all the friendly visits and computer keyboard tap dancing.

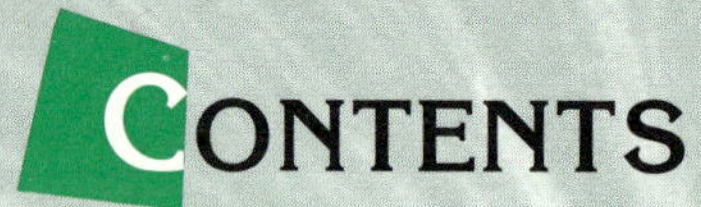

CONTENTS

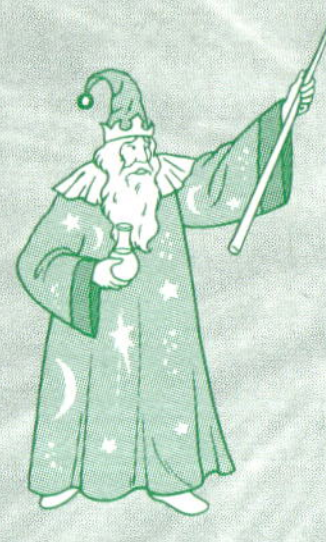

Part 1 Teaching Tips from the Wizard

Part 2 Getting Started

Part 3 Teaching Team Dynamics

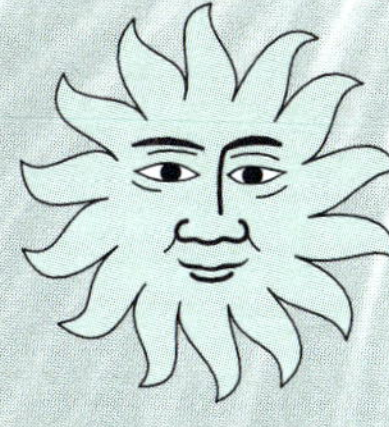

Part 6 Energizers

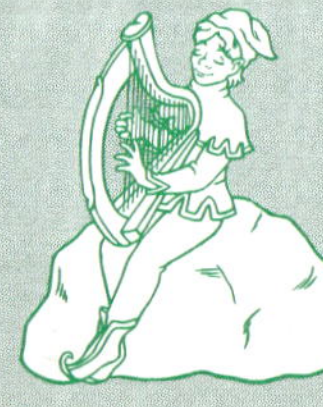

Part 7 Rewards and Recognition

Activities in this book are original or from an unknown source.

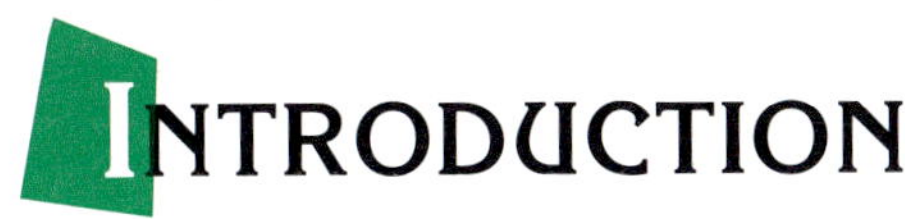

INTRODUCTION

The Real World, Or, Why Read This Book Anyway?

Perhaps you've been at this a while and may be remembering some teams for which the journey was not smooth, the people resented the assignment, and, even when working, the progress seemed slow and tedious. Or, perhaps you are new to the world of teams and want some tips to get started. Both of you are in the right place. These activities will help you liven up the process of working with people. They will help you honor differences in people's styles of working together.

The Challenge of Teams

Have you ever been given a tough assignment and told it was a "challenge"? Have you ever been assigned a difficult patient and been assured the work was "interesting"? You may have received these words with a sparkle in your eye and wheels turning in your mind, ready to give the situation your best shot. Whereas others may hear sarcasm and take a cynical view of fancy ways to say "hard work" or "you get to handle the worst assignment."

The challenge to the health care environment today is how to give quality care in a cost-effective way. This leads to new ways of looking at work and at the staff who perform the work. Consider how we enter this new era. Health care professionals have spent years developing an area of specialization and previously had been given almost free rein financially to buy the best equipment, practice the latest technology, and submit the bill to a private payer. Formal education or on-the-job training has led to a certain pride in independent practice. Departmental pride has driven work units.

But what is happening now? There are changes in how much money there is to spend—managed care with capitation, a way of budgeting expenses by allowing a fixed amount of money for providers for each client. There are changes in the composition of staff—staff reductions by attrition or layoffs, a change in the skill mix. There are changes in the nature of work—redesign has led to combining positions and cross-training to minimize the number of people with whom the client has contact. And there are changes in how staff work together—self-directed work teams and continuous quality improvement teams emphasize rewards for people working together rather than independently.

How does this affect staff? People are faced with rapid change, uncertainty about what their work will look like, what skills they will need for reinvented positions, and concerns about how they will be recognized for a job well done. If they work in teams, what will happen if everyone does not bring equal skill and commitment to the team effort? What does it mean to work smarter not harder? Is it an oxymoron?

This is the climate in which teams are being formed. Trust has been eroded. People are tired and frightened. The good news is that staff are in need of people who can stay open to change, who can model a positive attitude, and who will invest some energy in adding a bit of humor and creativity to the process of working together.

The Magic Wand

Don't you love a little something extra in life? The magic wand that accompanies this book is to add a magic touch to your work and to the activities in this book. Make it a part of your bag of wizard's magic tricks, your toolbox, for teams. I have distributed thousands of these wands to workshop participants around the country. Responses have been touching, heartwarming, wild, and exciting. We all need a bit of sparkle added to our lives. Thanks to the Continuing Education staff at Mosby who supported my request for this gift to you, for other Mosby staff who did a little something extra to honor such a request, and to you for having the courage to use it!

USE YOUR MAGIC WAND TO:

- Encourage participation—Place the magic wand in the center of the table; whenever there is a tense moment, any team member may pick up the wand and wave it over the group to lighten the tension.
- Request information—A gentle tap on the shoulder identifies the expert. "I dub you the pro. What do you think about this issue?"
- Relieve stress—"Abracadabra, we're fresh and ready to go."
- Stimulate creative thinking—Have team members pass it from one to another to start the ideas rolling.

The wizard's magic wand has touched each instructor's page to highlight key information and to provide a quick review of the exercises.

Look for the following magical icons:

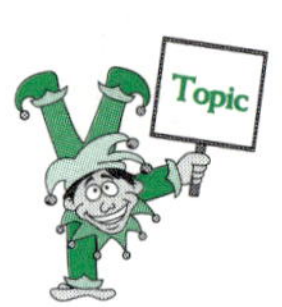

Exercise goal

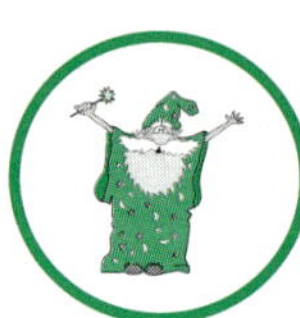
Tools needed to implement this exercise

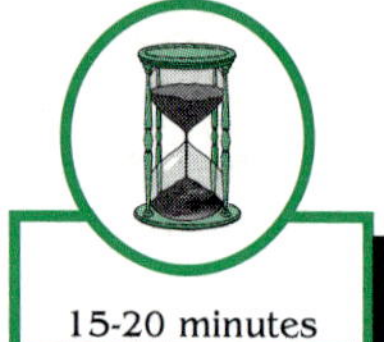

Time required

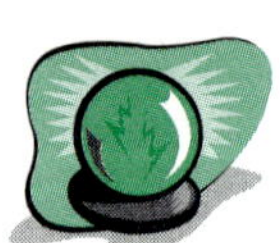
Debriefing

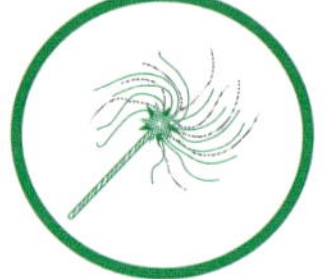
Suggestions that can provide a magic touch

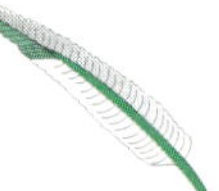
Reproducible pages

Your Mission . . . Should You Choose to Accept It

- To take the risk to be considered a person with a positive attitude.
- To be willing to try some activities with confidence—remember an old behavioral principle, you get what you expect.
- To be ready to evaluate what works and what doesn't and modify strategies to keep on keeping on.
- To set a goal to move teams from misery to the magic of working on problems and creating solutions that will provide improved quality care to clients and increase job satisfaction for staff.

Consider sharing your own activities and strategies for teams and meetings so we can build this book together. Your invitation to participate in the next edition is located at the end of this book.

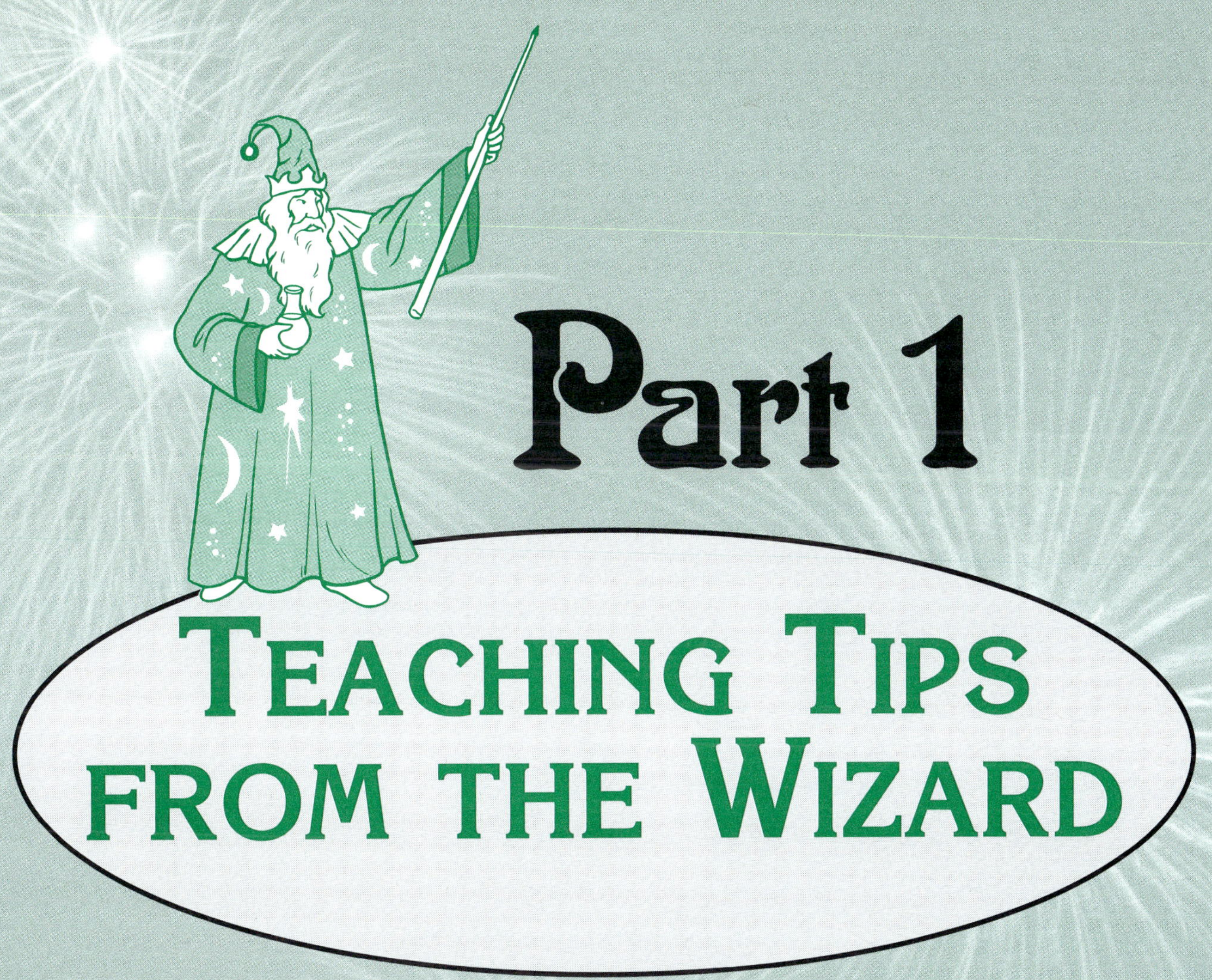

Part 1

Teaching Tips from the Wizard

Teaching tips give you strategies to add a magic touch to your work, to exceed your customers' expectations. Think of other staff as your internal customers. We spend many hours of our lives at work, too many to allow work to be serious all the time or boring. Use these tips to set the expectations that people are valued and work can be fun. Creative solutions to problems—here we come!

Abracadabra!

THE WIZARD'S MAGICAL TRAVELING TOOL KIT

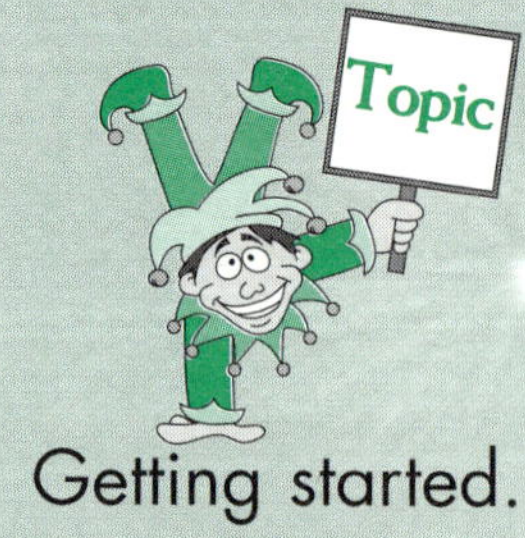

Getting started.

Consider collecting frequently used items to build a Wizard's Magical Traveling Tool Kit! Take your magical tool kit to each team meeting. Choose a convenient, easy-to-carry container for a tool kit, such as a toolbox, a make-up box, a beach bag, or a tote bag.

Tool Kit

Suggested items for a Wizard's Magical Traveling Tool Kit include:

The magic wand that accompanies this book
Scented markers
Colored markers
Colored Post-it Notes
Masking tape
Scotch tape
Scissors
Stapler
Pens and pencils
Whistles and noisemakers
Small toys to give away
Stickers and gold stars for agendas
A clown nose for tough times
A Koosh ball
Bubbles
Index cards (2 colors)

THE ART AND PLEASURE OF TEACHING

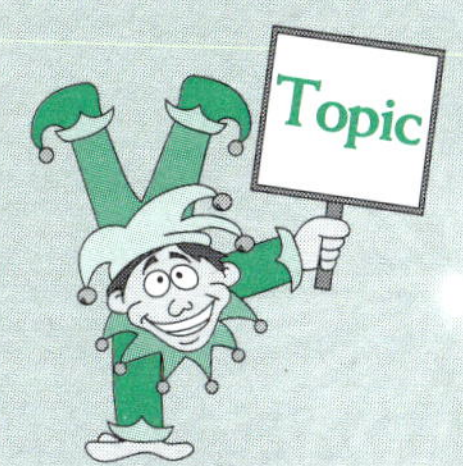

Thoughts for your reflection.

First Things First

- Use simple teaching whenever possible.
- Share your enthusiasm about work. It's contagious.

Keep Your Perspective

- Reframe problems as part of the story or issue that is missing. Consider yourself a detective whose goal is to solve a mystery rather than a problem, which may have a more negative connotation.
- Enter into the context of another's life. Health care employees come from different perspectives and different lives. Attend an event sponsored by another department in order to get to know them.
- Volunteer with other employees and observe them in a different setting. Several hospitals in Jacksonville, Florida, built houses for Habitat for Humanity. Another hospital has an annual bass tournament. Go to a community event of another culture represented in your staff.
- Take time to ask staff and volunteers to tell you about their work. Arrange to spend a few hours with employees from different departments to see their point of view.

Love a Challenge

- Treat each participant with respect. If a participant is angry, maintain your composure. Respect is a must, even under fire.
- Admit when you do not know an answer.

- Defer problematic questions by saying that is an interesting issue.
- Ask team members what they need to do their work.
- Ask the team members for their ideas.
- Ask for feedback. "What would make this meeting a better experience?"
- Listen to your instincts about the class's response to content or a member's involvement or lack of it. Deal with it.
- Refocus frequently on the goal of teams—to provide quality, cost-effective health care for the clients and families who have entrusted themselves to us.
- Keep your sense of humor about your own imperfections, and keep your sense of wonder about life and the client and family experience in health care.

Do Something Extra

- Provide extra reading material, articles that may be of interest. When you find a cartoon or an article that reminds you of someone on the team, give it to that person.
- Let your example be a teacher in a group setting.

Last but Certainly Not Least

- Have balance in your own life. Renew your energy outside the work setting so your life's meaning is more than work.

SOMEONE REMEMBERED MY BIRTHDAY

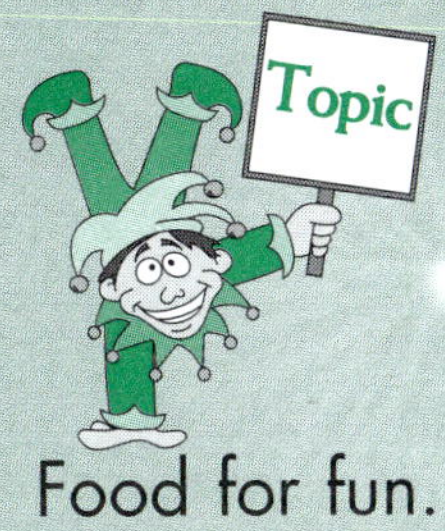

Food for fun.

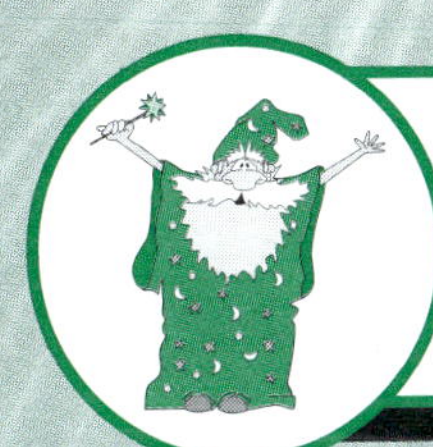

Wizard List List of birthdays of team members; birthday cake, cupcakes, or ice cream birthday cake; a birthday banner; noisemakers and hats, if desired

Preparation

1. Obtain birthday supplies listed above. Save extra paper products for the next celebration.
2. Consider buying superhero items or a theme you can relate to the team. Make your own, such as "Super Team Man of the Day" or "Quality Queen for the Day."
3. Make and hang a computer banner or a sign.

Implementation

1. Pick the team meeting day closest to the birthday. If no birthdays are on the horizon and the team needs a lift, have an "Unbirthday" party.
2. Sing "Happy Birthday" or "Happy Unbirthday to Us."
3. Serve refreshments.

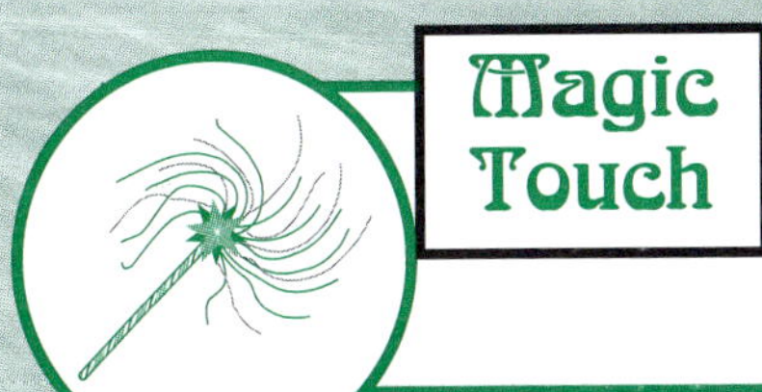

Magic Touch We all are unique contributors to the team, and a shared birthday celebration is a way of recognizing this.

IT'S A HOLIDAY—CELEBRATE!

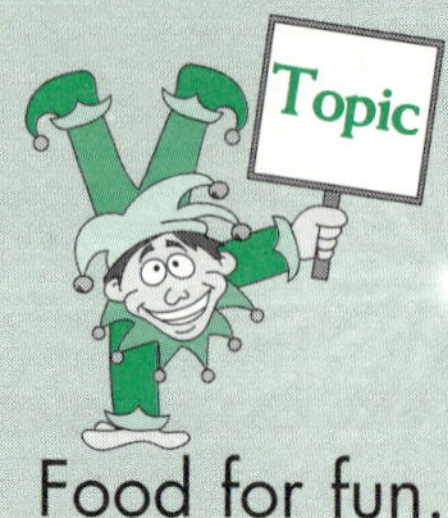

Food for fun.

Wizard List Refreshments of your choice, such as seasonal foods, decorated cookies (hearts for Valentine's Day, shamrocks for St. Patrick's Day), king cake near Mardis Gras, Easter bunny cake, ice cream cones for the first week of spring, popsicles for the first week of summer, ethnic foods for holidays from other cultures (check with team members or employees from other cultures for ideas); eating utensils; plates; napkins; beverages and ice; cups; garbage bag for clean-up

Preparation

1. Select the holiday.
2. Obtain food of choice.

Implementation

1. Serve with a smile. The celebration will be a welcome break in the routine.

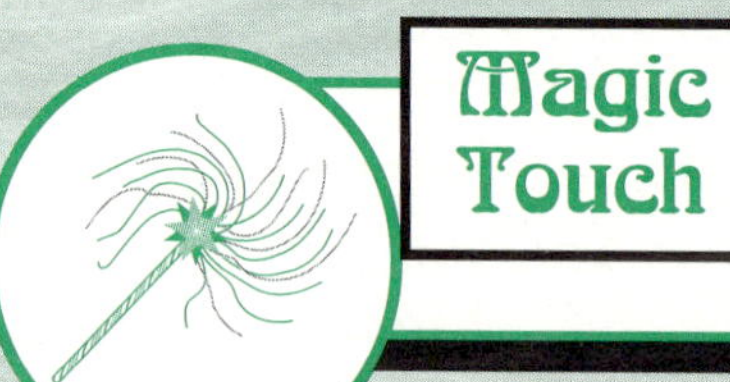

Interrupt a slump with an unexpected treat.

THE MUNCHIES

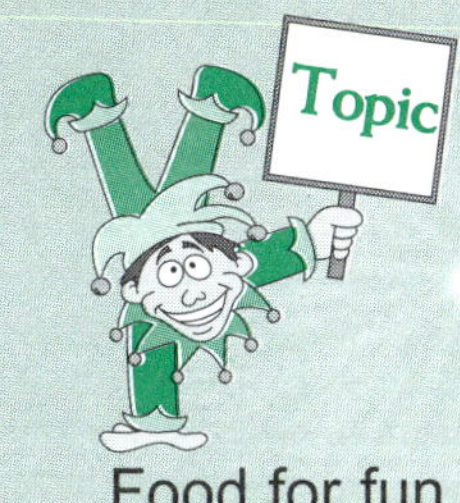

Food for fun.

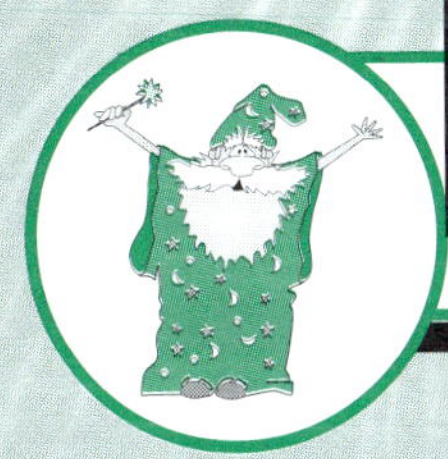

Wizard List

Popcorn, M & M's, or other light snacks; serving bowls (optional)

Preparation

1. Obtain snack food.
2. Provide serving bowls (optional).

Implementation

1. Serve the snacks and delight the crowd.

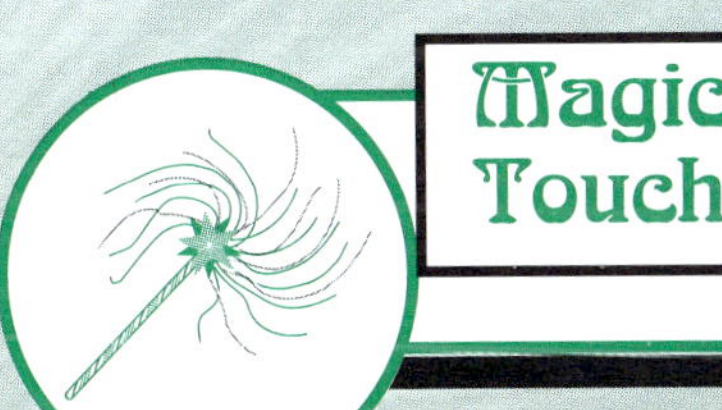

Magic Touch

Sharing food does more than feed the body.

By: Cheri Kilian-Hoffer

ELECTRONIC MOTIVATION

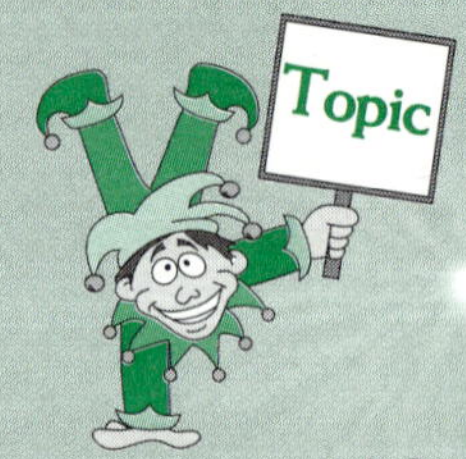

Use for fun and to give spirits a lift.

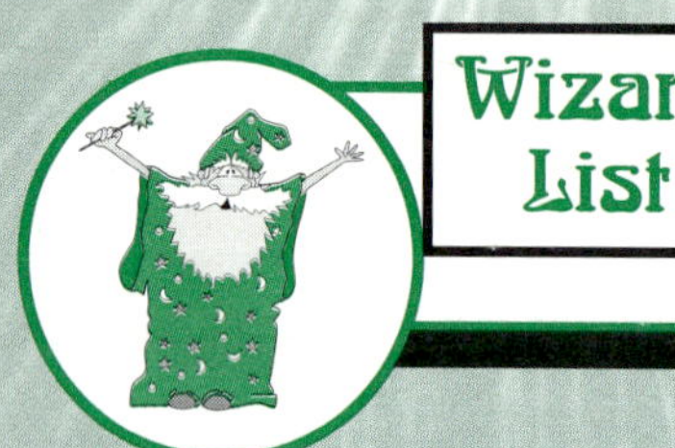

Wizard List

Access to E-mail

Preparation

1. Collect motivational sayings, and devise a play on words with the content of the message.

Implementation

1. Fill the airways with your charm. If you use E-mail for meeting notification or other memos, brighten the receiver's day with a motivational message or funny note at the end of each E-mail message.

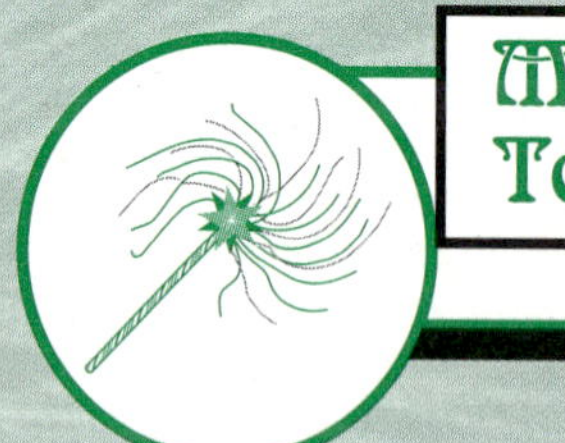

Magic Touch

Make a regular mailing list to save time.

By: Cheri Kilian-Hoffer

CELEBRATE THE DAY

Or, We Don't Have To Bore Our Class

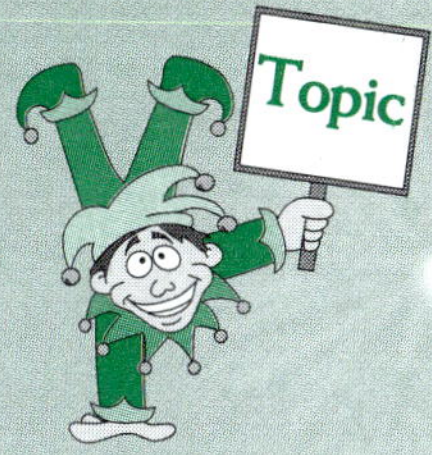

Use to add a creative touch to team training.

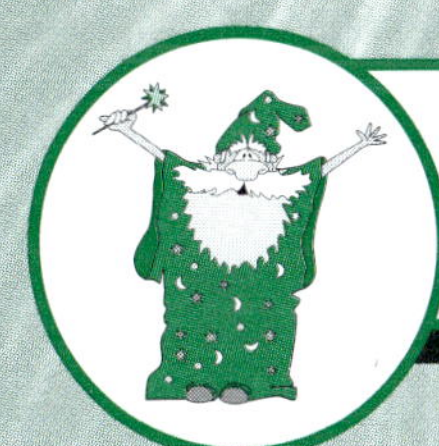

Wizard List

"Celebrate the Day" list, decorations and refreshments with a theme

Preparation

1. Select an appropriate holiday, or make up an occasion.

Implementation

1. Decorate the classroom for either a holiday that is commonly known or an obscure one, or have an "unholiday-but-everyday-is-special" day.
2. Use festive paper plates and napkins for refreshments.

Magic Touch

Team training and quality improvement training can be welcome or suspect. Staff may be assigned to training when they have other work priorities. When you teach, your class is your internal customer. You provide good customer service to them by being competent in your content and presentation modalities. Value-added customer service is to honor their need for an enjoyable, comfortable learning environment. Also, keep in mind that a little decorating adds a lot of pizzazz to any training session.

CELEBRATE 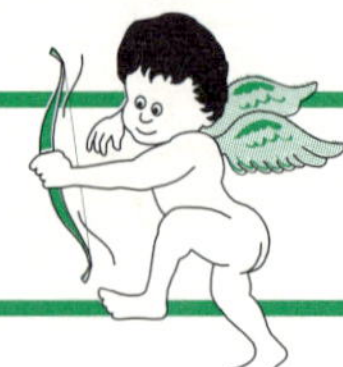 THE DAY

January 1	New Year's Day
January 9	Sherlock Holmes' birthday, 1854
February 14	Valentine's Day
March 2	Dr. Seuss' birthday, 1904
March 17	St. Patrick's Day
April 1	April Fool's Day
May 1	May Day
June 14	Flag Day
July 4	Independence Day
August 13	Alfred Hitchcock's birthday, 1899
September 8	Star Trek's first episode, 1966
October 31	Halloween
December 5	Walt Disney's birthday, 1901

Add your own!

It's Transparent

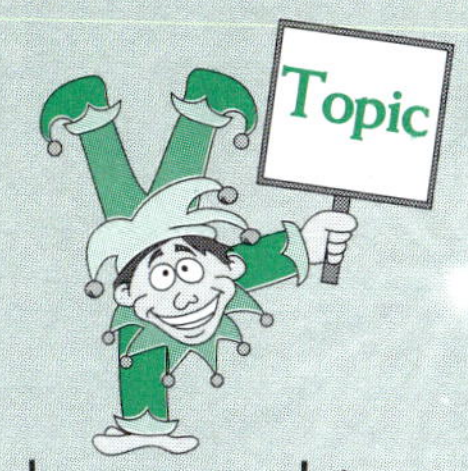

Use to add a creative touch to teaching.

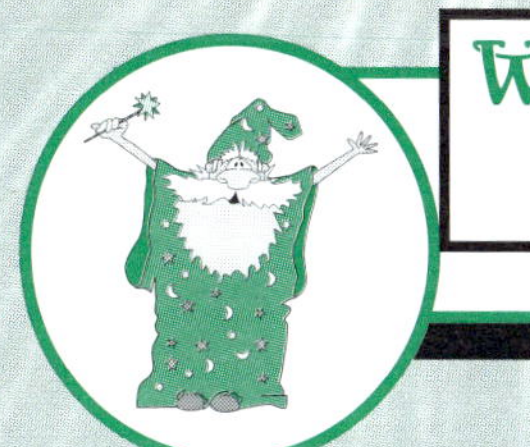

Wizard List

"Many Faces" worksheet, markers, transparency sheets

Preparation

1. Review "Many Faces" worksheet to select the face or faces you want to use.

Implementation

1. Make a transparency of each face on a separate transparency, placing the face in one corner so you can use it over other transparencies with content.
2. Collect your own clip art and make your own "Content Connector" transparencies.

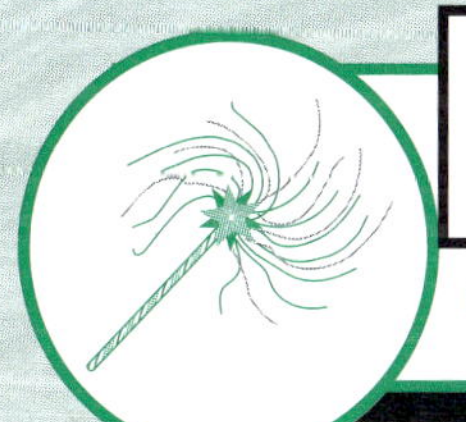

Magic Touch

When teaching content of team dynamics or tools, or presenting data, use simple faces to capture the team's attention or refocus their attention as minds wander.

Inspired by: Evelyn Lewis

MANY FACES

Wow!
Yikes!
Tough
Well, maybe
Don't bore me
What?
Suspicious
Terrified
Here we go again
Try your own
OK, I'm thinking about it

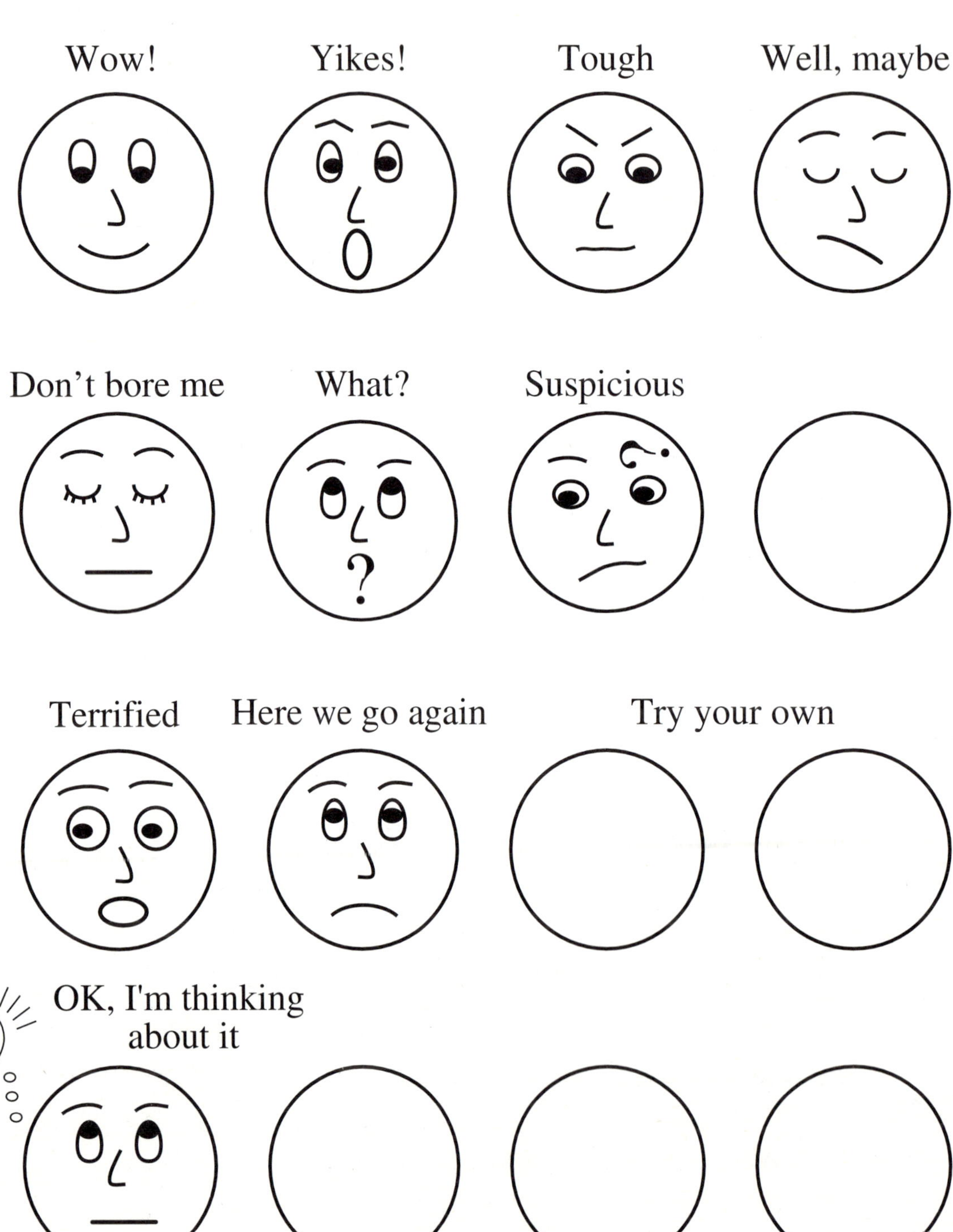

RING THE BELL

Fighting the Tangential Temptation

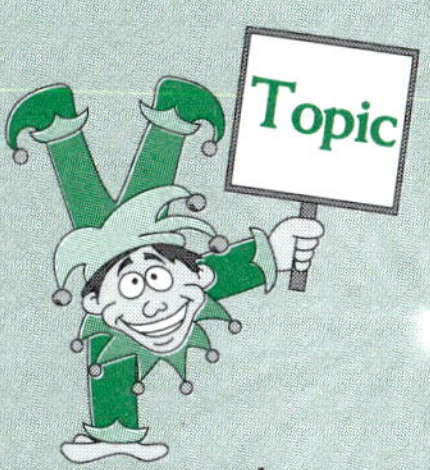

Focus reminder. Use if team members have difficulty staying on the subject.

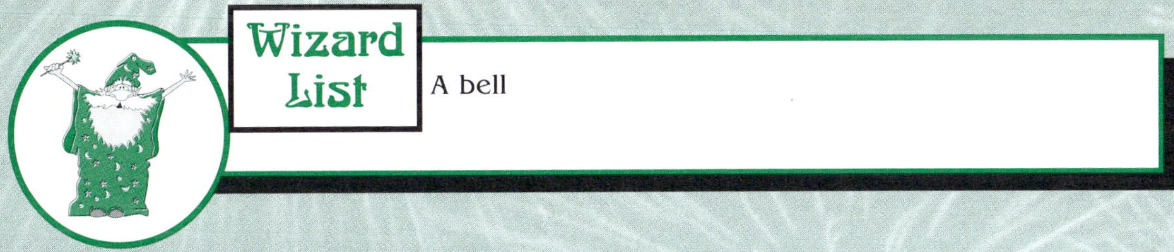

Wizard List

A bell

Preparation

1. Obtain a bell.
2. Make mental notes of the bell's purpose.

Implementation

1. Ring the bell and explain that the bell can be a useful tool to gently refocus the group when team members are tempted to wander from the problem to be solved or when the group needs to refocus.
2. Explain that if the team agrees to use the bell, it will be brought to each team meeting. Any team member can ring it when the group is getting off task.

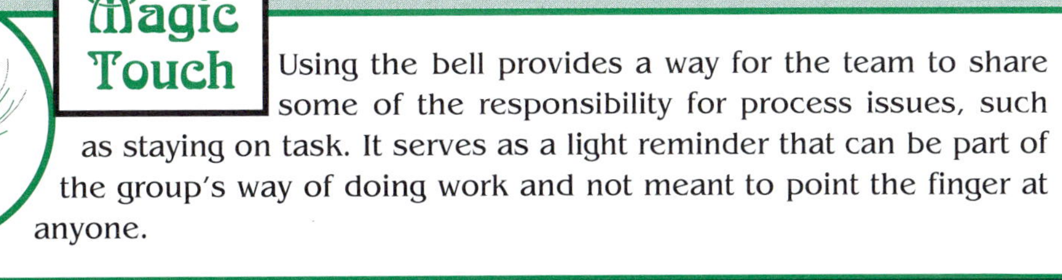

Magic Touch

Using the bell provides a way for the team to share some of the responsibility for process issues, such as staying on task. It serves as a light reminder that can be part of the group's way of doing work and not meant to point the finger at anyone.

By: Frances Coltrane, RN, MSEd

Lateness Does Not Pay!

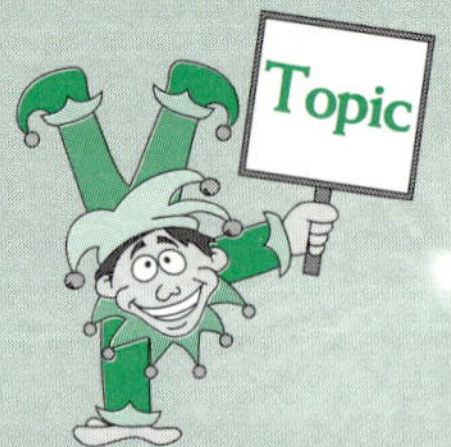

The importance of time. Use to encourage arriving on time.

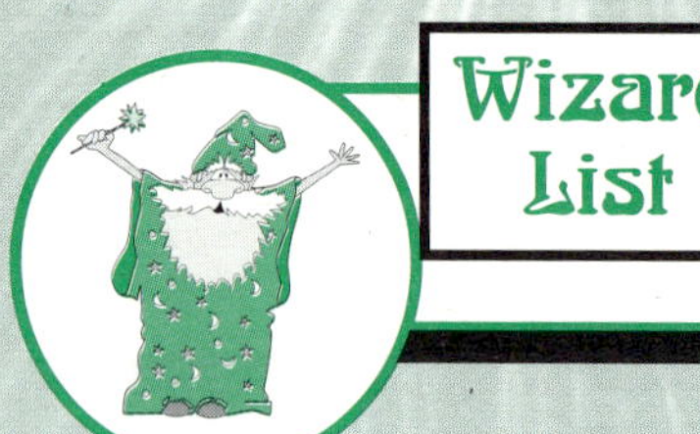

Wizard List

No supplies needed

Preparation

1. Make mental notes for discussion on the importance of being on time.

Implementation

1. Explain to the group that starting on time is important to honor the task at hand and the time of all members.

Magic Touch

Setting team norms will help establish positive group dynamics. To serve as a gentle reminder of the importance of being on time, the *last one in has to take the minutes!* (Use this when the duties of recorder are rotated.)

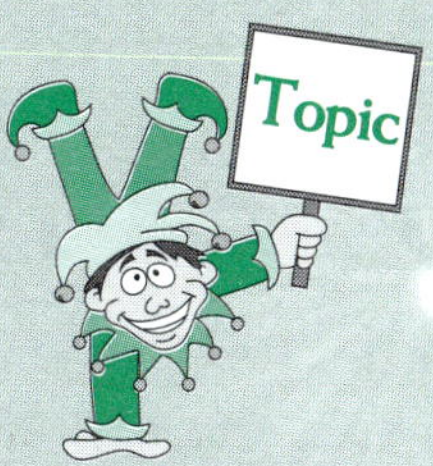

Use to add a creative touch to team training.

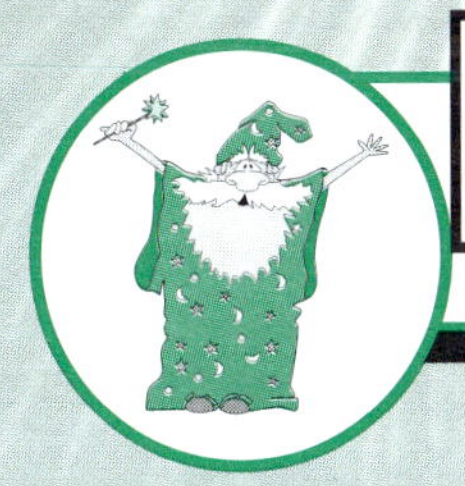

Wizard List

"Coach Talk," flip chart, marker

Preparation

1. Select a quote from "Coach Talk."
2. Write the quote on a flip chart.

Implementation

1. Display the selected quote from "Coach Talk" on the flip chart in front of the room or directly outside the meeting room entrance.
2. Mention the quote and apply it to the training session, if appropriate.

Magic Touch

Check the library for other quote sources. People come to expect these and are influenced by them in surprising ways. Do you ever look for quotes on a business or church sign as a pick-me-up? Or, make up your own quotes.

COACH TALK

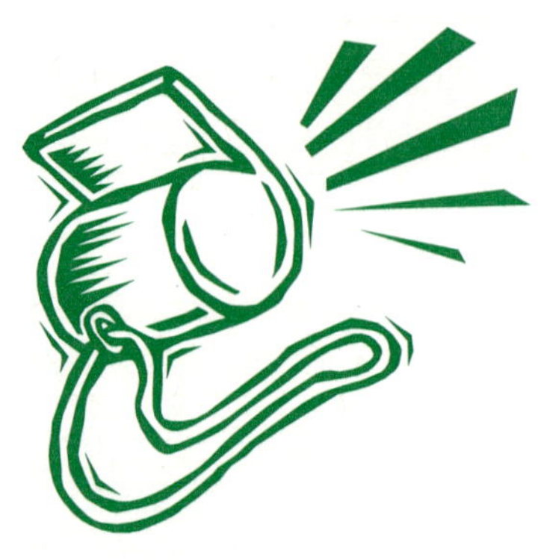

"In baseball and in business, there are three types of people. Those who make it happen, those who watch it happen, and those who wonder what happened."

—Tommy Lasorda
Former manager, Los Angeles Dodgers

"Do what is right, do the best you can, and treat others like you want to be treated. First we will be best, then we will be first."

—Lou Holtz
Former football coach, Notre Dame

"If you accept losing, you can't win."

—Vince Lombardi
Former football coach, Green Bay Packers

"There is no substitute for work. It is the price of success."

—Earl Blaik
Former football coach, West Point

(Martin, 1993.)

CHOOSING THE AMUSING

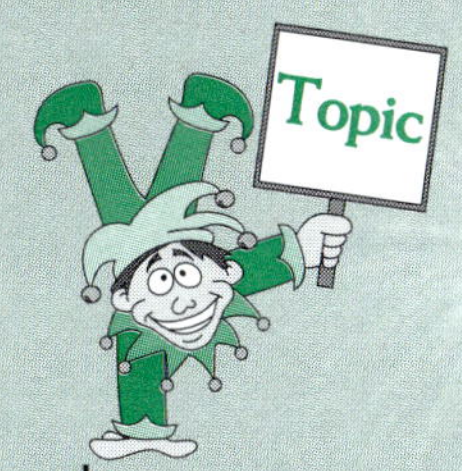

Tradition. Use to personalize a team.

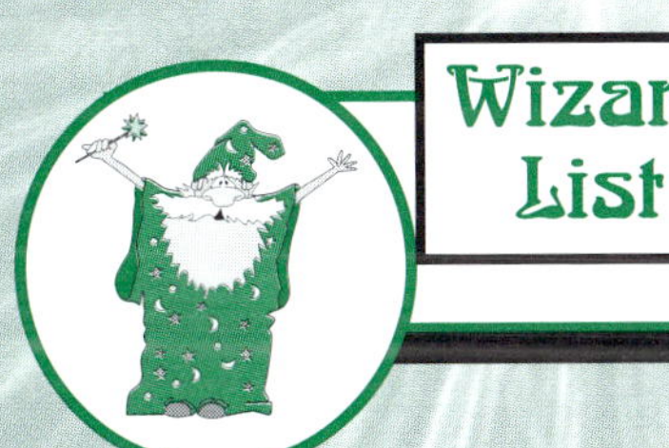

Wizard List

No supplies needed

Preparation

1. Pay attention in team meetings to one-liners used by teams or funny off-handed comments that can be reintroduced during tough times. You are looking for comments that become a recognized part of that team's history.

Implementation

1. Listen for such comments.
2. Remark on them at the time to reinforce appropriate use of humor.
3. Reintroduce comments, giving the original speaker credit. For example, one team working on customer service came up with the word *fussified* to identify an irritated customer; the team worked to decrease *fussified* behavior. In another case, one nurse while working on the team's mission statement had a sudden "Ah ha" and said, "Is this 'What's it all about, Alfie?'"

   You can introduce one-liners, too. When a team member demonstrates special talent, dub him or her the "Guru," such as the "Guru of Data Collection" or the "Flow Chart Meister."

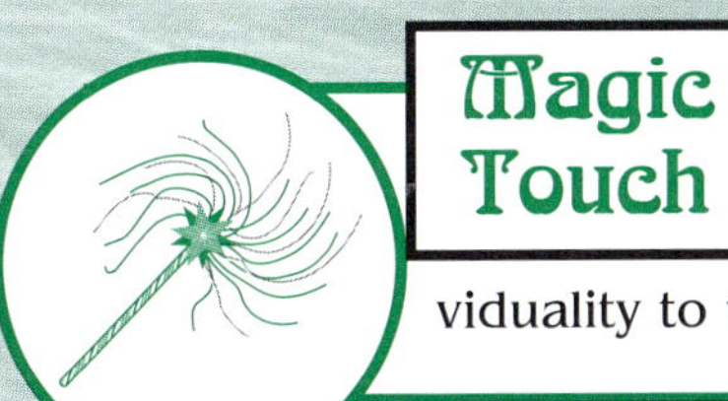

Magic Touch

Allowing a team to create unique terms or words inspires creativity and brings a sense of their own individuality to the group.

TAKE ME TO YOUR LEADER

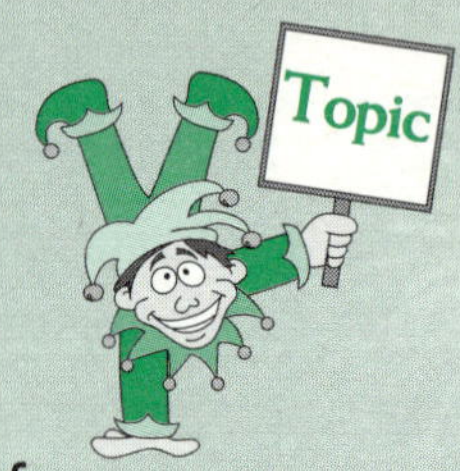

Use to choose a leader for an activity.

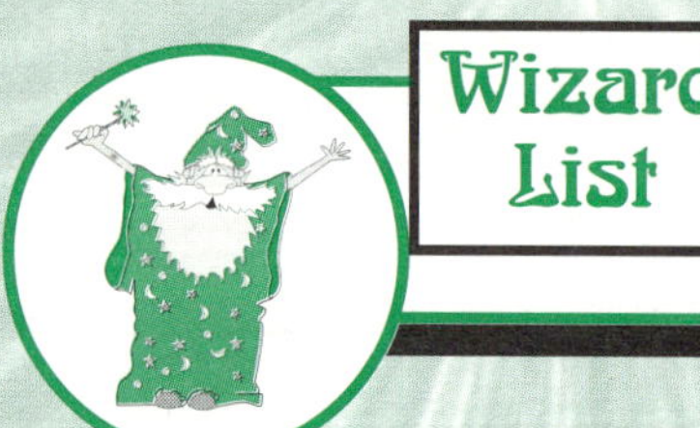

Wizard List

No supplies needed

Preparation

None

Implementation

To select a leader for an activity or who goes first in a small group activity try one of the following activities:

1. The leader is the team member who graduated from the largest, or the smallest, high school class.
2. The team member who looks most like the President of the United States goes first.
3. Everyone is asked to point at the same time to the team member who should be the leader. Whoever is chosen most often is the leader or goes first. Or, the team member sitting to the right of the selected member is the leader or goes first.
4. The leader is the team member who travels the farthest to work.
5. The leader is the team member with the most recent speeding ticket.
6. The leader is the team member with the shortest hair.

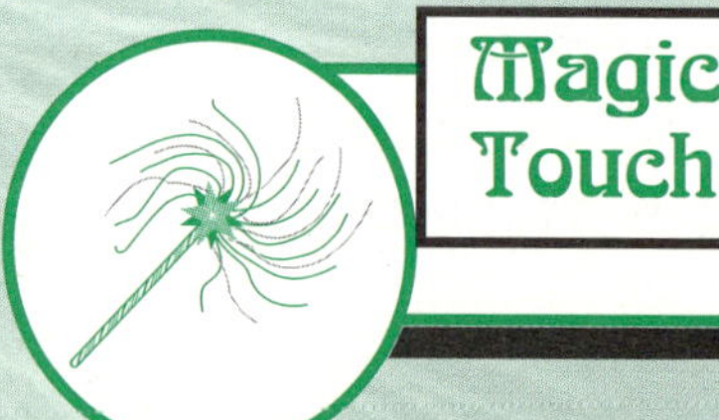

Magic Touch

Nonthreatening, novel ways to choose leaders can lighten the process and share the responsibilities.

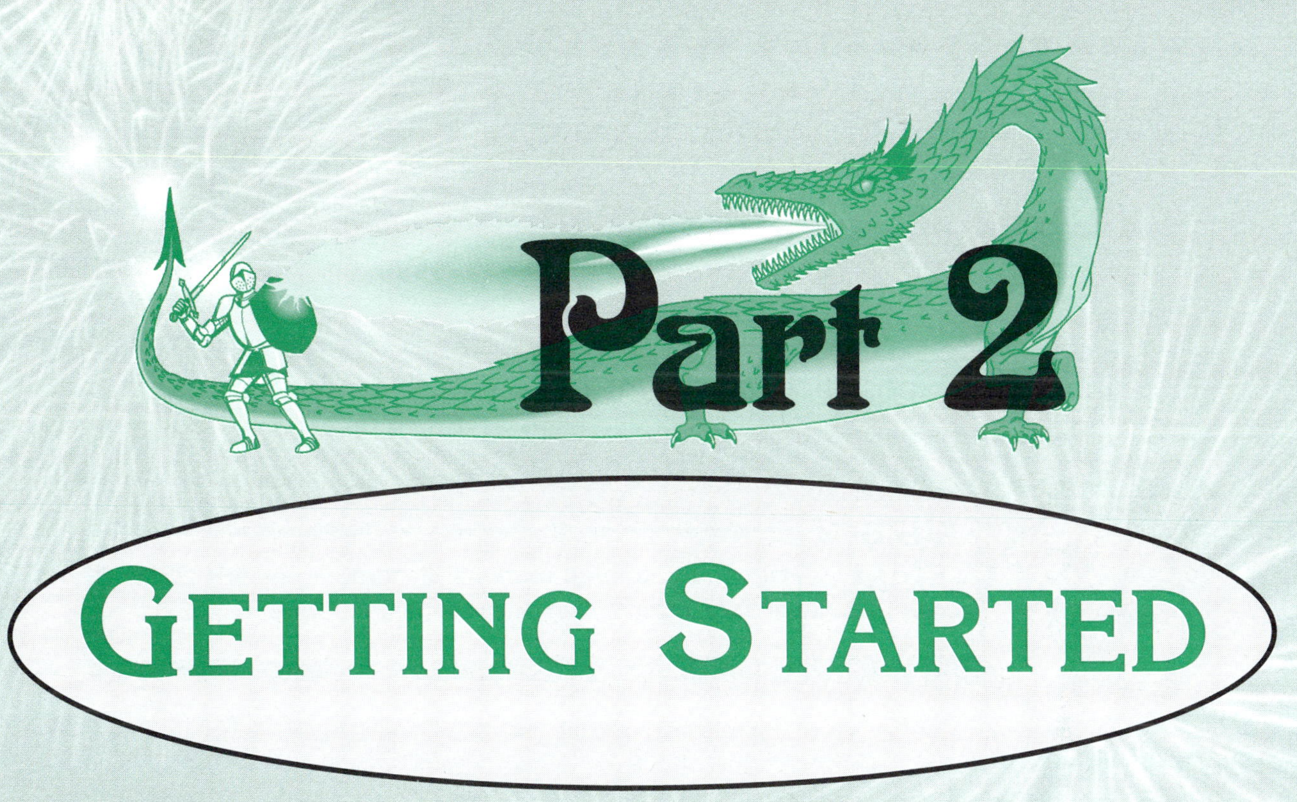

Part 2

Getting Started

Think of a time when you were assigned to attend a new committee or arrived at the first meeting of a new team. What were your concerns? Did you bring with you memories of past uncomfortable experiences? What were your expectations?

What have you heard and read about teams? Some people cringe at the word. Others, with positive experiences, enter eagerly into a new team. Some think of teams as boring and uninspired, another dreaded committee! Teams don't have to be dull! Staff welcome an opportunity to work together when someone has the courage and creativity to lighten the meetings and energize the team players. This book provides a variety of exercises to use at various stages of team development and to deal with a variety of impasses or slow times.

Perhaps you have been selected to facilitate a quality improvement team or you are managing staff that needs to become a team to solve problems together more efficiently. This first section of the book provides exercises to get started in a positive direction, to learn more about the people on the team and the experiences they bring with them to a team that may influence their work. Try some of the following exercises to get your team meeting started off in a positive direction!

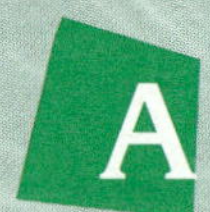

A TALE OF TWO TEAMS

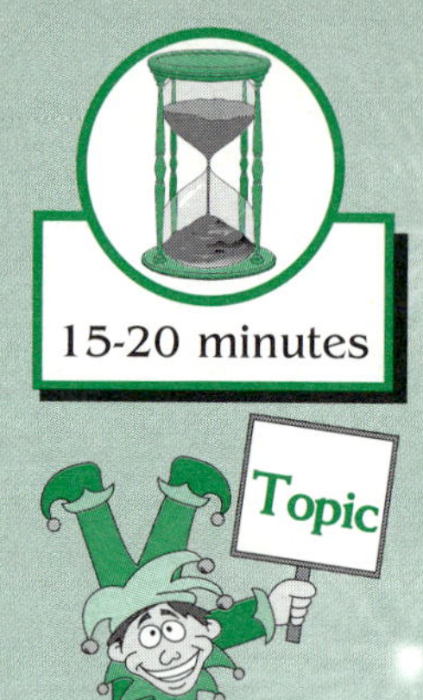

"It Was the Worst of Teams, It Was the Best of Teams" . . . with Apologies to Charles Dickens

Team member expectations. Use this at an early meeting to learn about past team experience.

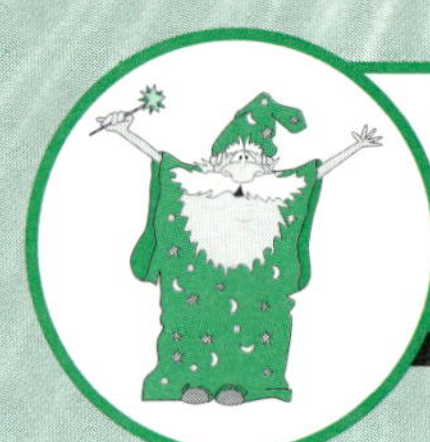

Wizard List

Flip chart, colored markers, decorated pencils, "Tale of Two Teams," index cards (two colors)

Preparation

1. Before the meeting, write the title of this exercise on a flip chart to display at the front of the meeting room.
2. Copy "A Tale of Two Teams" and affix it to the flip chart or make a poster or a transparency.
3. Write "The Worst of Teams" on one flip chart page and "The Best of Teams" on another page.

Implementation

1. Welcome the members to the team.
2. Ask members to think about other meetings, committees, or teams they have experienced. Give them 60 seconds.
3. Invite team members to share these experiences in order to build a better team. Distribute one index card in each color and a pen or pencil to each member. Ask members to use one color (specify which color) to briefly list things they have found nonproductive or not liked in former teams or meetings, such as lateness or no agenda. Ask members to use the other colored card to list things they liked or found useful. Ask team members to consider what helps them make their best contribution to a team. Allow 3 to 5 minutes.

4. Collect the cards and ask for two volunteers each to take one color of cards, review the cards briefly, and write the answers on the appropriate flip chart.

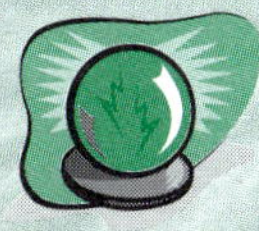

Debriefing

Lead a discussion of the ideas and ask team members to think about how this information could be used to establish ground rules for the team. Keep the information and share it again when the team writes their ground rules. Thank team members for their participation and tell them that the pencils are theirs to keep to remind them that the team is in their hands.

Magic Touch

If you decide to distribute decorated pencils, you might choose pencils that fit the theme of the debriefing, such as pencils with stars ("Each of you is a star in this production.") or with a seasonal design if the meeting is close to a holiday ("We celebrate holidays and we celebrate the initiation of a successful team.").

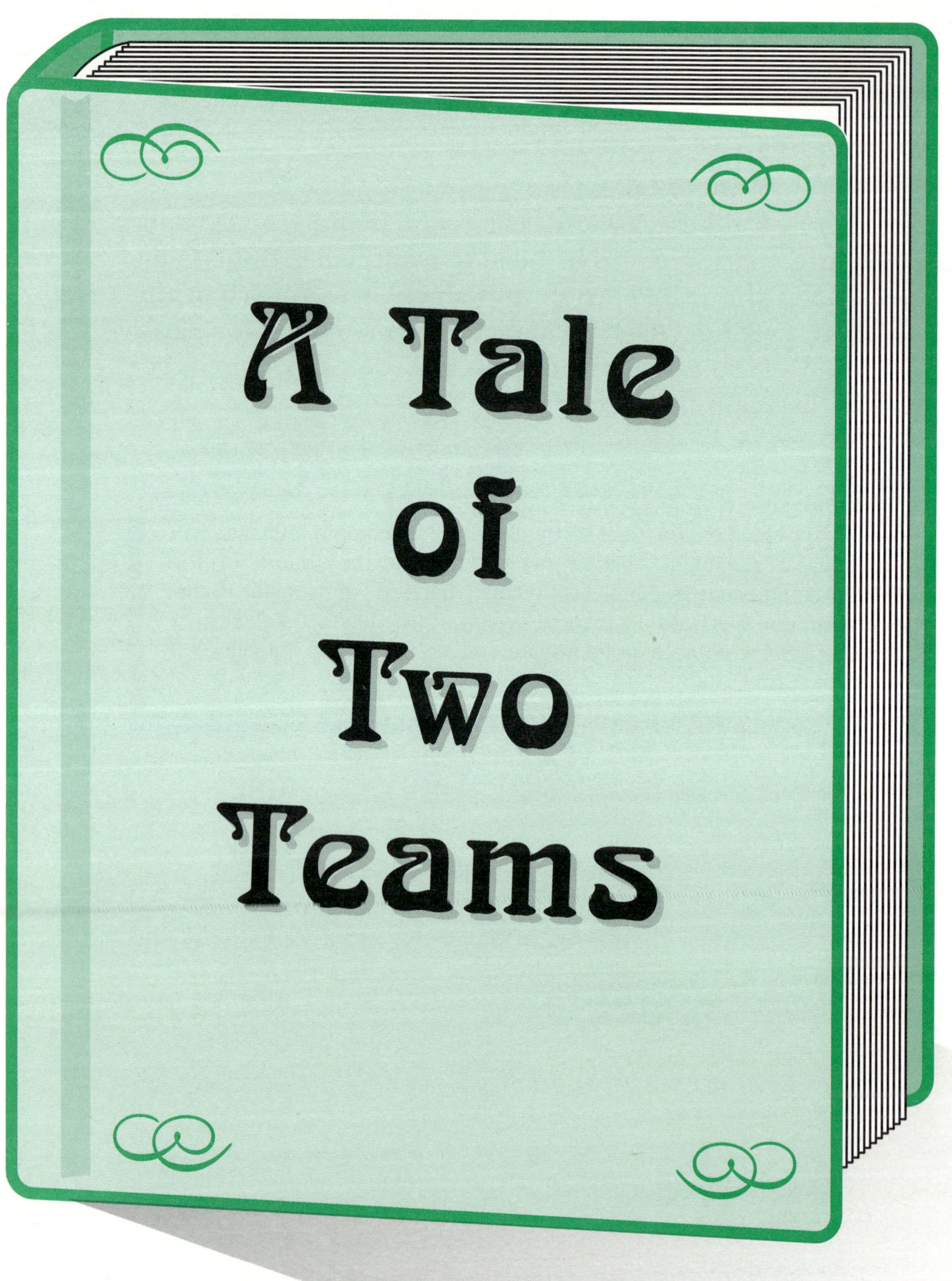
A Tale
of
Two
Teams

HELP WANTED

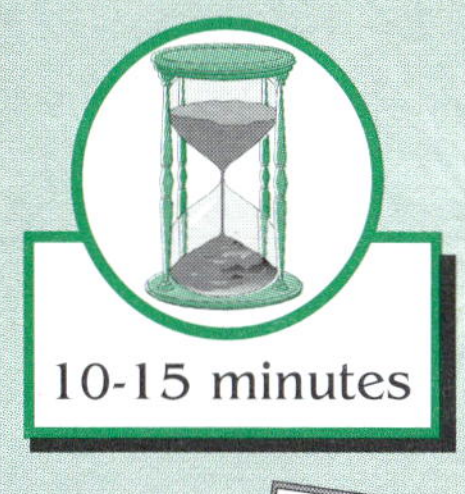

World's BEST Team Member

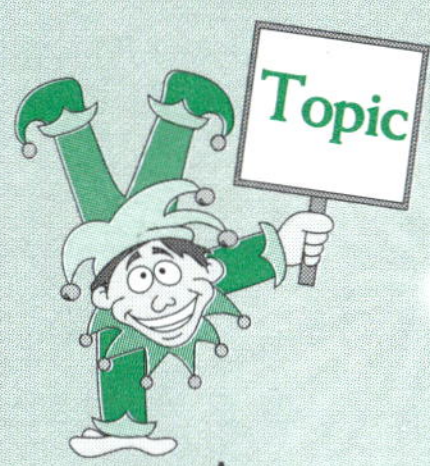

Team member characteristics and behaviors. Use this at an early meeting to learn about past team experience.

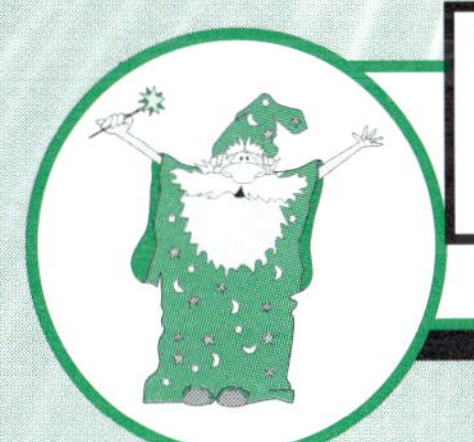

Wizard List

"Help Wanted" worksheet, flip chart, marker, pens or pencils, basket or box

Preparation

1. Copy "Help Wanted" worksheet for each team member. Use brightly colored paper, if possible.
2. Write boldly on a flip chart "Wanted: World's BEST Team Member" or make a poster of the "Help Wanted" worksheet.
3. Provide pens or pencils.

Implementation

1. Distribute "Help Wanted" worksheet and pens or pencils.
2. Instruct team members to write a classified ad in 25 words or less to describe the BEST team member possible.
3. Request that they write clearly, because you will be collecting the ads and distributing them for another member to read.
4. Ask for a volunteer to write on the flip chart titled "Wanted: World's BEST Team Member."
5. Collect the ads in a basket or box. Mix up the ads and have each team member draw one and read it out loud.
6. Ask the volunteer to note briefly on the flip board the team member characteristics that are mentioned. List each characteristic only once.

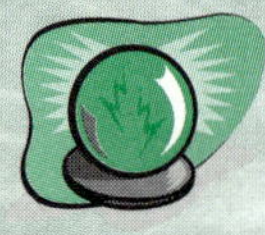

Debriefing

Explain that people have different ideas about teams and different experiences that can influence expectations and can be used to build a better team.

Magic Touch

Have each team member read his or her own if you think someone is likely to take the task less seriously if the ads are anonymous. This also saves time. End the exercise by waving the magic wand. "Abracadabra. This team will work together like magic."

Classified Help Wanted 1000

WANTED

World's BEST Team Member

come
help
go call

d but
ducts
ole lot
ction
ation a
oplied

and
eeded
y go

Start wo
the job y
wanted

Bring yo
but still r
on doub
of app
and info
artistic r

Work e
like to r

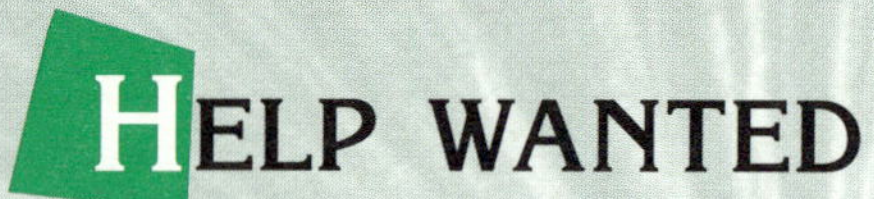

HELP WANTED

World's WORST Team Member

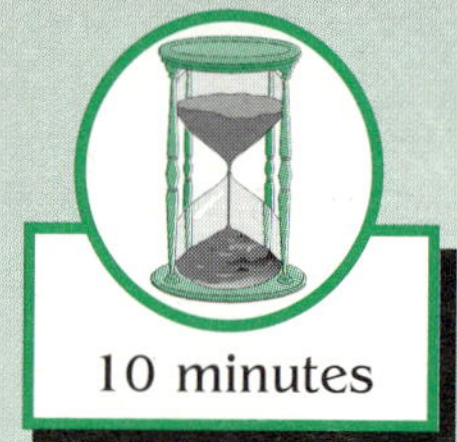

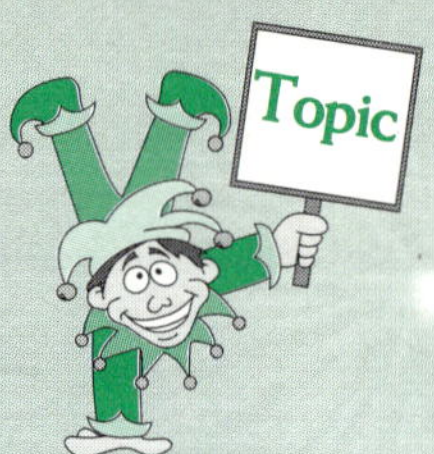

Team member characteristics and behaviors. Use at an early meeting to learn about past team experience.

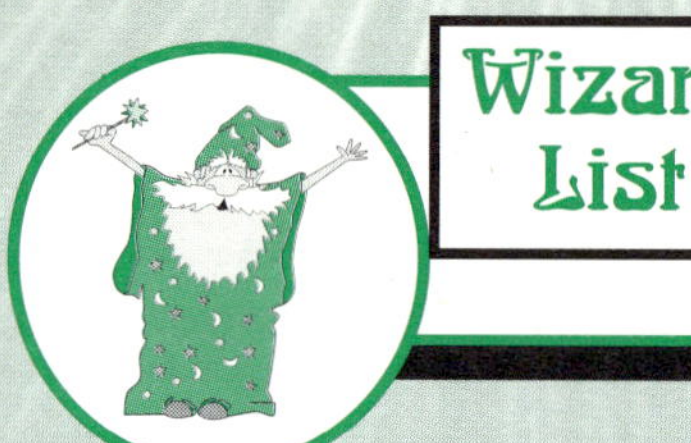

Wizard List

"Help Wanted" worksheet, "Help Wanted" example, flip chart, marker, pens or pencils, basket or box

Preparation

1. Copy "Help Wanted" worksheet for each team member. Use brightly colored paper, if possible.
2. Copy "Help Wanted" example.
3. Write boldly on the flip chart "Wanted: World's WORST Team Member!"

Implementation

1. Distribute "Help Wanted" worksheet.
2. Instruct team members to write a classified ad in 25 words or less to describe the WORST team member possible.
3. Read aloud "Help Wanted" example. Have fun; be dramatic.
4. Have each person read his or her ad, and request that it be done dramatically just for fun.

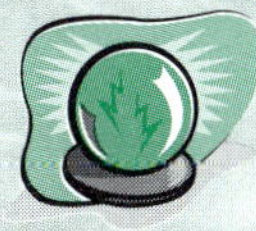

Debriefing

Explain that people have different experiences with groups, and some are nightmarish. Explain that exposing these concerns to the light of day and laughing at them can help teach us what not to do!

Magic Touch

Offer a silly prize or a mystery prize for the worst description and let the group vote. Award a funny certificate for "Most Observant of Crummy Behavior in Groups," "One Honest Person Award," "Most Likely To Keep a Humorous Perspective," or "Quick Wit Award."

Classified Help Wanted 1000

WANTED

World's WORST Team Member

Classified | Help Wanted | 1000

WANTED

World's WORST Team Member

Wanted: Obnoxious, know-it-all expert, team member who is consistently late, interrupts other members, refuses to do these great exercises, and never brings refreshments.

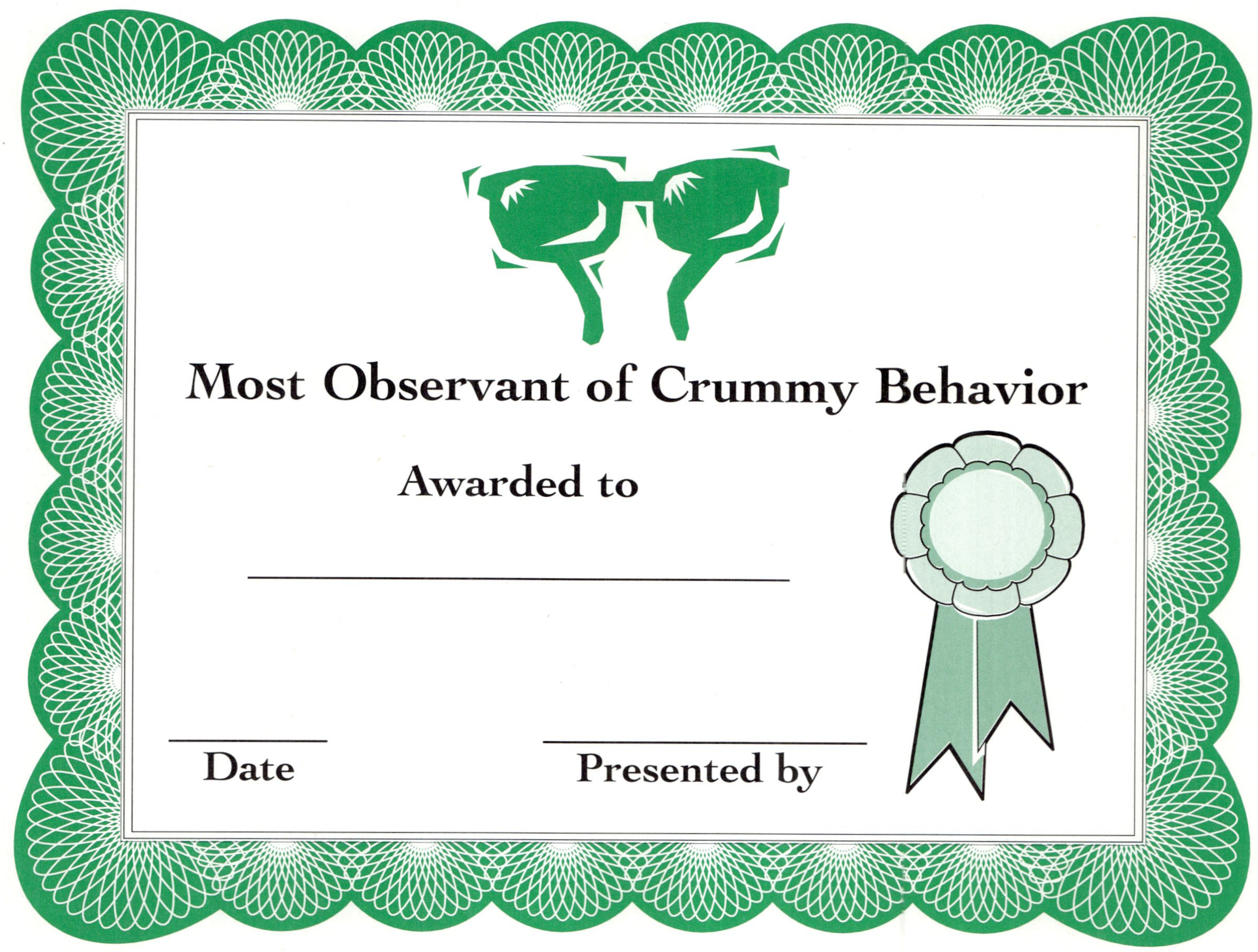
Most Observant of Crummy Behavior
Awarded to
Date
Presented by

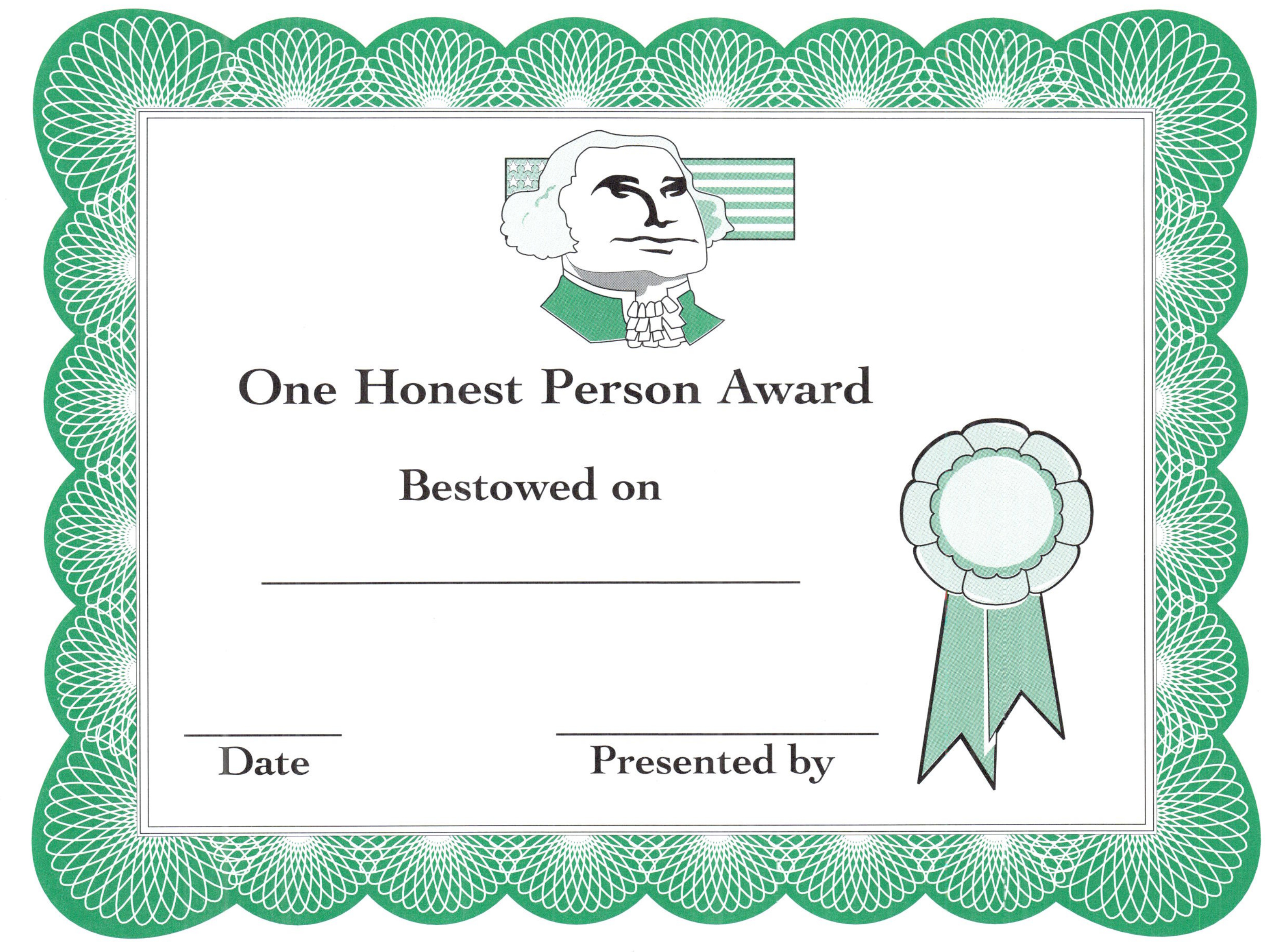
One Honest Person Award
Bestowed on
Date
Presented by

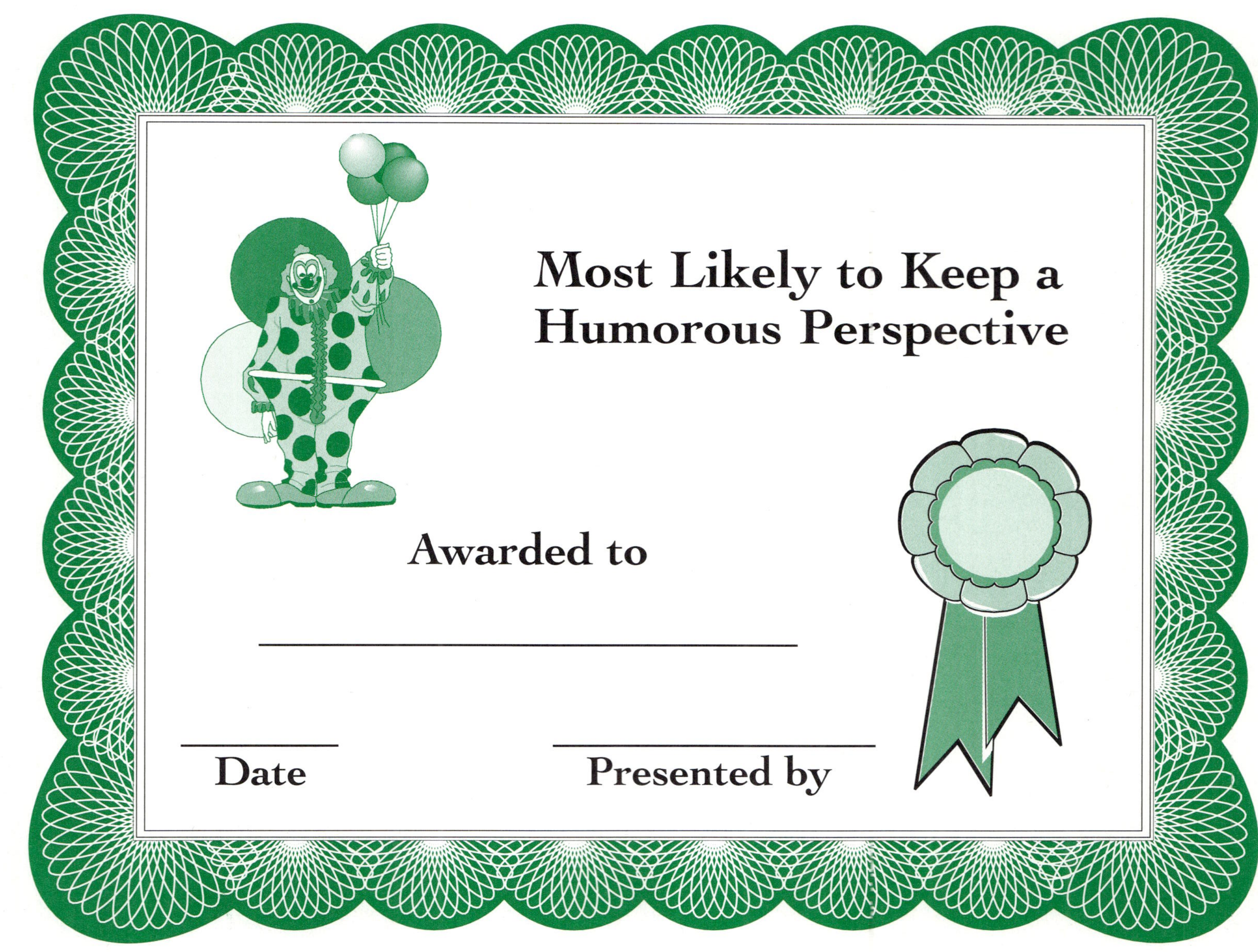
Most Likely to Keep a
Humorous Perspective
Awarded to
Date
Presented by

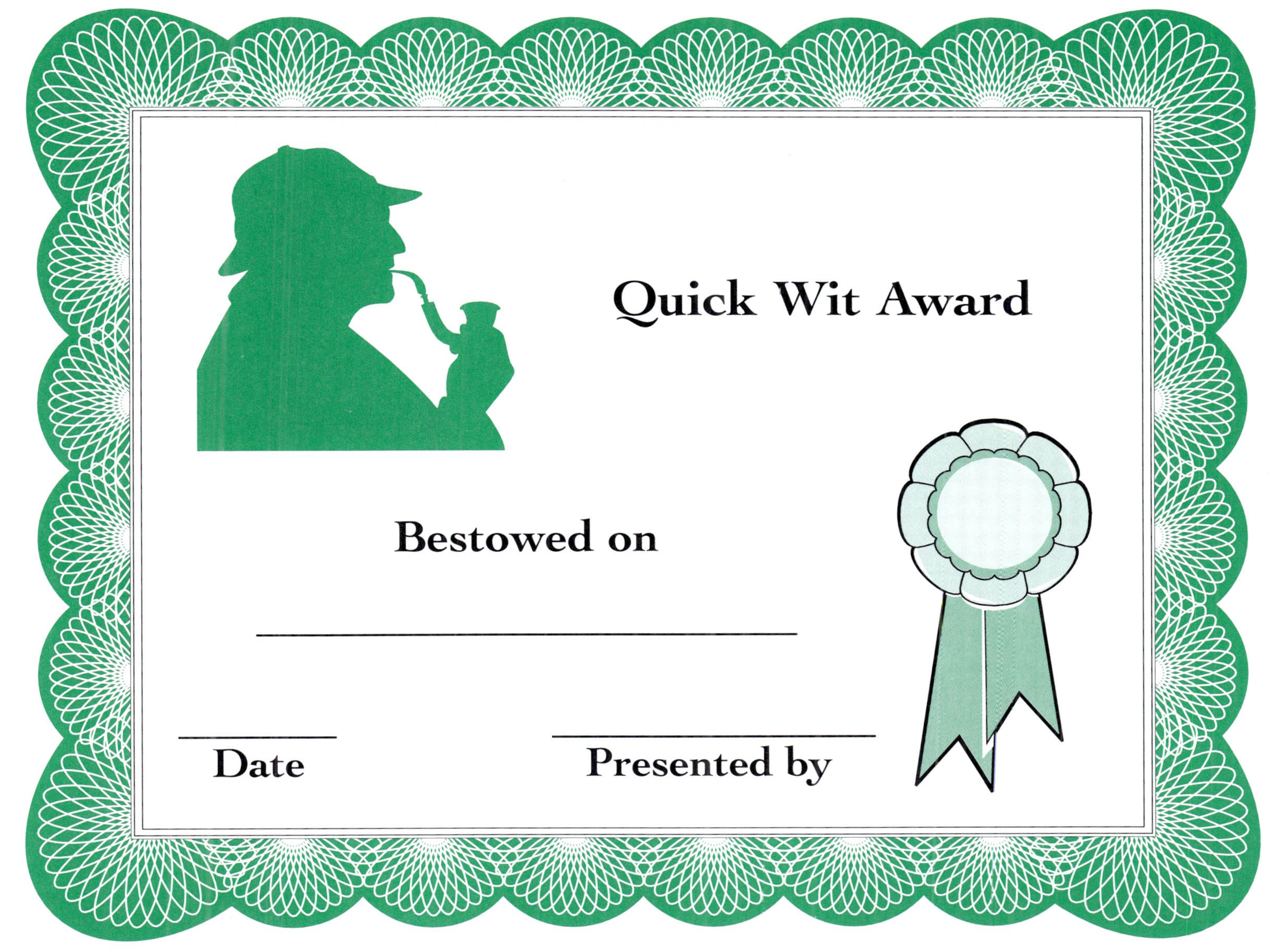
Quick Wit Award
Bestowed on
Date
Presented by

TEAMS I HAVE KNOWN

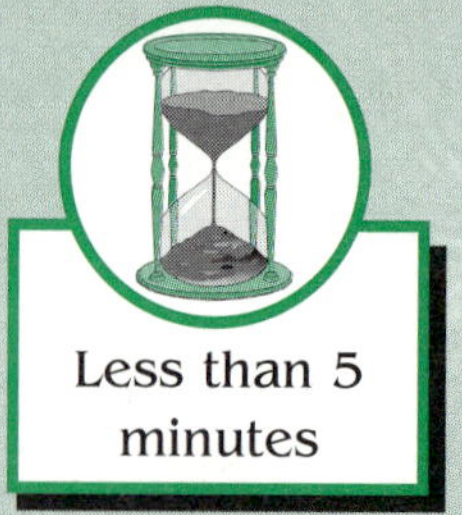

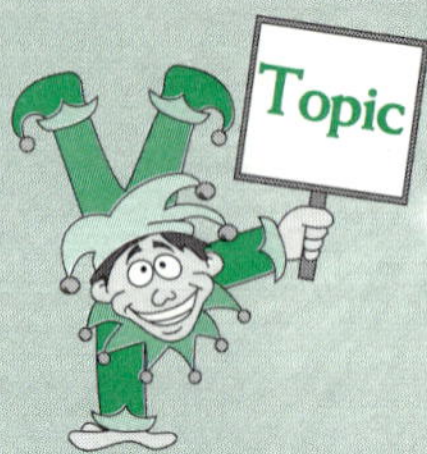

Use early to learn amount of members' team experience.

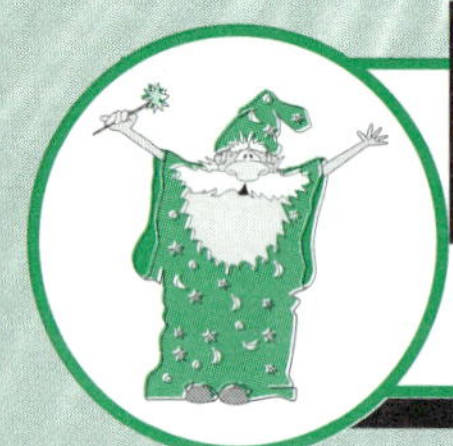

Wizard List

"Teams I Have Known" worksheet, timer or watch with second hand, whistle or noisemaker, prizes, pens or pencils

Preparation

1. Copy "Teams I Have Known" worksheet for each team member.
2. Provide a prize (small toy, eraser) for each team member.
3. Provide pens or pencils for each team member.

Implementation

1. Distribute the "Teams I Have Known" worksheet to each member.
2. Explain to the team that they will have 1 minute to get as many worksheet squares as possible initialed by team members with the experience described in each box. The goal is to get at least one person's initials in each square. Depending on the experience of the group, some boxes may have one set of initials, some more than one, and some none. One person can initial more than one box, but try to have contact with each team member.
3. Say "Ready . . . get set . . . GO!" and blow the whistle.
4. At the end of 1 minute, blow the whistle again to signal the allotted time has elapsed.
5. Have team members share what they learned about one another's group experience.
6. Distribute prizes for participation.

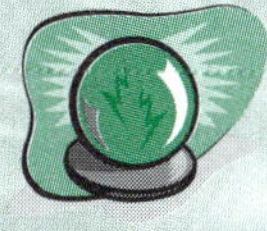

Debriefing

This is a simple way to learn more about the group member's experience with groups. This information adds to the team's knowledge of its resources.

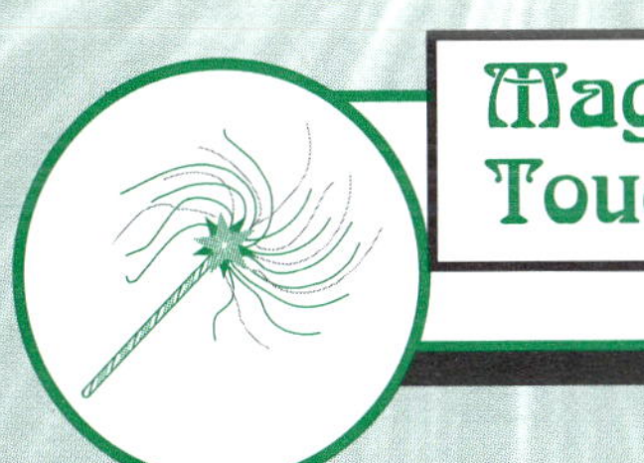

Magic Touch

Prizes are a great way to encourage participation and add some zip to the activity.

TEAMS I HAVE KNOWN

Have You . . .

Been on 1-5 teams?	Facilitated a team?	Led a team?
Been recorder or secretary of a team?	Been on more than 5 teams?	Never been on a team at work?
Been a member of a quality improvement team?	Been a member of a self-directed team?	Decided you want to be here today!
Not decided whether you know why you are on the team?	Decided you would rather be in the mountains?	Decided you would rather be in a tropical paradise?

WE COME BEARING GIFTS

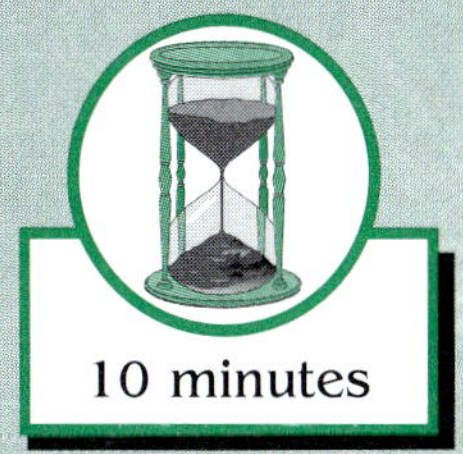

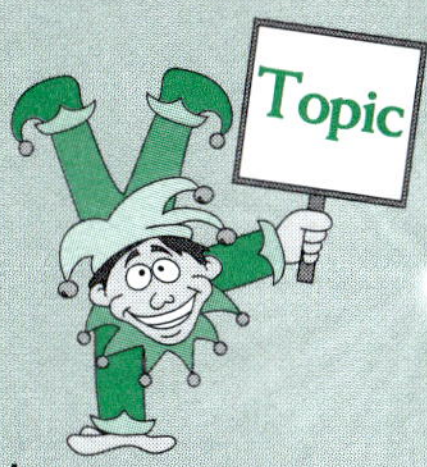

Recognize skill and talent. Use this when people do not know one another well.

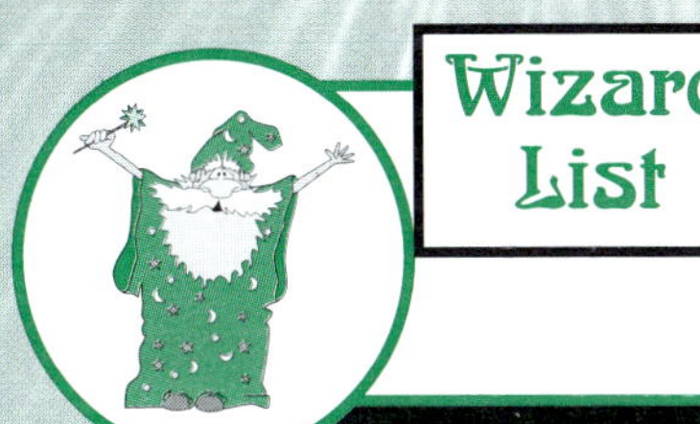

Wizard List

Small gift (wrapped), "Gifts I Bring" worksheet, large bowl or gift-wrapped box with removable lid, pens or pencils

Preparation

1. Copy "Gifts I Bring" worksheet for each team member.
2. Gift wrap a small gift to give to one team member.
3. Provide pens or pencils for each team member.

Implementation

1. Discuss briefly the uniqueness of every individual and the importance of each team member's contribution. Acknowledge that it is not easy for some people to talk about their own strengths, but that it is important to know what all have to offer in the work setting for the team to be successful.
2. Show the gift-wrapped box and mention that it illustrates the gifts each of us can bring to a team if we are willing to participate fully.
3. Distribute the "Gifts I Bring" worksheet and ask team members to think about the gifts they bring to the work at hand.
4. Ask team members to select four strengths, skills, or personal characteristics that they are willing to use to help the team meet its mission and write them on the worksheet.

5. Have each team member read the gifts listed or ask them to exchange worksheets.
6. Have each team member fold the worksheet and put it into the bowl or gift-wrapped box.
7. Explain that you never know when one person's contribution can be just the gift the team needs to succeed and that you want to give a surprise gift to illustrate this.
8. Award the gift by drawing one "Gifts I Bring" worksheet from the bowl.

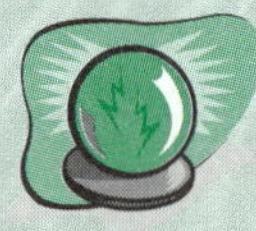

Debriefing

Ask team members why such an exercise might be useful. If they are not covered, mention:

- You are being asked to do your best here.
- You are here for the very gifts you have.
- Commitment is essential to success in team problem solving.

Magic Touch

Gifts might include: colored paper (to recognize differences), colored paper clips (to link us together), bottle of bubbles (to stimulate creativity), candy (to recognize how good we are), Post-it notes (to help us stick together), any fun office supplies.

GIFTS I BRING

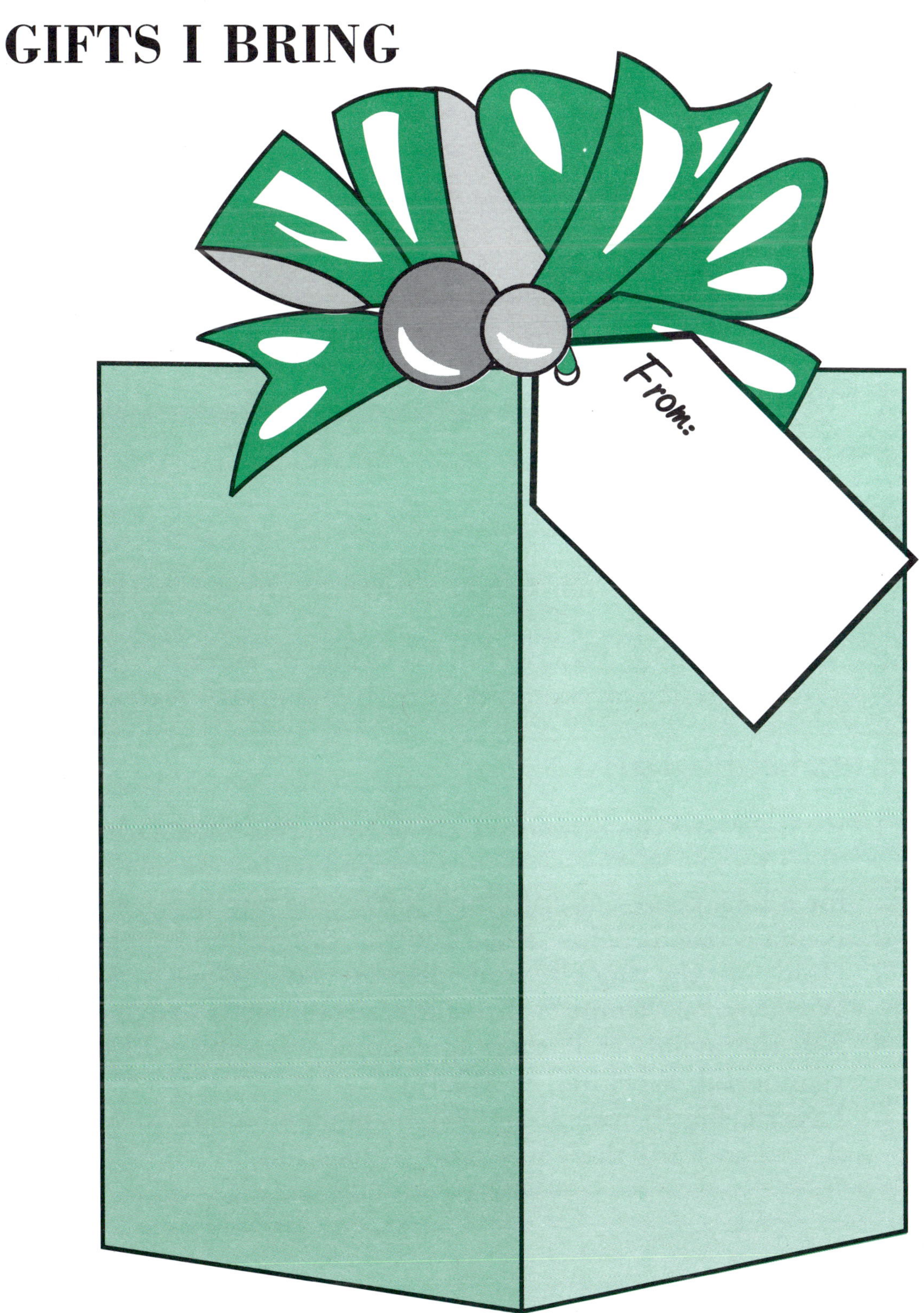

WACKY, WONDERFUL, WORKING, OR WIMPY WEEKENDS?

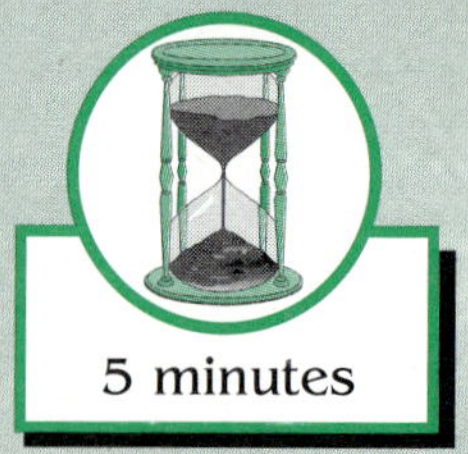

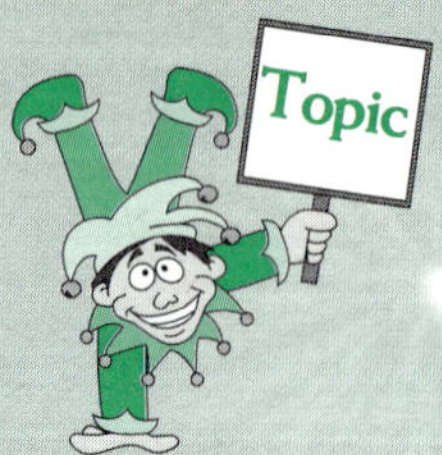

Icebreaker. Use this to help people relax.

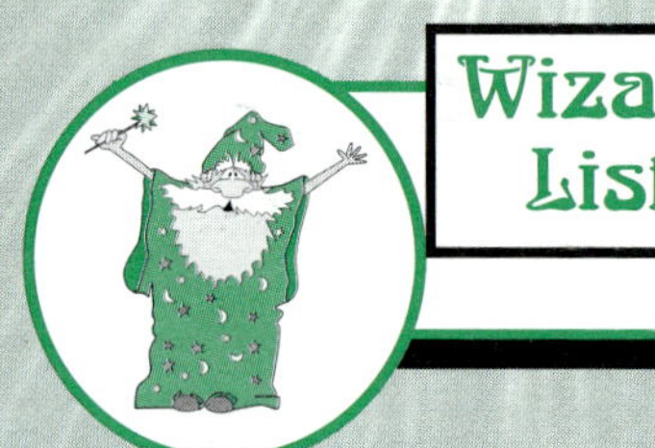

Wizard List

The big W pattern, poster board, "Wacky, Wonderful, Working, or Wimpy"

Preparation

1. Make a big *W* from bright poster board using the supplied pattern.
2. Make a "Wacky, Wonderful, Working, or Wimpy?" sign, either a transparency or poster, or copy it and attach it to a flip chart.

Implementation

1. Explain how sometimes we are thrown together with people we don't know. Perhaps we have worked with some team members for a long time, but still don't know one another.
2. Explain that it helps to see another dimension of a person.
3. Hold up the big *W* and display the "Wacky, Wonderful, Working, or Wimpy?" flip chart, poster, or transparency.
4. Ask the members if their upcoming weekend will be Wacky, Wonderful, Working, or Wimpy?
5. Pass the big *W* around and ask team members to identify which *W* category fits their weekend plans and why.

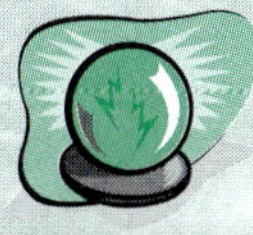

Debriefing

Ask people if they learned anything new about their coworkers. If it seems as though people enjoyed the exercise, and you notice laughter, remind them that a light touch makes the work easier and adds energy to the process. Be sure to mention that to prevent burnout, staff in a medical setting need life balance.

Magic Touch

Share something personal. Describe your own plans. If you haven't any plans, say you are in danger of having a Wimpy weekend. Point out that such a weekend spent just relaxing and resting may be just right sometimes, especially for people who are restored by time alone.

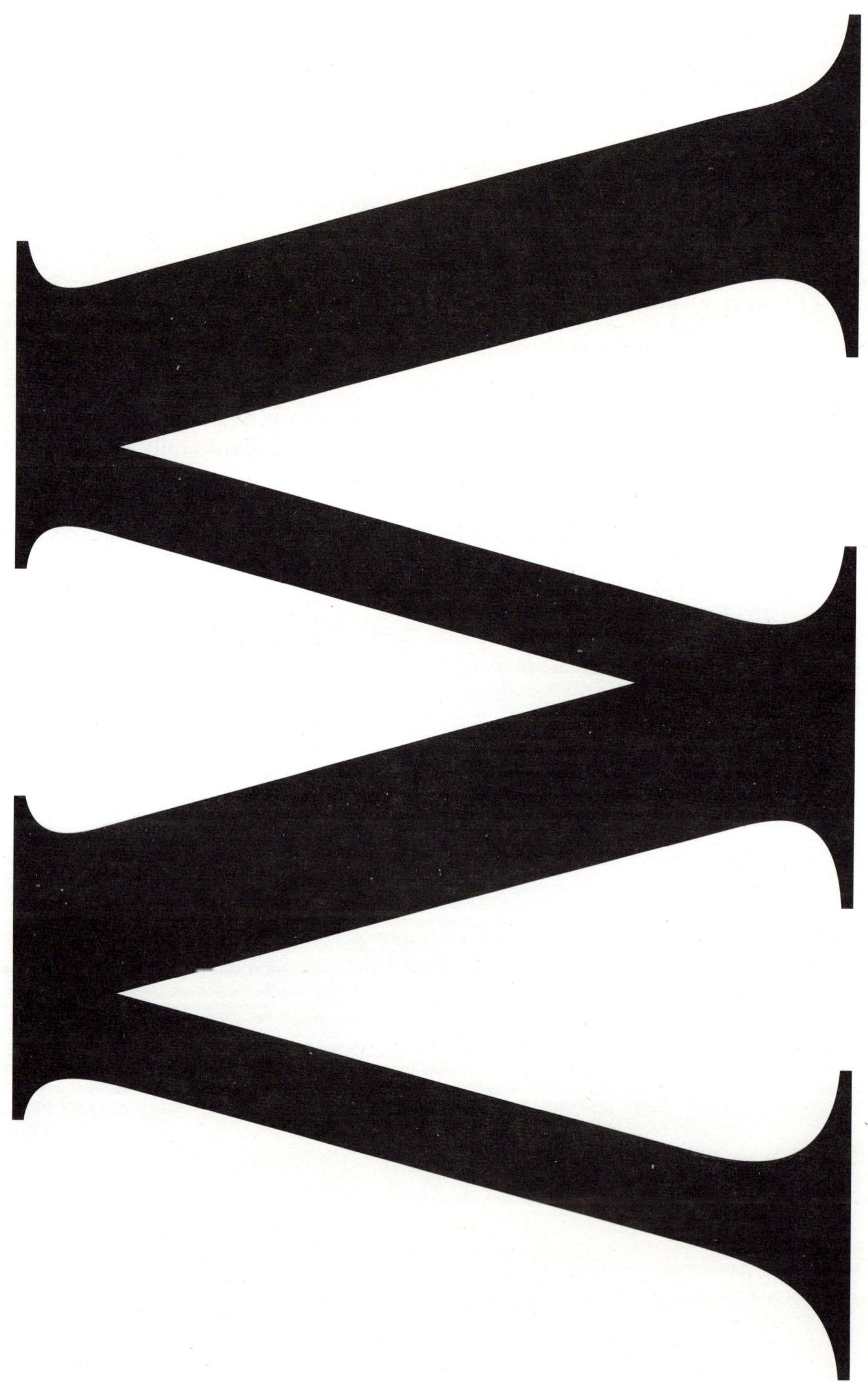

Wacky, Wonderful, Working, or Wimpy?

ON A MUSICAL NOTE

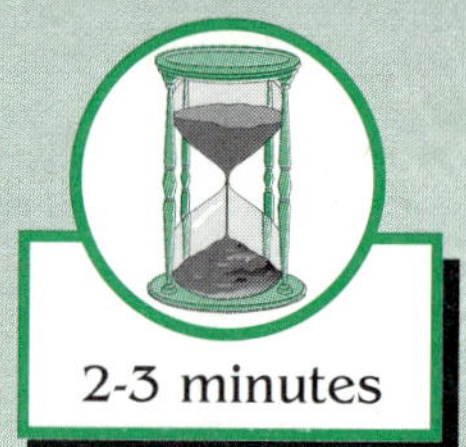

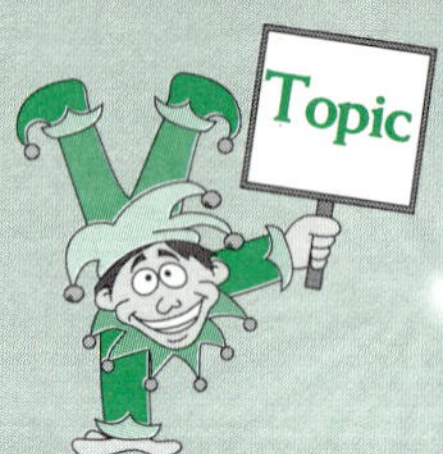

Ice Breaker. Use as a prelude to meetings as team members assemble or during breaks.

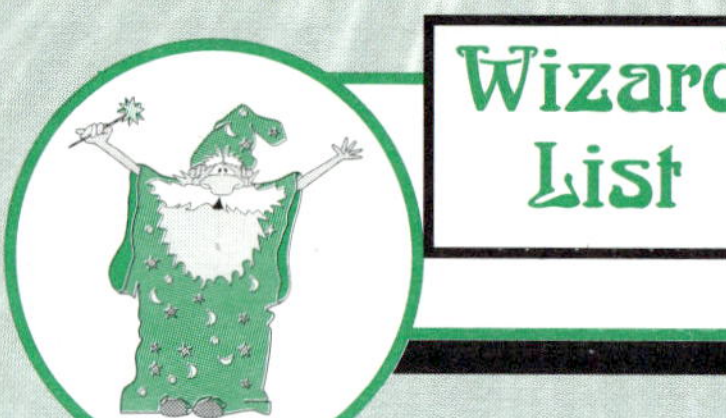

Wizard List

Music and audio equipment

Preparation

1. Collect songs or lyrics to songs that are old favorites. *Remember that copyright law prohibits using copyrighted music without permission at paid events.*
2. Include a variety of music styles. Choose musical arrangements that are catchy or silly, or that illustrate a point.
3. Review the suggestions for music selections on page 46.

Implementation

1. Play music to set a tone as the team members convene.
2. If appropriate, wave the magic wand that accompanies this book to the beat of the music.
3. Ask for volunteers to provide musical selections for future meetings.

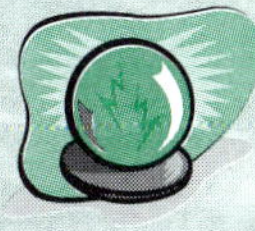

Debriefing

Ask the team if the music works. Try to get a feel for how the music is received. Involve the team members in selections for upcoming meetings. Ask team members to bring in a song with lyrics or a theme that they think applies to the team.

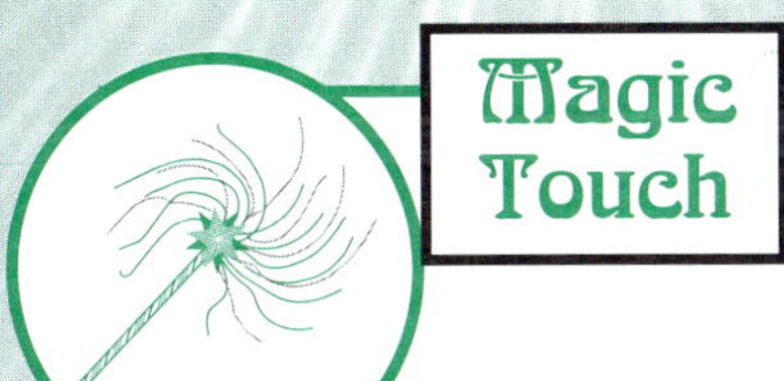

Magic Touch

Call a member before the meeting to ask for suggestions. Choose music that will energize, amuse, and inspire.

Adapted from: Judy K. Scott, RN, MSN

SUGGESTIONS FOR MUSIC SELECTIONS

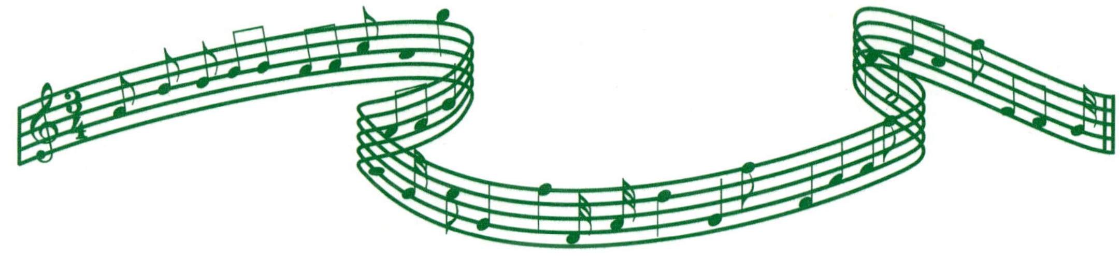

Pachibel's Canon, in times of stress.

William Tell Overture, to energize.

"He's Got the Whole World in His Hands," when the team is overwhelmed.

"The Hokey Pokey," to give the team a stretch break. Yes, you'll have to do it, too!

"Fly Me To the Moon," when everyone wants to abandon hope.

"Whistle While You Work" or "Whenever I Feel Afraid," as pick-me-ups.

"This Little Light of Mine, I'm Going To Let It Shine," when empowerment is an issue.

"Sixteen Tons," by Tennessee Ernie Ford, when money is an issue. (Someone on your team is bound to be old enough to remember this!)

TEAM ANALGESIA

For Quick Relief, Laughter Is the Best Medicine

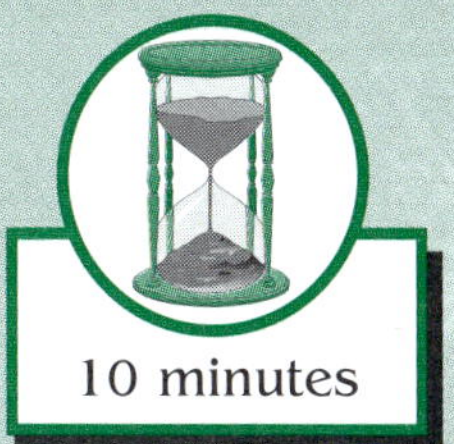
10 minutes

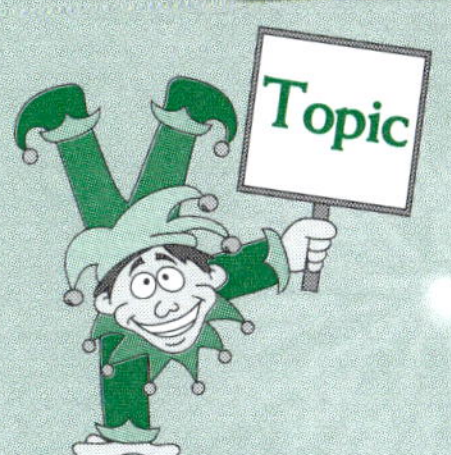

Icebreaker. Use to illustrate that life and teams don't always go smoothly.

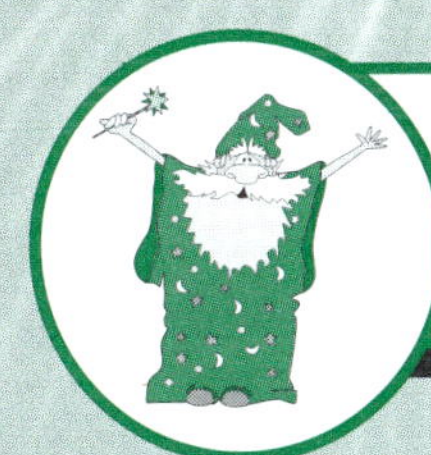

Wizard List

Clown nose, "Laughter ℞," transparency or poster material or flip chart

Preparation

1. Make "Laughter ℞" sign, either a transparency or poster, or copy it and attach it to a flip chart.
2. Purchase a clown nose or use the magic wand included with this book.
3. Prepare a real-life embarrassing moment of your own to read aloud.

Implementation

1. Put on the clown nose and explain that laughter can be the best medicine for tired teams. If you are using the wand, add that laughter adds a magic touch.
2. Mention that Steve Allen, the famous comedian, said that there is no need to make up jokes, because real life provides humor.
3. Share your embarrassing moment with the team.
4. Ask members to think of an embarrassing moment—something that might not have been funny when it happened, but makes a great story now.
5. Ask the team members to divide into small groups; 3 to 4 people make a nice group.

6. Ask each member to share a personal embarrassing moment with his or her individual group. Allow 5 minutes.
7. Ask each group to nominate one person to share his or her story with the whole team. If you have more time, make the groups larger.
8. Reconvene the entire team and ask each group's volunteer to share the embarrassing moment.

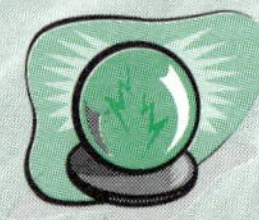

Debriefing

Ask what lessons they have learned. Remind the group that we are all in this together. Things don't always go smoothly in the life of a team, but embarrassing moments or lessons learned teach us not to take ourselves too seriously. Besides, they can make a good story.

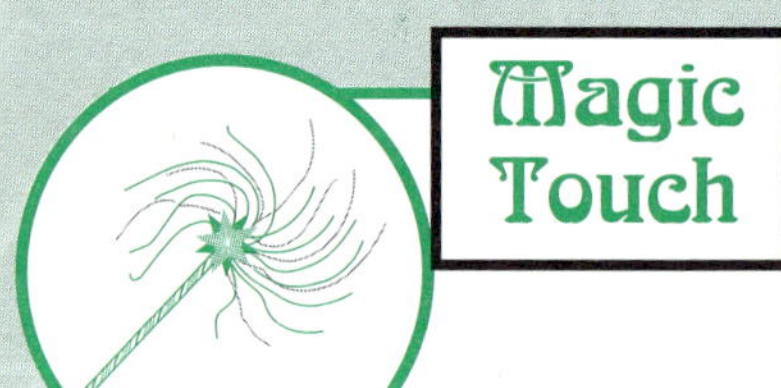

Magic Touch

Sharing your own embarrassing moment with the team really helps get the ball rolling and puts everyone at ease.

LAUGHTER ℞:

To decrease team pain . . . increase levity.

LAUGHTER IS THE BEST MEDICINE!!!

STRESSED FOR SUCCESS

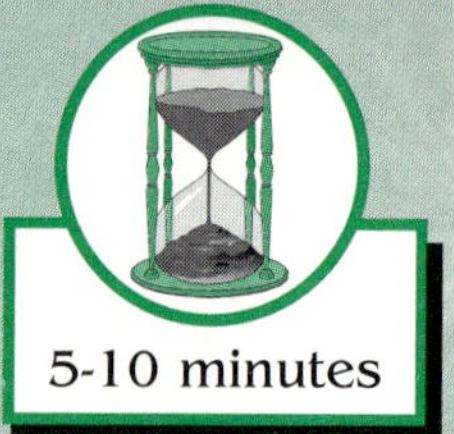

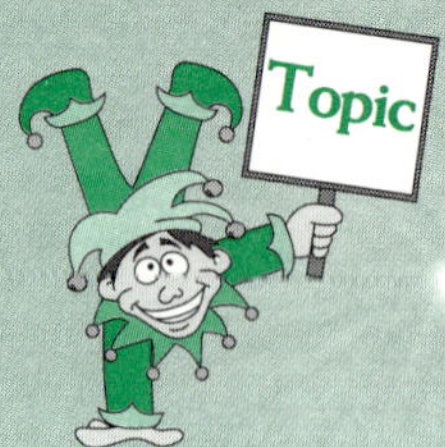

Icebreaker. Use to demonstrate that we all have stress.

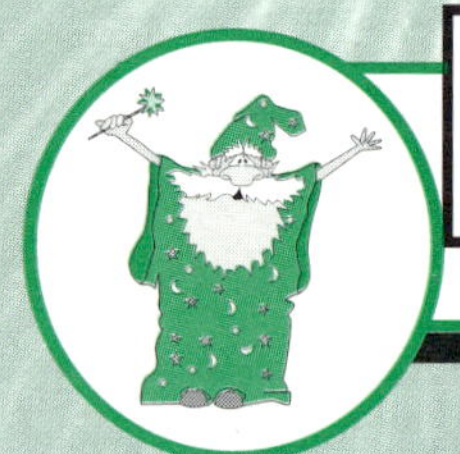

Wizard List

Plain shelf paper, masking tape, colored markers, watch with a second hand, whistle, toy tops

Preparation

1. Cut shelf paper into two 5-foot pieces of paper.
2. Lay the shelf paper lengthwise. At the top of one write "Stressed for Success! Stressors I Know" and at the top of the other write "My Secrets for Successful Coping . . . or, How I Am Able To Be Here Today!"
3. Provide markers for each team member.
4. Provide a small toy top for each team member.

Implementation

1. Tape each piece of shelf paper lengthwise on separate walls to permit everyone to write at the same time!
2. Remind the group that we come to meetings with lots of other priorities in our lives and stressors that distract us. We also come with wisdom we can share.
3. Ask the team to spend a few minutes sharing their thoughts.
4. Place colored markers where everyone can choose one.
5. Tell the group that when you say "GO," everyone is to grab a marker and write their responses on the posted "Stressed for Success" and "My Secrets for Successful Coping." Remind

members that prizes might be involved. Announce that they have 2 minutes.

6. Say "Ready . . . get set . . . GO!" and blow the whistle.
7. In 2 minutes blow the whistle again to signal the time has elapsed.
8. Ask one team member to read all the stressors and another to read all the coping strategies.
9. Ask the team to discuss what they have learned.

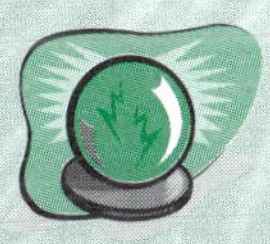

Debriefing

Summarize the discussion and identify any special points you want to make. Thank team members for their willingness to play along.

Magic Touch

Award each a small top, saying, "Keep this with you so when you are upset, rather than BLOW your top, you can SPIN this top." Collect and use unusual whistles; the funnier, the better.

THE WEATHER IN MY LIFE TODAY IS . . .

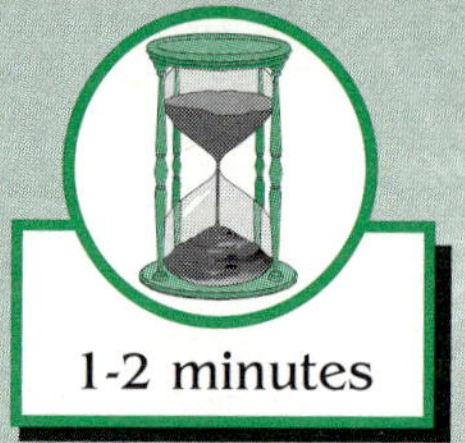

Icebreaker. Use to refocus attention on the team. This is an activity you can use periodically at the beginning or end of the team meeting for a quick mood check.

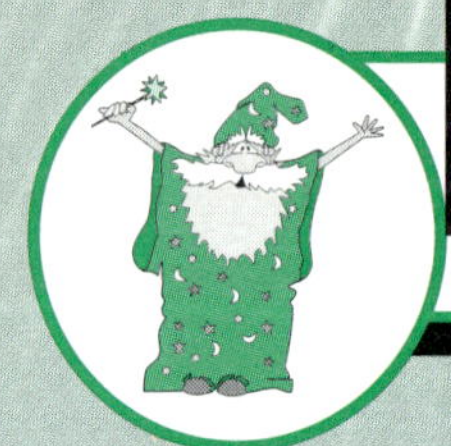

Wizard List

"The Weather in My Life Today Is . . ." sign, weather cards, flip chart, colored 3″ × 5″ index cards (optional)

Preparation

1. Copy "The Weather in My Life Today Is . . ." sign to make a transparency or poster, or make a flip chart drawing.
2. Copy the weather card worksheet, making enough copies for each team member to have a choice of one of each card. Place the cards together to make a deck of cards.

Implementation

1. Ask the group to look at the cards, remove the one that best represents their mood, put it face down in front of them, and pass the cards to the next person.
2. After everyone has chosen a card, ask one person to collect the cards without seeing who chose which card, to shuffle these, and then record the results on the flip chart.

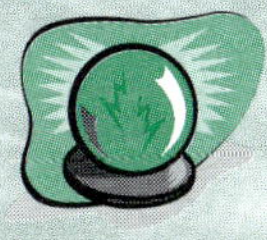

Debriefing

Point out that recognizing our moods and acknowledging them to ourselves can help us regroup and get ready for the meeting. If you implement this exercise at the end of the meeting, ask the team to give a weather report for this meeting.

Magic Touch

As a variation, write on colored 3″ × 5″ index cards "Cloudy," Stormy," "Steady Drizzle," and "Sunny." Match the color of the card with the appropriate weather. For example, use purple for "Stormy" and yellow for "Sunny." Laminate the cards to keep them fresh.

THE WEATHER IN MY LIFE TODAY IS . . .

CLOUDY

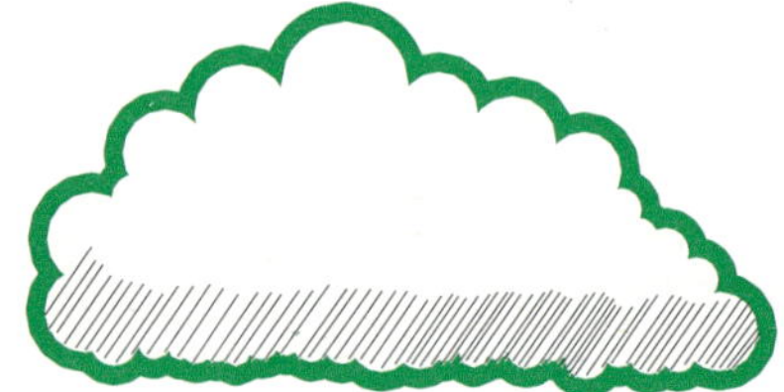

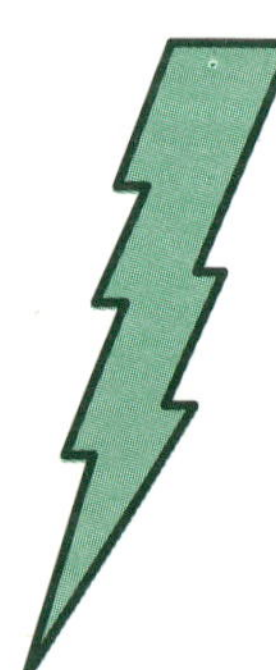

STORMY

STEADY DRIZZLE

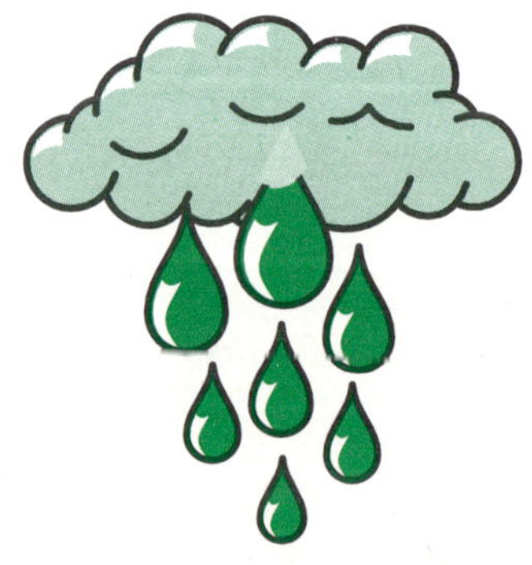

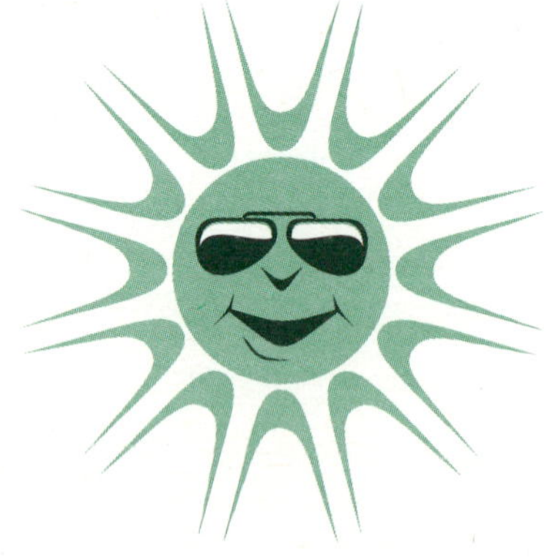

SUNNY

WEATHER CARDS

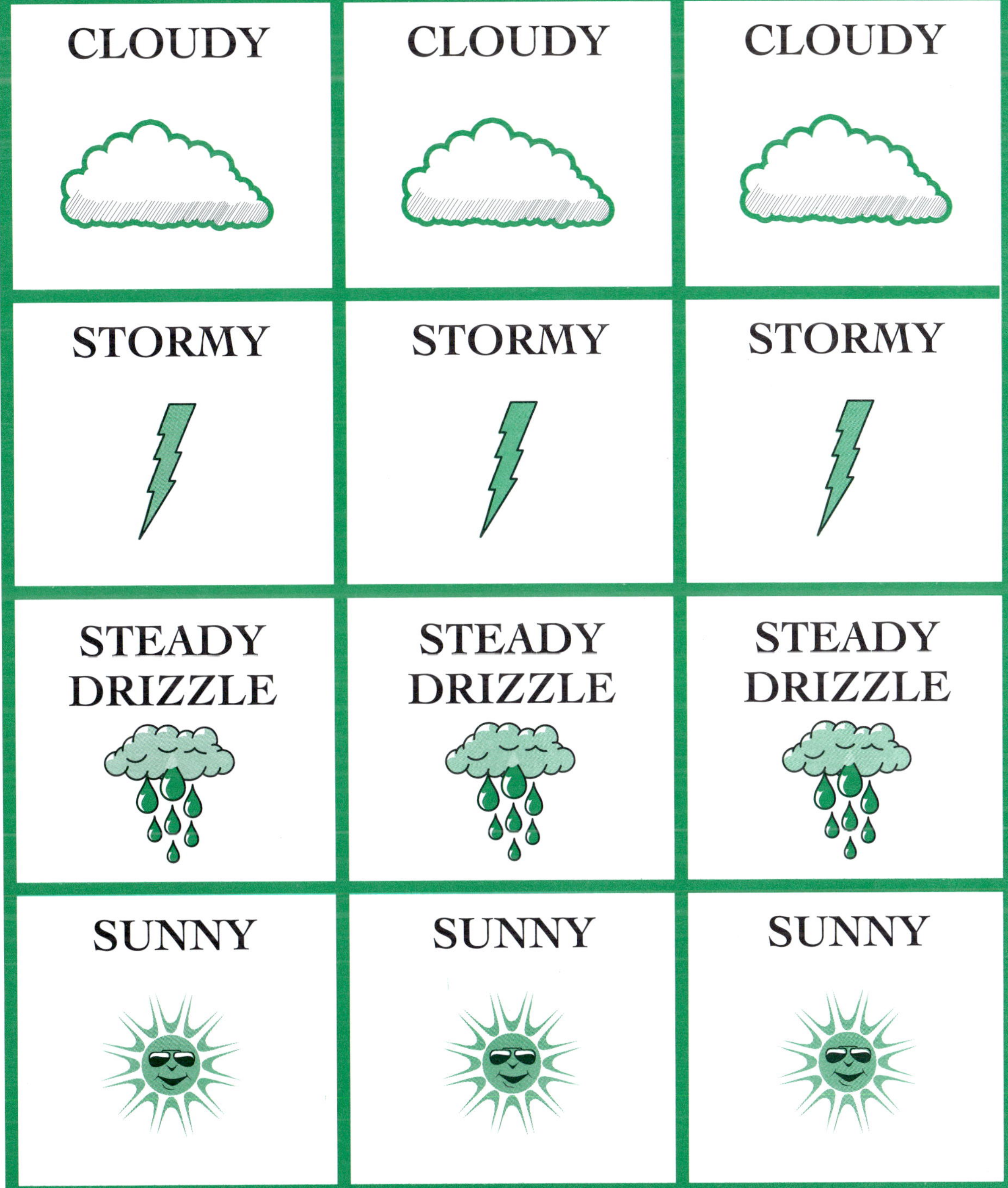

Squaring Off

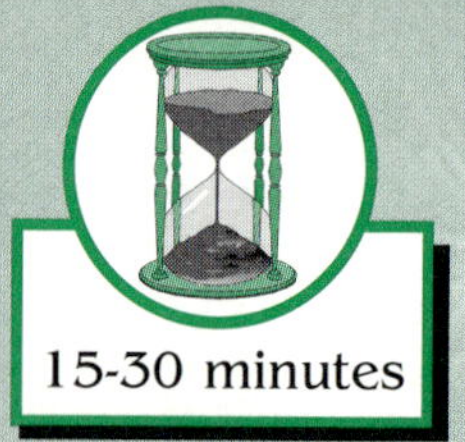

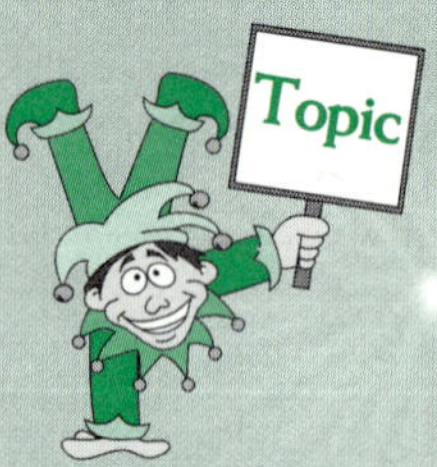

Team member expectations.

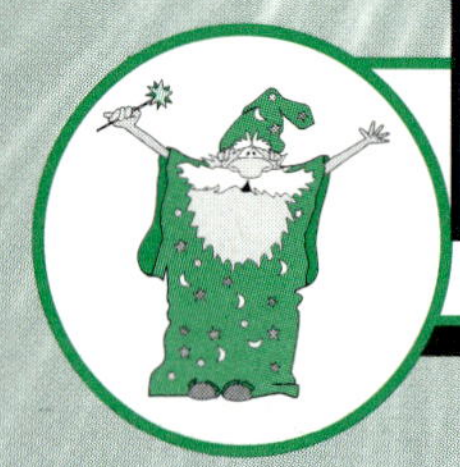

Wizard List

Flip chart paper, colored markers, masking tape, "Squaring Off," pens or pencils

Preparation

1. Make "Squaring Off" transparency or poster.
2. Provide one piece of flip chart paper for each team member.
3. Provide one marker for each team member.

Implementation

1. Give each team member one piece of flip chart paper and a colored marker. (For a large group, you can use 8½″ × 11″ paper and have team members share results in small groups.)
2. Instruct members to copy "Squaring Off" onto their flip chart paper.
3. Ask each person to:
   a. In the first row, draw three pictures of things they enjoy doing, such as walking, cleaning, sewing, biking.
   b. In the second row, draw three pictures of things they hate to do, such as mowing, cooking, repairs.
   c. In the third row, write three things they hope to accomplish through the team, what they hope to learn, and what they hope the team will accomplish.

4. When all pictures are completed, ask all team members to come to the front of the room one at a time and tape their picture to the front wall or flip chart.
5. Have the team members introduce themselves, tell how long they have worked at the facility, in what department, and then explain their pictures.

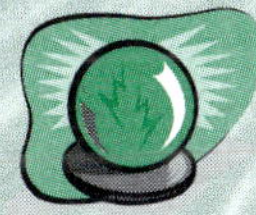

Debriefing

Refer back to pictures at the end of the meeting to see if individuals are beginning to meet their goals.

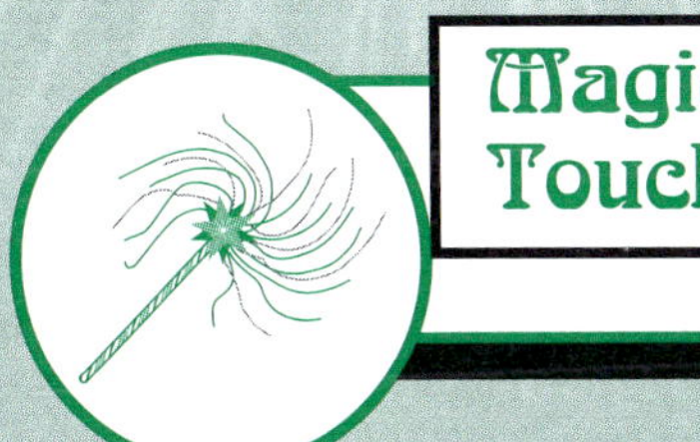

Magic Touch

This exercise can be used later in the life of the team to check progress toward goal achievement.

SQUARING OFF

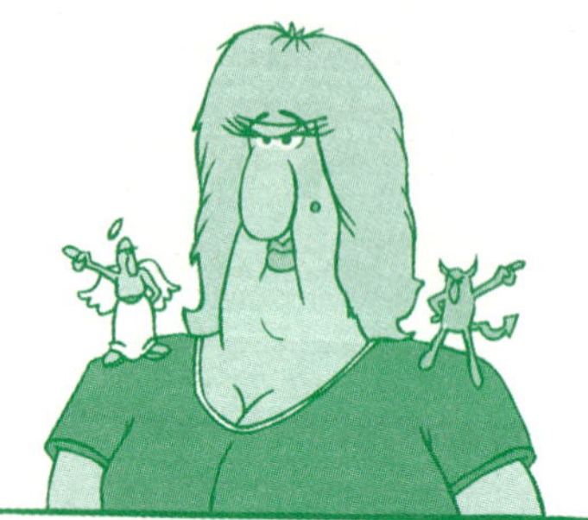

LIKES			
DISLIKES			
GOALS FOR TEAM MEETING			

THE NEXT STEP

. . . For the Second Meeting

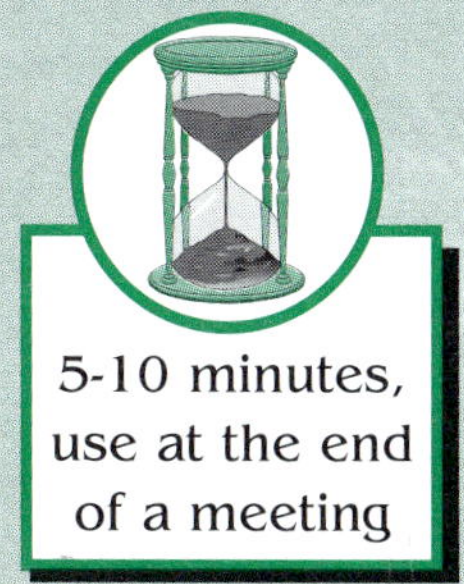

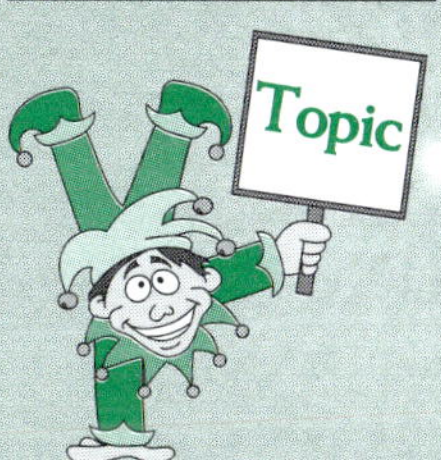

Feedback, Part 1. Use at the second meeting for feedback about team expectations.

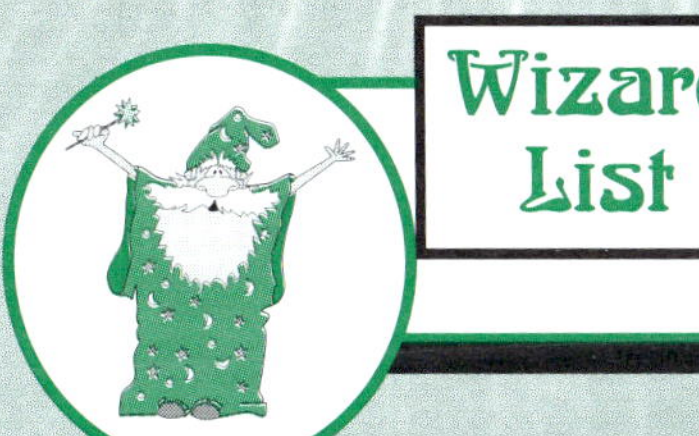

Wizard List "The Next Step," pens or pencils

Preparation

1. Make copies of "The Next Step" for each team member.
2. Provide pens or pencils for each team member.

Implementation

1. Ask team members to reflect on the previous meeting, consider how it went compared with their expectations, and think about where the team needs to go from here.
2. Distribute "The Next Step."
3. Ask team members to quickly fill in the "steps" on the worksheet and be prepared to read their responses.
4. Have each member read their responses aloud.
5. Collect the worksheets, explaining they will have a chance to use the information in the next meeting and that their responses are team business and confidential.

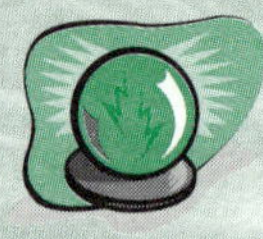

Debriefing

Ask if team members saw any differences in their teammates' point of view. Point out that people have different perceptions and that those differences can enrich the team if they are openly considered. We need to be honest, open, and nonjudgmental. Explain this is the first of many times they will be asked to give feedback and to accept responsibility for the work and growth of the group. "We are busy in our work lives, focused on doing our part in patient care. Meeting time must be well spent. We can't afford to waste time."

Magic Touch

If you choose to use this exercise and offer the promise of further opportunities to give feedback, be sure to follow through with this commitment. Use "Step Back" in your next meeting.

THE NEXT STEP

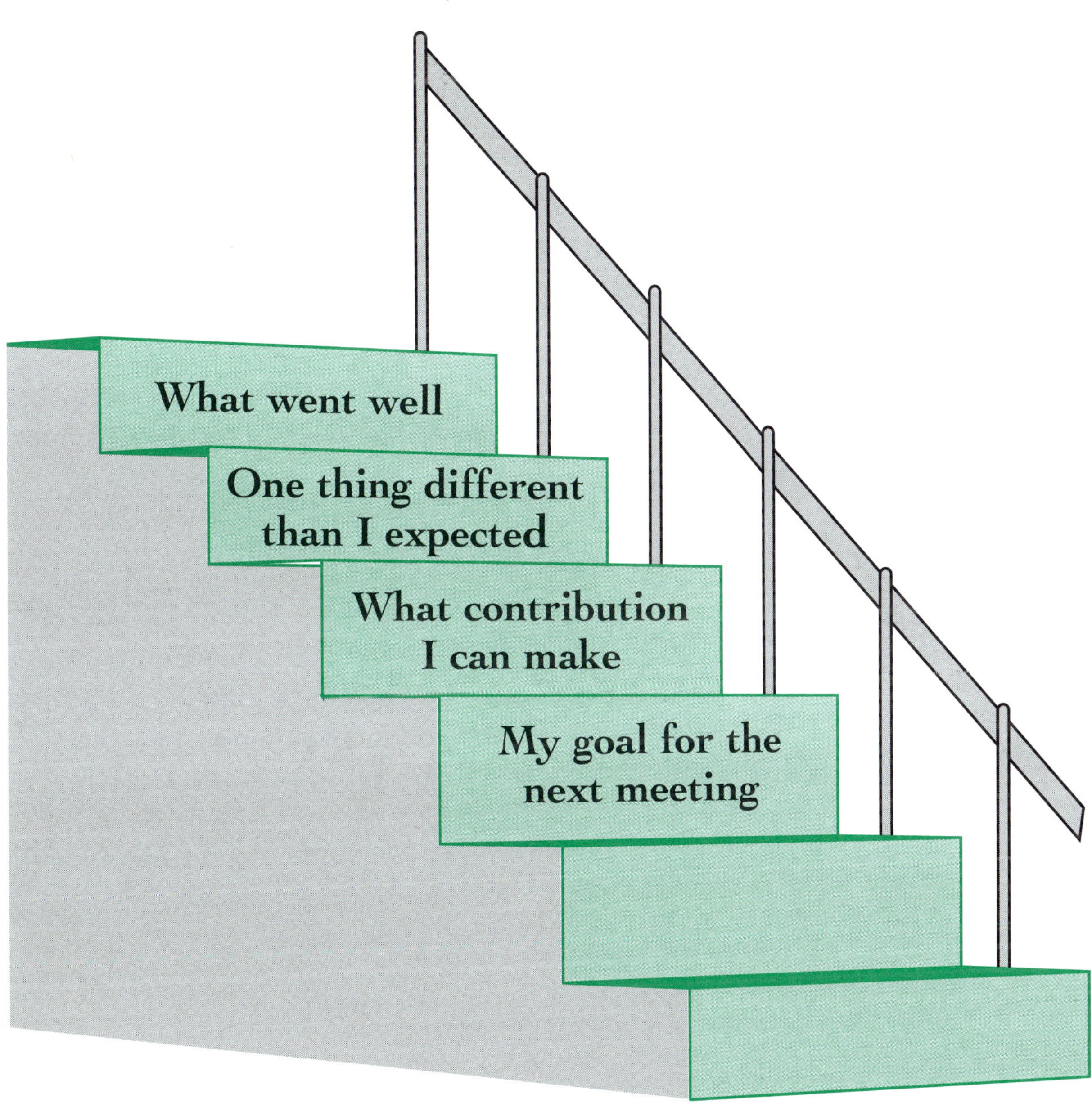

STEP BACK!

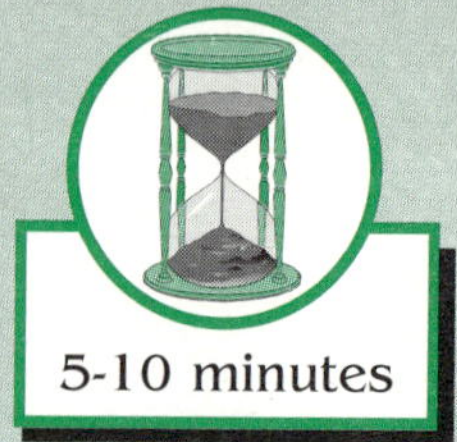

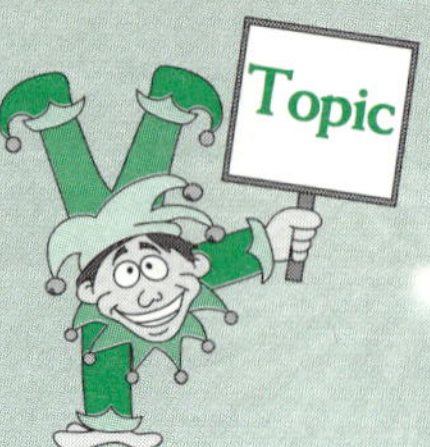

Feedback, Part 2. Use in the meeting after "The Next Step."

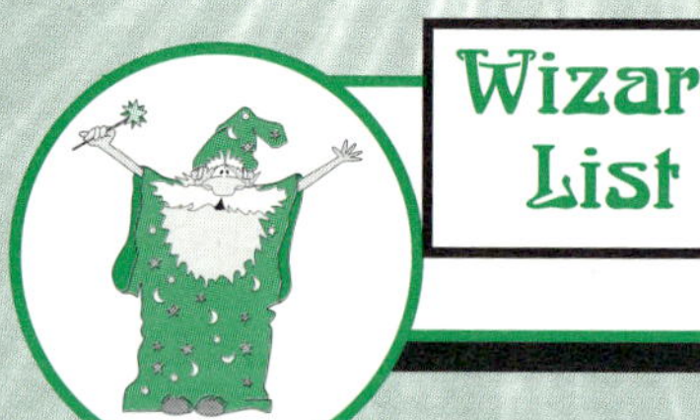

Completed "The Next Step" (Feedback, Part 1), pens or pencils

Preparation

1. Bring the completed "The Next Step" worksheets to the meeting.
2. Plan to implement this exercise 5 to 10 minutes before the end of the meeting.
3. Provide pens or pencils for each participant.

Implementation

1. Explain to the team that you are going to pass out their completed "The Next Step" worksheets from the last meeting.
2. Ask each member to review "The Next Step" worksheets and comment on the team's progress and their own involvement.

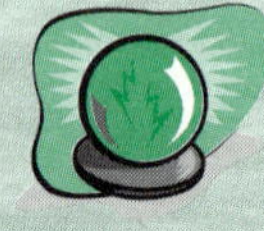

Debriefing

Ask for discussion of their evaluation of the team so far. Is the team focused? Are they meeting their commitment to the team so

far and are they meeting their goals? Identify how this is taking place.

Magic Touch

You might choose to use this in later meetings, after the team has experienced some of the different stages a team goes through. See Part 3 of this text "Yes, We'll Form, Storm, Norm, and Perform" for material on stages. If the team is moving into the storming phase, things may not be going smoothly. After you teach the team about the behaviors found to occur in teams in the storming stage, it is easier to surface conflict and discuss important differences of opinion.

STAND UP AND BE COUNTED!

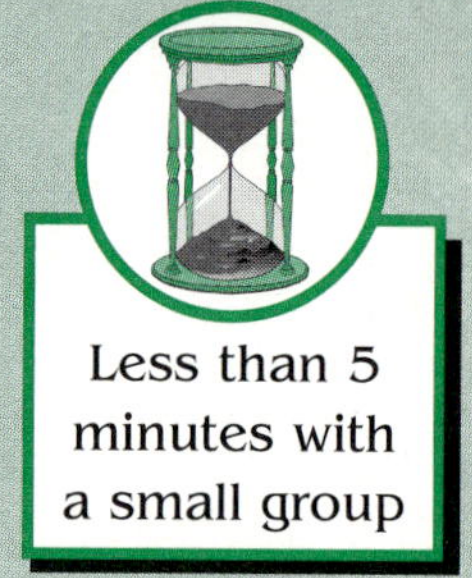

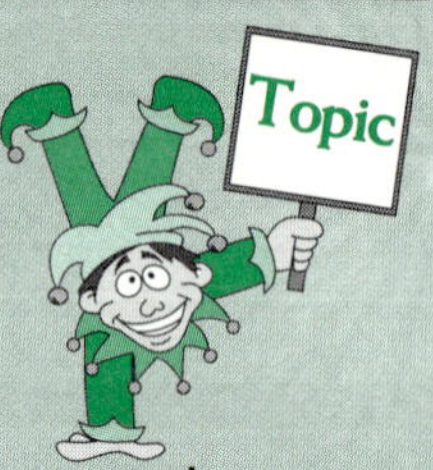

Feedback with exercise. Use to get feedback about team members' expectations about teamwork. This one requires people to move; sometime this is helpful after much sitting or for a group that is less likely to do a written exercise.

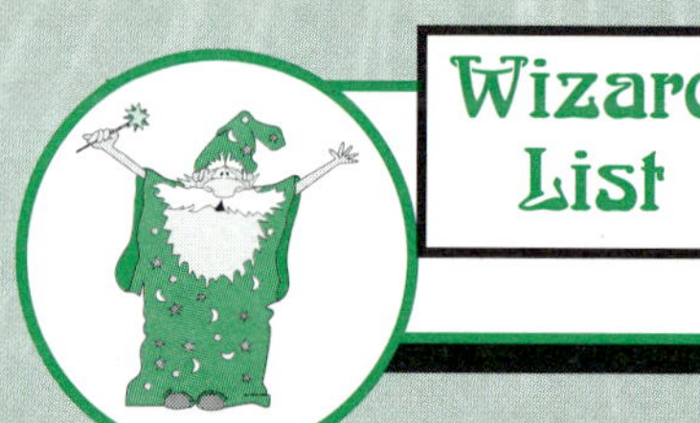

Wizard List "Efficiency, Accuracy, Enjoy, I want it all" posters, masking tape, candy

Preparation

1. Copy "Efficiency," "Accuracy," "Enjoy," and "I Want It All" signs. Use 8½″ × 11″ paper or make posters.
2. Tape one sign in each corner of the room.

Implementation

1. Ask team members to choose the sign that most indicates what they want in a team.
2. Instruct team members to go stand in front of the sign they have chosen and be prepared to explain their choice.
3. When all have moved, ask them to explain their choice. For a large group there can be a consensus discussion and a spokesperson can be appointed to announce the group's feeling.

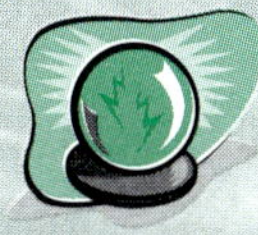

Debriefing

Explain that it helps to get physical and practice taking a stand . . . get it?

Magic Touch

You might choose to give treats such as miniature candy bars or gum or hard candies as a reward for "standing up." Additional topics for discussion may include the influence of peers in proclaiming an opinion and the chances you take when speaking out for an idea.

Efficiency

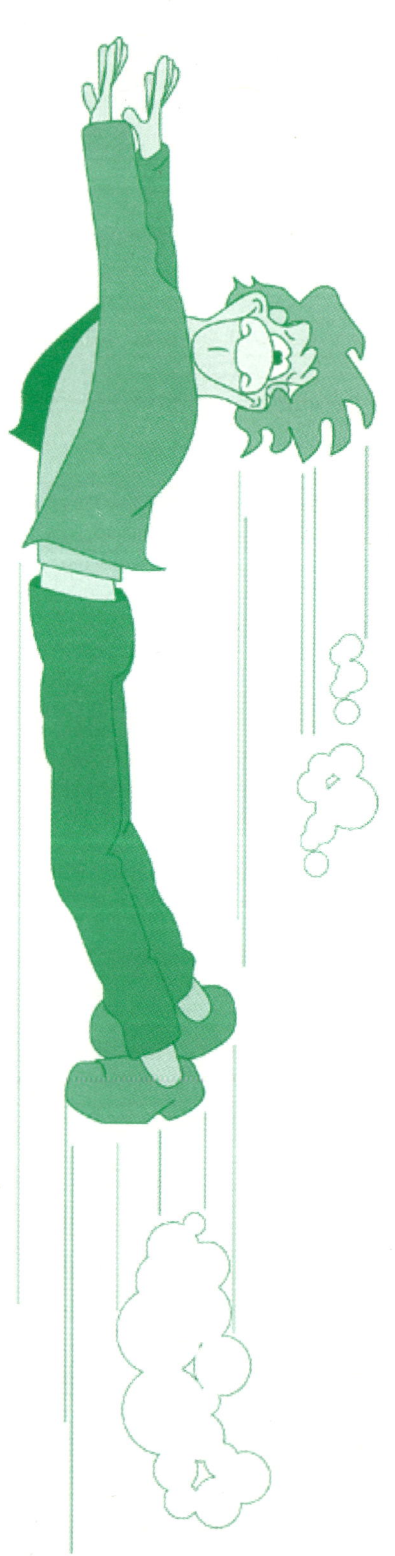

Accuracy

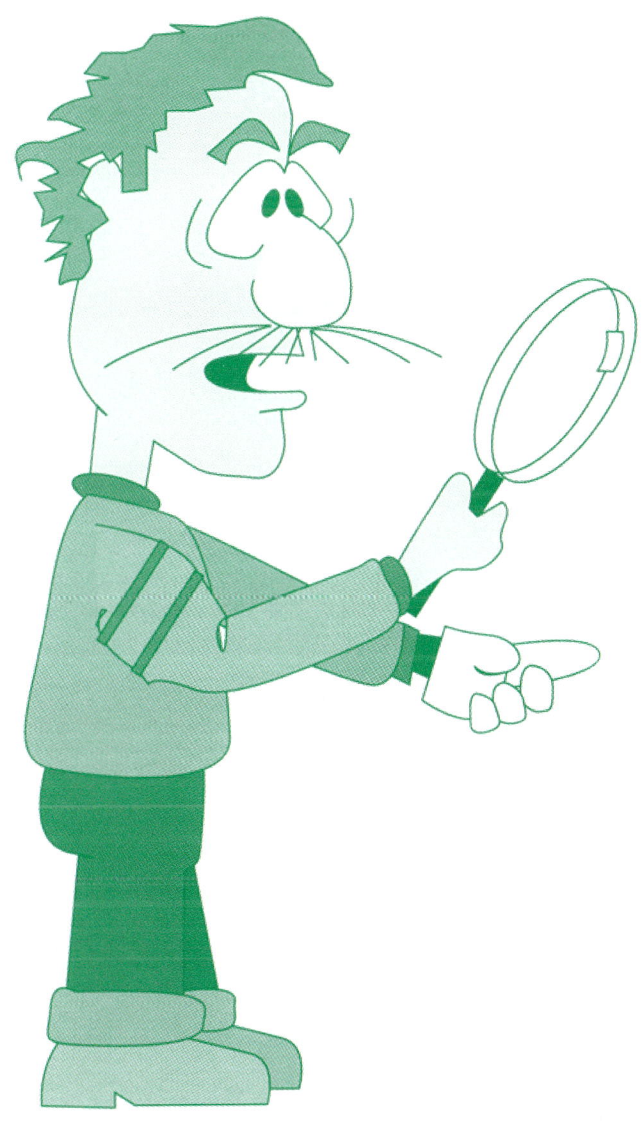

Enjoy

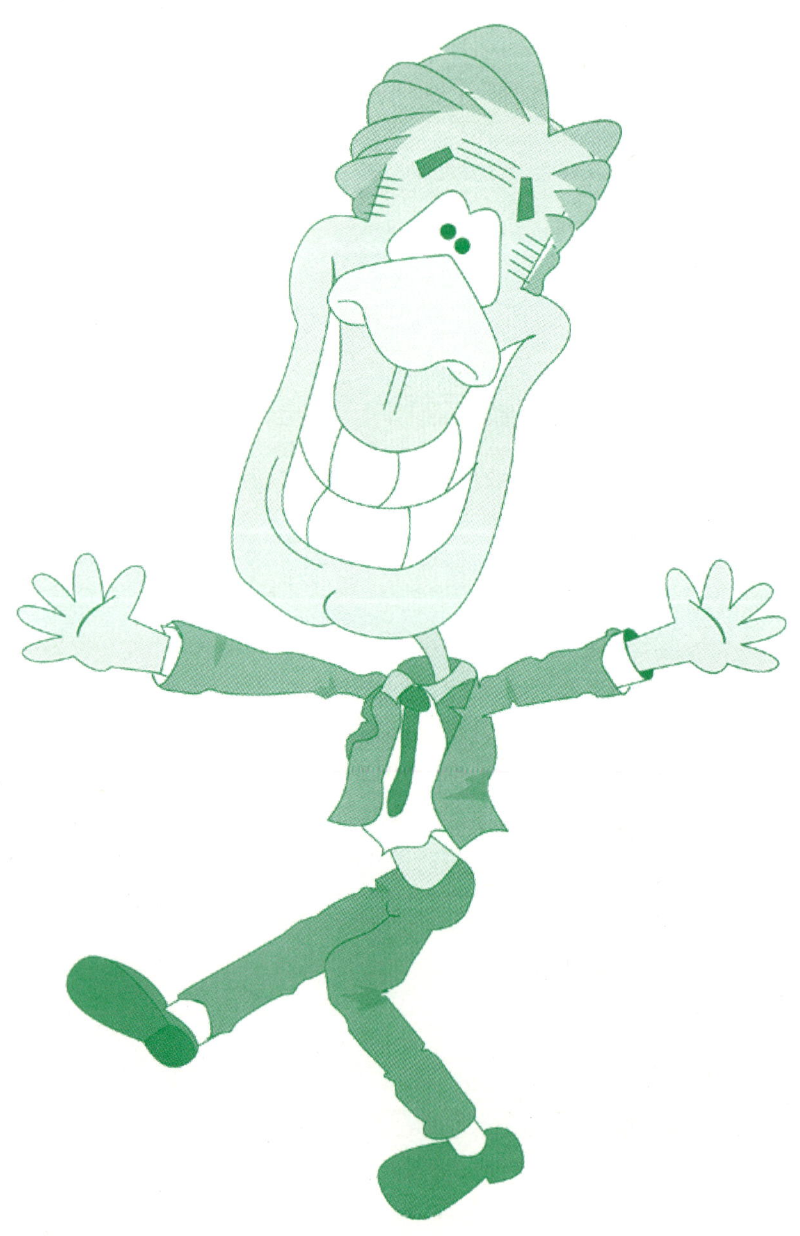

I want it all!

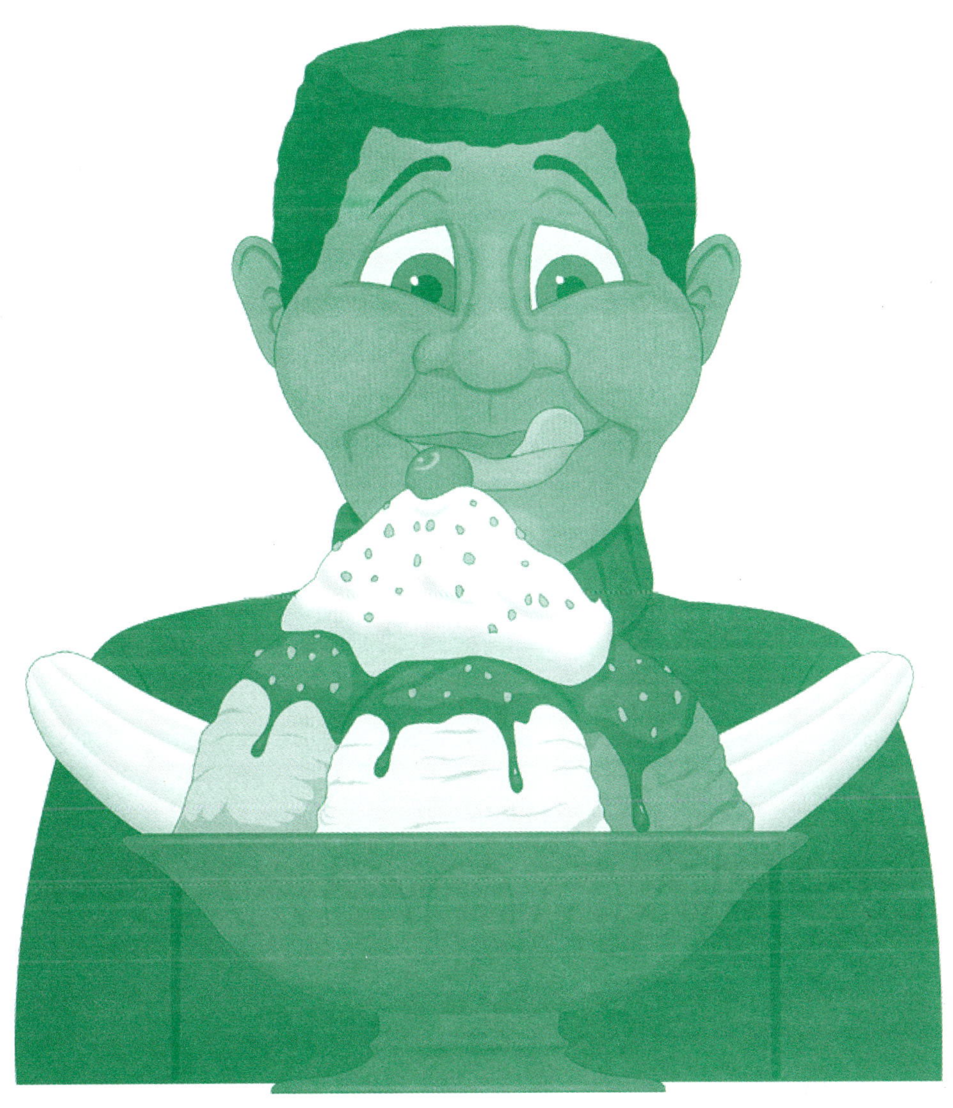

YOU'RE ON MY AGENDA

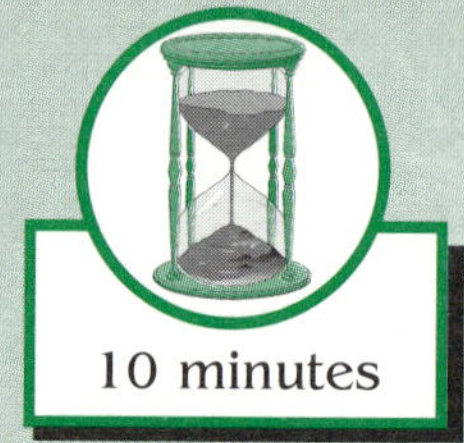

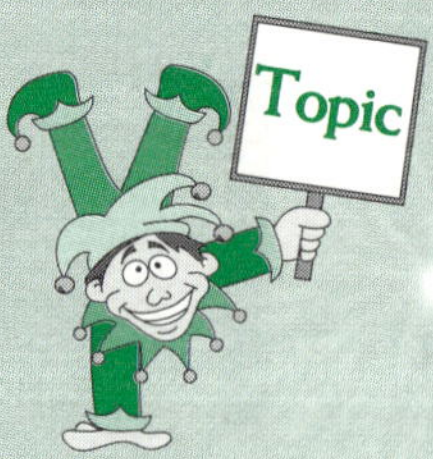

Agendas. Use when teaching team training or for making your personal agendas effective and interesting. This is not a team exercise.

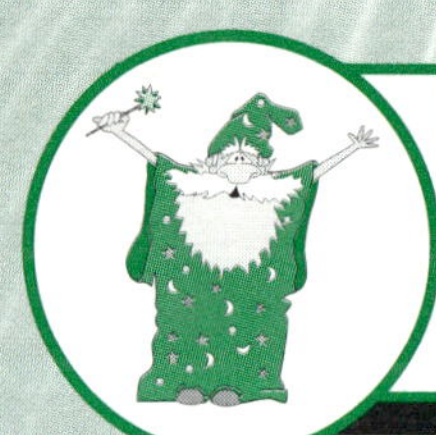

Wizard List

"Create an Agenda . . . Who, Me?," "Make Sense of This!," "Make Sense of This! Answer Key," "There's a Poet in Each of Us," pens or pencils

Preparation

1. Copy "Create an Agenda . . . Who, Me?," "Make Sense of This!," "Make Sense of This! Answer Key," "There's a Poet in Each of Us."
2. Provide pens or pencils for each team member.

Implementation

1. Distribute "Create an Agenda . . . Who, Me?"
2. Explain the importance of an agenda. Point out the scrambled word at the top of the agenda and mention how this activity gets members involved.
3. Distribute "Make Sense of This!" and ask class members to unscramble the words listed. Allow 3 minutes.
4. Distribute "Make Sense of This! Answer Key" and ask that each member be on their honor to correct their own papers.
5. Provide the winner with a small prize.
6. Distribute copies of "There's a Poet in Each of Us" to provide an additional example of creative approaches. Try writing one of your own!

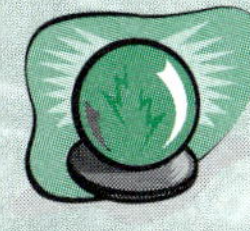

Debriefing

Distributing an agenda before a team meeting gives members a chance to prepare to make their best contributions and serves as an assignment reminder. Adding a creative touch to each agenda sets up the expectation that this is one memo worth reading.

Magic Touch

Wave your magic wand and create an impressive agenda using some of the following suggestions: seasonal or motivational stickers and clip art, gold stars when the team is making progress, a scrambled word that is specific to the life of the team, colored paper.

CREATE AN AGENDA . . .
WHO ME?

AGENDA

Start thinking now!! Make sense of this: **stapient**
The first person to arrive at the meeting with the right answer gets a prize.

Date:

To:

From:

Location:

Start Time: 1:00

End Time: 2:00

Team goal: To provide effective patient teaching at discharge

Meeting goal: Review of process

Topic	Presenter(s)	Time
Update/review	Jim Johnson	5 min.
Responsibility	Molly Green	15 min.
Existing process	Dianne Reid	15 min.
Data collection	Glenn Tye	15 min.
Legal issues	Guy Framptom	5 min.
The next step/summary	Jim Johnson	10 min.

MAKE SENSE OF THIS!

Scrambled words

1. sepdoolakeic
2. suasionper
3. rageousout
4. knihtpuorg
5. texper
6. logueaid
7. senconsus
8. sionsim
9. ponsresibility
10. stapient

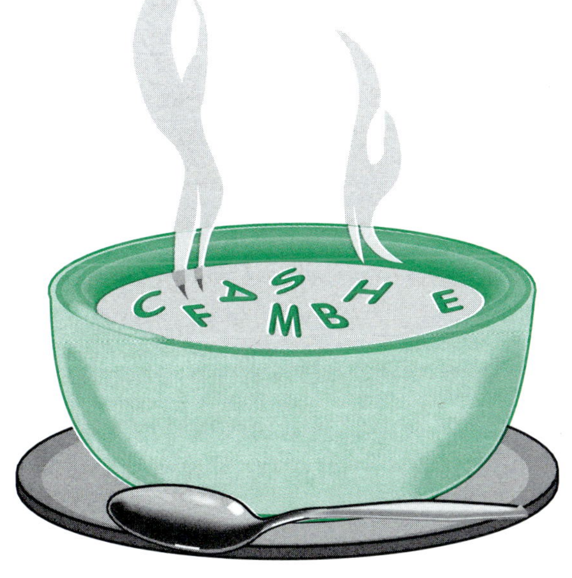

MAKE SENSE OF THIS!

Answer Key

1. kaleidoscope Give a small kaleidoscope for the prize and explain that it represents the changing nature of the health care scene and the need to solve problems efficiently, in a timely manner for quality care.
2. persuasion Give a small gift such as a funny memo pad from a card shop printed with some office humor. Remind the team that they will need their powers of persuasion in the implementation phase of a solution to the team.
3. outrageous Give an outrageous gift like bubbles or pick-up sticks. Use this when you will be brainstorming in the meeting to illustrate that contributions can be off the wall. Some outrageous ideas have led to creative solutions to problems. Are you old enough to remember when a computer took up a whole city block? (UNIVAC in Washington, D.C.) Who would have thought that the same computing power could be in a small personal computer in millions of homes?
4. groupthink Give a roll of Life Savers in all the same flavor. Use this when group members seem to agree all the time, look for easy solutions, and hesitate to confront one another. Explain that although candy that is all the same shape and flavor is good, variety is appreciated.
5. expert Use this to initiate a discussion about each team member's importance on the team. You can give a sheet of small gold star stickers to each team member and instruct that the stars should be used as rewards when someone

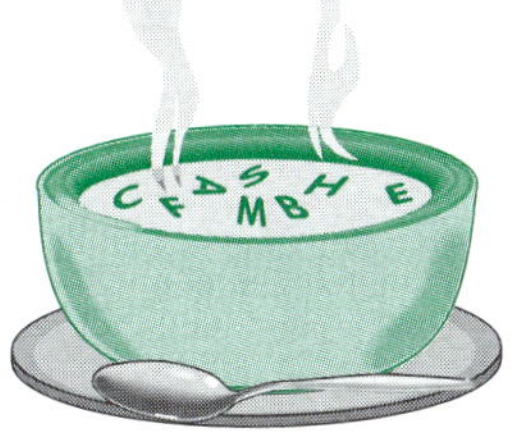

does something extra or just when someone needs a lift. Give the person who first unscrambled the word two sheets!

6. dialogue   Dialogue is a true sharing of thoughts and ideas. Just the ticket for positive teamwork. Give a movie pass: "Just the ticket!"
7. consensus   A high-level skill in teams is the ability to reach consensus. Sometimes a tool, such as a decision-making grid, is necessary to weigh the options and have a more objective method of making a decision. We don't want quick-fixes (no "Band-aid" solutions). Give a box of decorative Band-aids. There are some great Band-aids that feature various cartoon characters.
8. mission   Use this word when the team seems to be losing its focus. Remind the group that the mission is the focus of the meetings. Give a small magnifying glass or toy telescope.
9. responsibility   Tell them if they want to see who is responsible for the team, use this—and give the winner a small mirror. Then give mirrors to all members and tell them they are all winners when they all are involved. Remind the group that the sign of a true professional is one who does the best he or she can even when he or she doesn't feel like it.
10. patients   Patients are the reason we are here. Give heart stickers or a heart-shaped eraser.

THERE'S A POET IN EACH OF US!

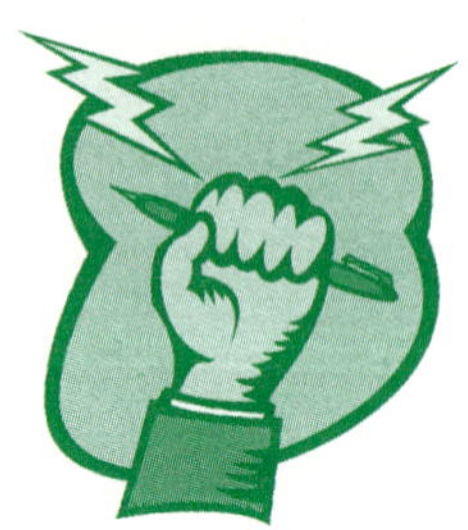

Roses are red,
Violets are blue.
I thank you for all
the work that you do.

Please read this agenda,
Come ready to work.
Within all this data
A solution does lurk!

We've been on this team
For such a long time.
Stay tuned for a solution
That's truly sublime.

GREEN VEGETABLES

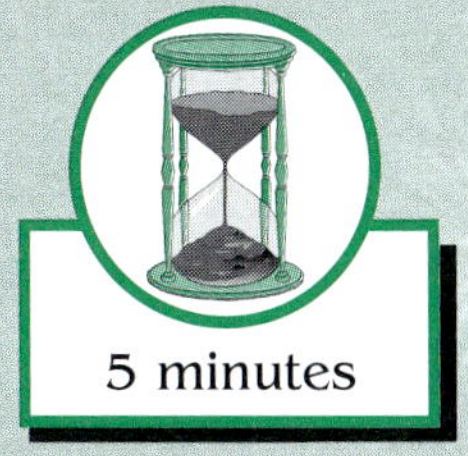

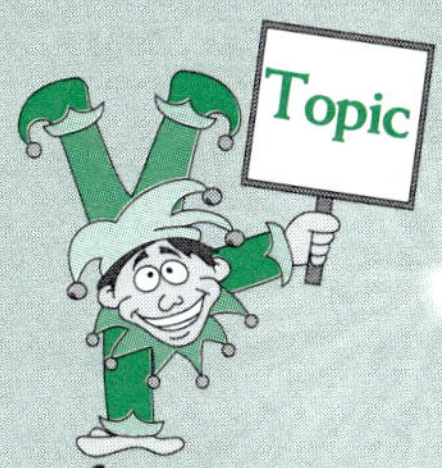

Group problem solving. Use to illustrate the effectiveness of team problem-solving as compared with an individual approach.

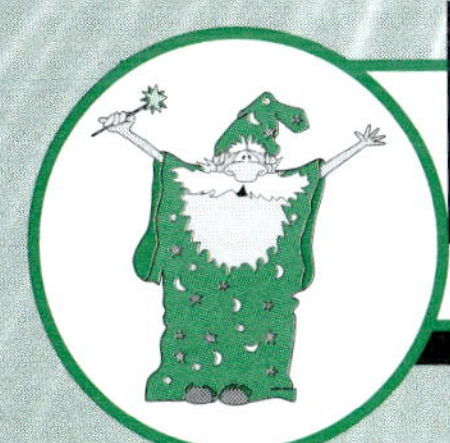

Wizard List

Green vegetable (real, silk, or plastic), flip chart, markers, green paper, pens or pencils

Preparation

1. Obtain a green vegetable to use as a visual aid. The vegetable can be real, silk, or plastic.
2. Title a flip chart page "Why Teams Are Better."
3. Provide one sheet of green paper for each team member.
4. Provide pens or pencils for each team member.

Implementation

1. Ask the group to participate in an experiment.
2. Distribute a sheet of green paper and a pen or pencil to each team member.
3. Hold up the green vegetable and ask each member to think of as many green vegetables as possible. Instruct them to write the vegetable names on the green paper. (Allow about 30 seconds.)
4. Ask members to count the number of vegetables on their sheet and write that number at the top of the paper.
5. Ask how many had 1 to 5, 6 to 10, or more than 10. Ascertain the highest number and write it on the flip chart.

6. Divide the team members into small groups and have each group select a recorder.
7. Instruct the members of each group to work together to record their list of green vegetables. (Allow about 30 seconds.)
8. Ask how many each group listed and record each group's total on the flip chart.

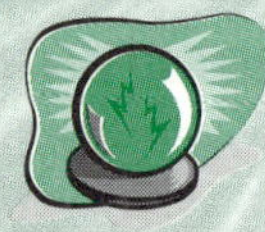

Debriefing

The groups should have generated a longer list than any individual did. (Of course they will!) Ask the group to explain what this illustrates. For example, more ideas are generated from teams and more can be accomplished in the same, or shorter, period of time.

Magic Touch

Sometimes, either in an effort to help or due to anxiety, leaders or facilitators will answer their own questions. When this happens, the group will expect all questions to be answered; this can lead to feeling uninvolved. Be sure the comments cover the purpose, that the team can do more work than an individual working alone.

SHORT CLIPS

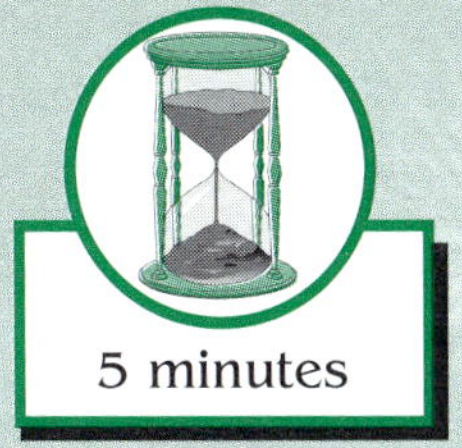

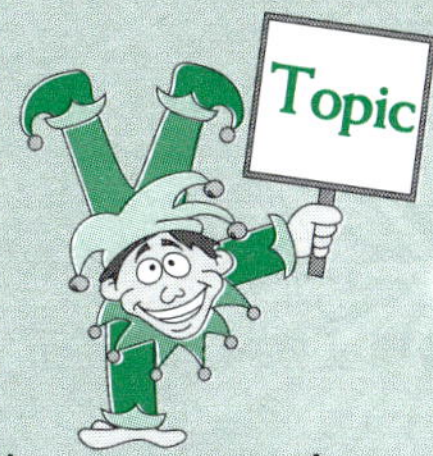

Working together. Use this to illustrate the benefits of working together.

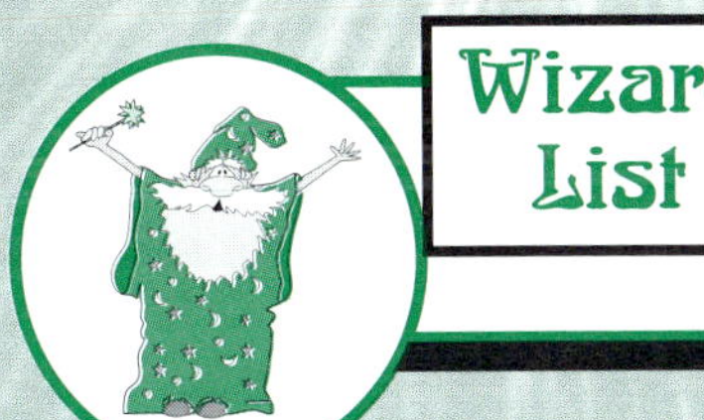

Wizard List

Colored paper clips (2 boxes of 100 clips each), watch with a second hand

Preparation

None.

Implementation

1. Ask the team to give you 5 minutes for a demonstration that is important to the team.
2. Explain you need one volunteer to put 100 paper clips together in a chain as quickly as possible and one volunteer to time the event.
3. Have the timer say "Start" and then record the time it takes the other volunteer to build the chain. Announce the time.
4. Next, tell the group that they can work together to put the 100 paper clips in a chain. You time them and tell the group the time it took.

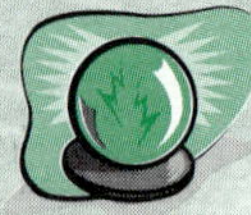

Debriefing

Ask the group what they learned. If no one mentions that teamwork is more efficient and more fun, add these!

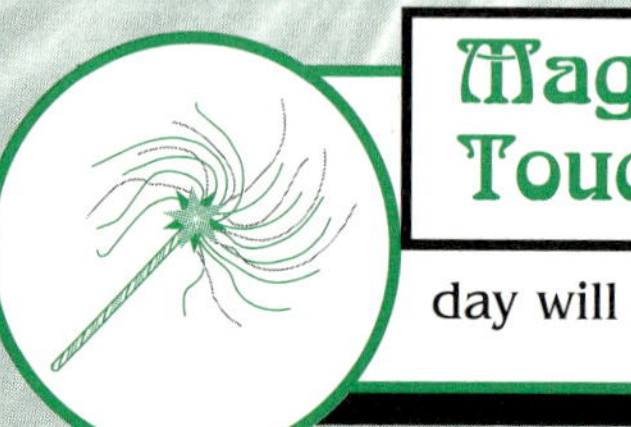

Distribute a box of color paper clips to each team member. Wave the wand. "When you use these, your day will be brighter."

By: Diane Raines, RN, MSN

AN APPLE IS THE TEACHER!

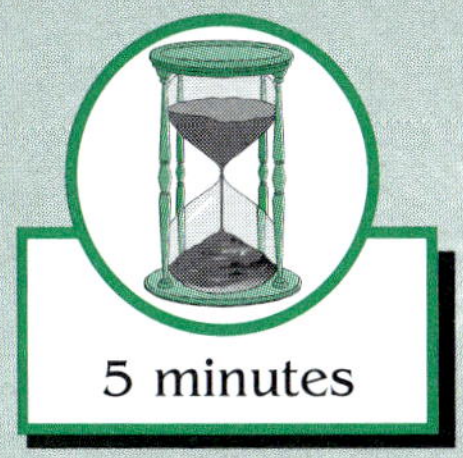

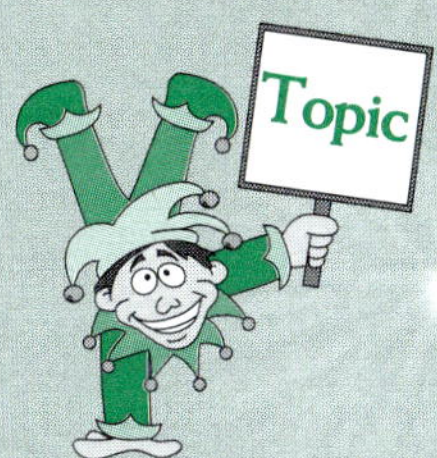

Details. Use to illustrate the importance of observation to detail and closer examination before assuming processes are alike in different departments. Also use when problem-solving tools become tedious.

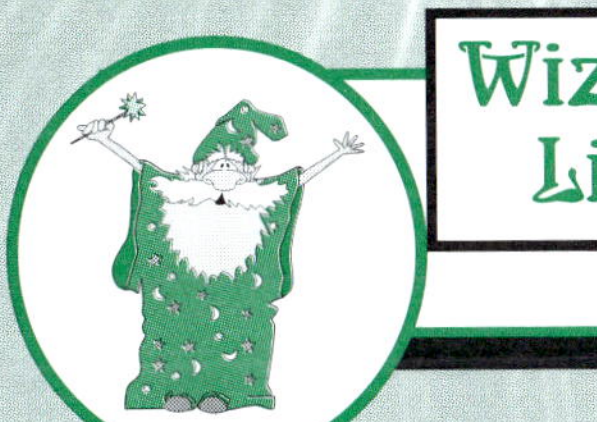

Wizard List

Apples (enough for everyone and all the same variety), basket

Preparation

1. Bring apples, all the same variety and similar in size, in a basket to the meeting.

Implementation

1. Ask all team members to come up and choose an apple.
2. Explain that they have one minute to observe their apple and notice all its characteristics. Tell the members to "get to know their apple."
3. Instruct the members not to mark their apple or change its appearance in any way!
4. When one minute has elapsed, collect the apples in the basket and mix them up.
5. Ask each group member to go to the basket and find his or her apple!
6. Ask the members to talk about what they learned.
7. Tell team members the apples are theirs to keep.

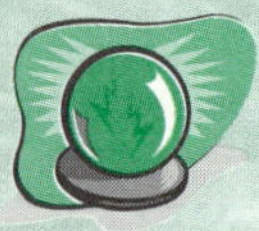

Debriefing

Admit that you expect some members are wondering why they did this activity and what it could possibly have to do with the team. Point out that the power of observation, attention to detail, and not making the assumption that staff, equipment, or processes in different departments are the same.

Magic Touch

If you are at a time in the life of the team when a celebration is in order . . . or if it just seems like a time the team would be responsive, have someone wash the apples. (This is HEALTH care, you know.) Provide thinly sliced cheddar cheese, chocolate fondue (if you use an electric fondue pot), or a caramel fruit dip as a gourmet treat!

THE BAKER'S DOZEN

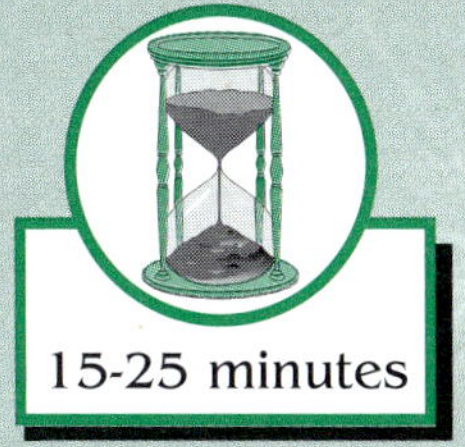

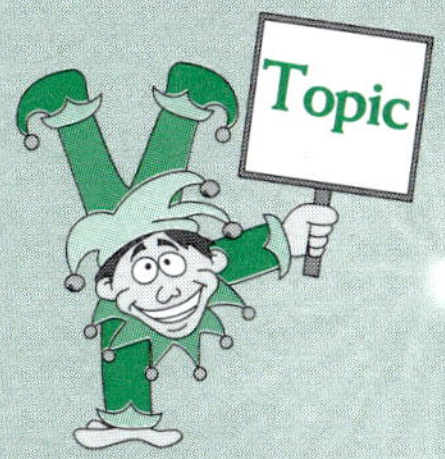

Icebreaker. Personalizing team building. Due to time requirements, use in a half-day or all-day meeting or team training session or use fewer questions for a shorter meeting.

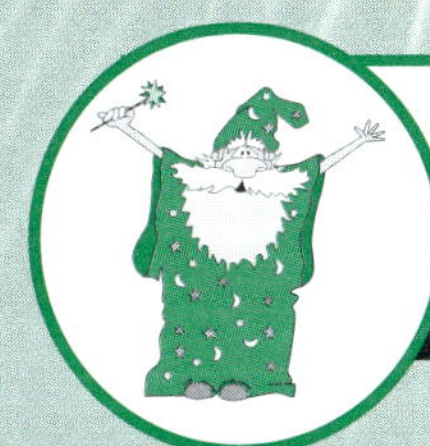

Wizard List

"Baker's Dozen" worksheet, "The Baker's Dozen" sign, pens or pencils, doughnuts or cookies for all

Preparation

1. Copy "The Baker's Dozen" worksheet for each team member.
2. Copy "The Baker's Dozen" sign.
3. Purchase doughnuts or cookies—make sure you have enough for everyone.
4. Provide pens or pencils for each member.

Implementation

1. Set up a table to display the doughnuts or cookies and "the Baker's Dozen" sign.
2. Ask the team to answer the questions on "The Baker's Dozen" worksheet and be prepared to share their answers. (Allow 10 minutes.)
3. Distribute "The Baker's Dozen" worksheet and pens or pencils to each team member.
4. Ask members to pick a partner, someone they don't know well if possible, and share their answers. Allow 5 minutes.

5. Ask for volunteers to share something interesting they have learned about their partner.
6. Invite the team to share in the Baker's Dozen, the food you provided.

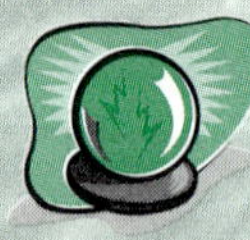

Debriefing

Explain that we do icebreakers such as "The Baker's Dozen" to make people more comfortable and to build trust for the work ahead.

Magic Touch

Sharing food after the members have had a chance to share personal information helps continue the "getting acquainted" process.

THE BAKER'S DOZEN

1. My first job was ______________.
2. My favorite job was ______________.
3. I have been in health care ______________ years.
4. My idea job would be ______________.
5. My favorite part of my job is ______________.
6. One thing that irritates me at work is ______________.
7. If I were to describe my experience with teams, I would say ______________
   ______________.
8. I hope this experience will be ______________.
9. One strength I bring to this team is ______________.
10. One concern I have about this team is ______________
    ______________.
11. My goal for myself in this group is ______________.
12. What I'd like to see the team accomplish is ______________
    ______________.
13. One thing I have always wanted to do is ______________
    ______________.

Fold Here

THE BAKER'S DOZEN

THE TIME CAPSULE

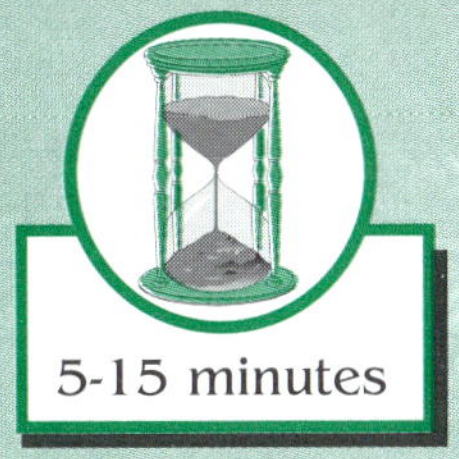

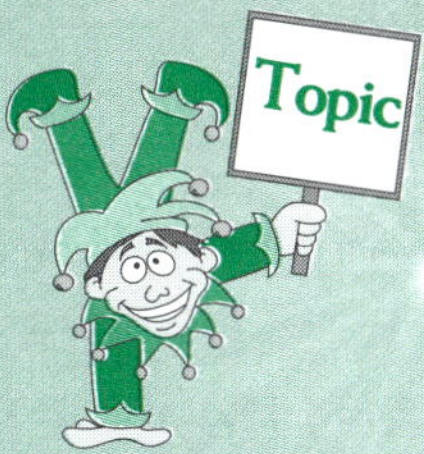

Icebreaker or energizer. Use to give perspective.

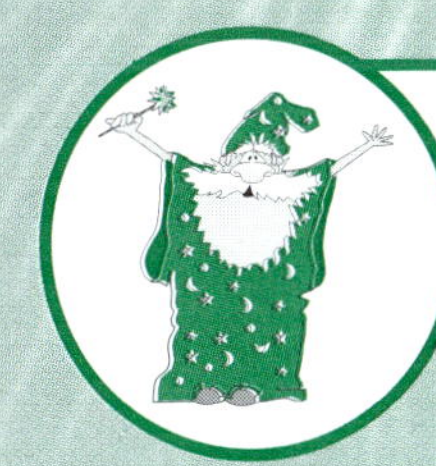

Wizard List

"The Time Capsule" worksheet, colored markers

Preparation

1. Copy "The Time Capsule" worksheet on brightly colored paper for each team member.
2. Provide a marker for each team member.

Implementation

1. Distribute "The Time Capsule" worksheets and read the scenario aloud.
2. Ask the group to take a few minutes to think of their department's important, memorable contributions.
3. Ask the members to choose a memorable item and write it in the time capsule.
4. Ask each member to share their memorable items.

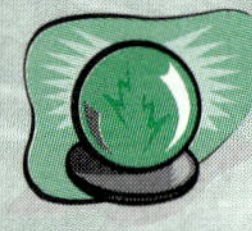

Debriefing

Explain that spending a few minutes to reflect on positive events adds perspective to our work, allows us to be proud of our accomplishments, and refreshes us for the work ahead.

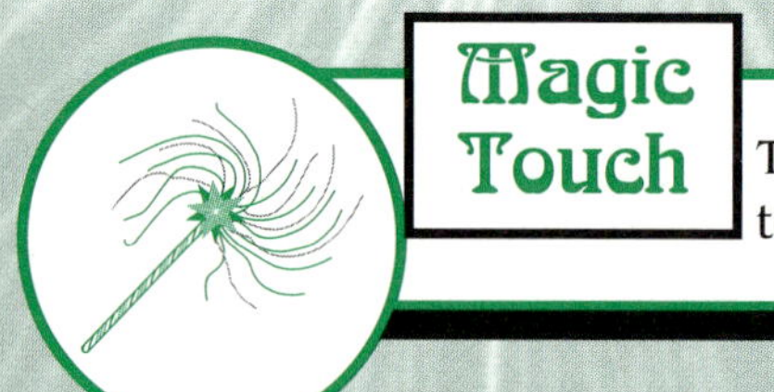

Magic Touch

Thinking about where we have been encourages us to think about where we should be or want to be.

THE TIME CAPSULE

Your health care organization has just merged with another. To commemorate the occasion, each department has been asked to contribute one item, or a facsimile of it, to a time capsule to represent its contribution to the delivery of health care in this year. The capsule will be opened in 5 years—change is too rapid to wait 100 years!

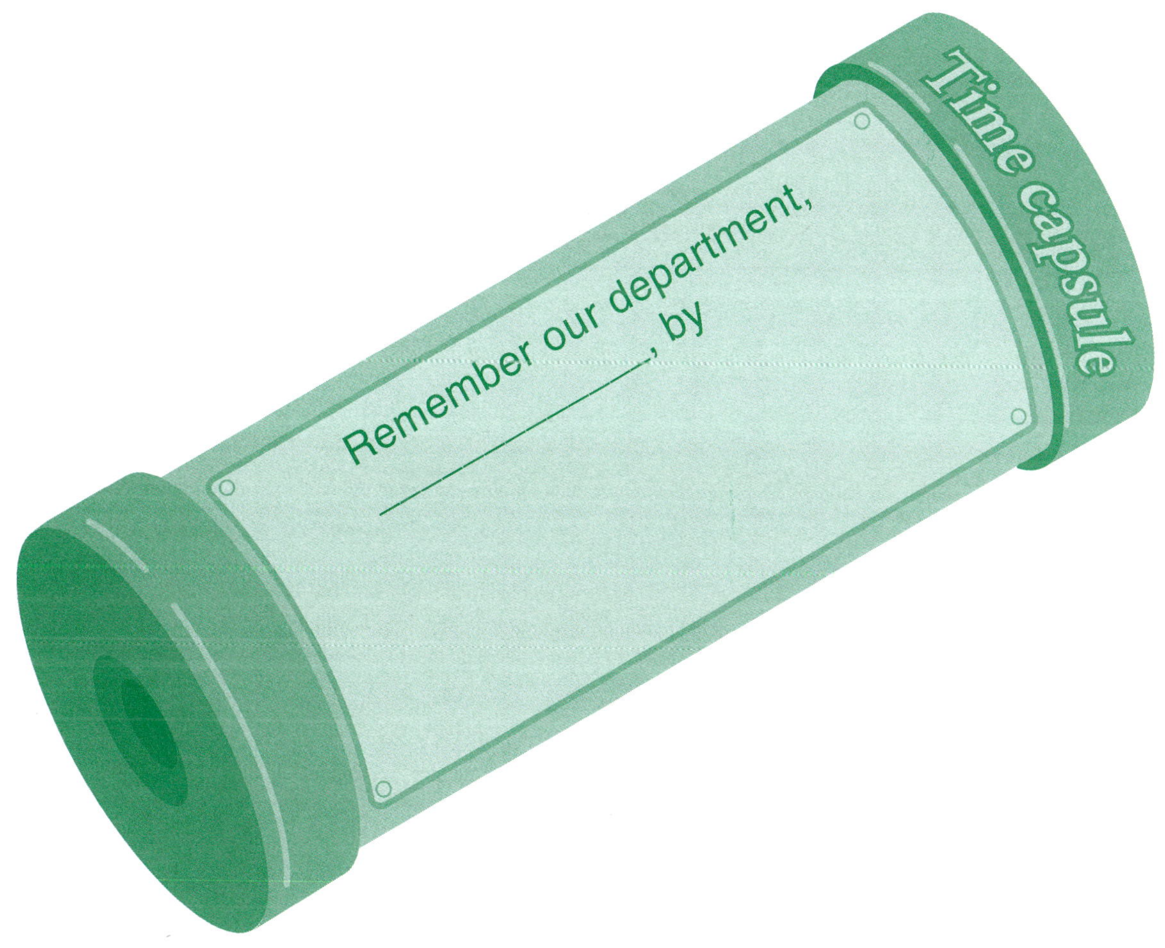

ART IN PROGRESS

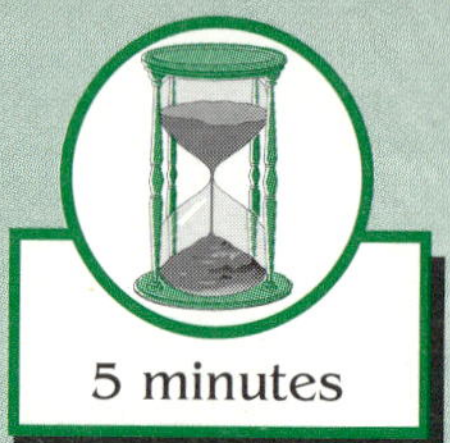

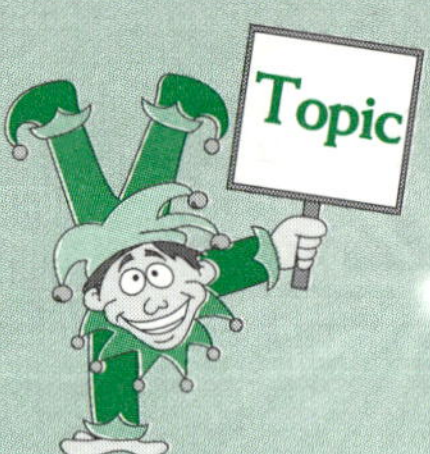

Focused behavior. Use to encourage members to have meeting goals.

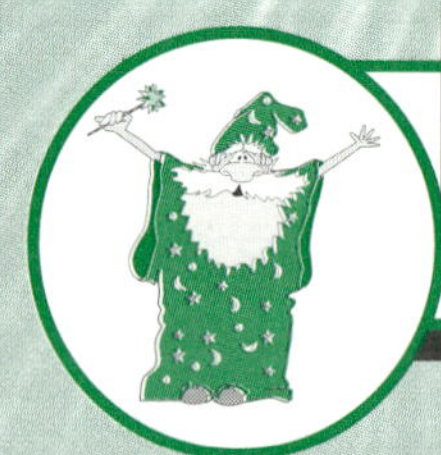

Wizard List

Butcher paper or plain white shelf paper 5-10 feet long, masking tape, colored markers, flip chart

Preparation

1. Cut butcher paper or plain white shelf paper 5 to 10 feet long.
2. Write on the flip chart, "Before you sit down, draw a picture to depict your goal for this meeting."
3. Provide markers for the team members.

Implementation

1. Tape the paper to a flat wall at a height that is easy to reach.
2. Display the "Before you sit down draw a picture to depict your goal for this meeting" near the entrance.
3. After the first member to arrive has drawn a picture, ask that member to point out the sign to the others as they enter. (Some members may have trouble conceptualizing a picture for this. Writing the goal is okay. The main idea is to get members to consider the idea of having such a goal.)
4. Draw your own! You may want to do this first to get the thought process moving in the right direction.
5. Before the meeting starts, ask members to explain their drawings.

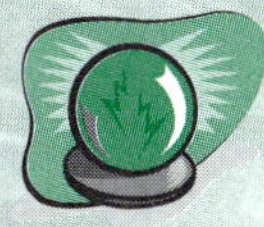

Debriefing

When we force ourselves to think about a goal for the meeting, rather than just showing up, it helps us to be more productive and to share responsibility for progress. Encourage members to establish this habit.

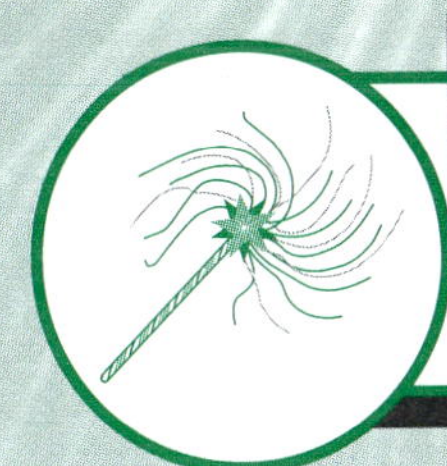

Magic Touch

Suggest using this exercise in staff/committee meetings to help people set goals for what they want to accomplish.

BE A GROUPER

A Fishy Tale

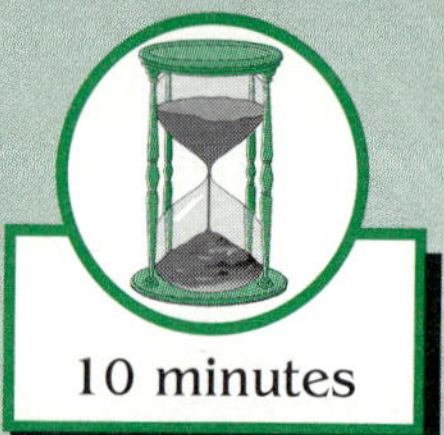

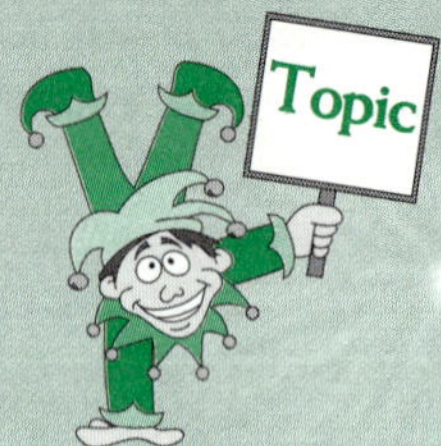

Team characteristics. Use to think about ingredients of a successful group.

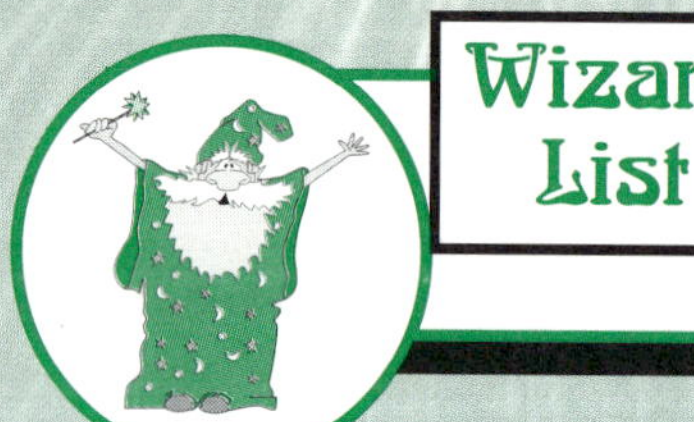

Wizard List

"Be a Grouper" handout, magic wand, cookies and milk (optional)

Preparation

1. Copy "Be a Grouper" for each team member.
2. Supply magic wand.
3. Provide cookies and milk.

Implemenation

1. Ask team members if they remember having a story time in school, and cookies and milk, and a rest time? Tell the team you're setting the stage for your story time and the cookies and milk are atmosphere enhancers.
2. Serve the cookies and milk.
3. Read aloud "Be a Grouper."
4. Explain that many cultures use storytelling to teach a lesson. Wave the magic wand and say, "One magical ingredient to a team's success is everyone's participation."
5. Ask who will take the wand first, to share one thing that the group in the fishy tale need to win the coveted "I'm a Grouper" award.

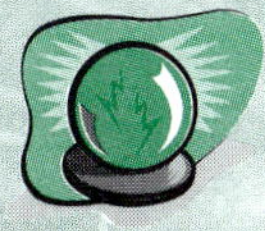

Debriefing

Allow time for team members to respond. To encourage response, mention the importance of dealing openly with conflict, being open to member's ideas, giving feedback to each other, and so forth. Thank the team for being willing to play.

Magic Touch

Ask a team member to read the story aloud to the group. Allow a few minutes for a silent review. Storytelling is a great way to teach a lesson or illustrate a specific point.

BE A GROUPER

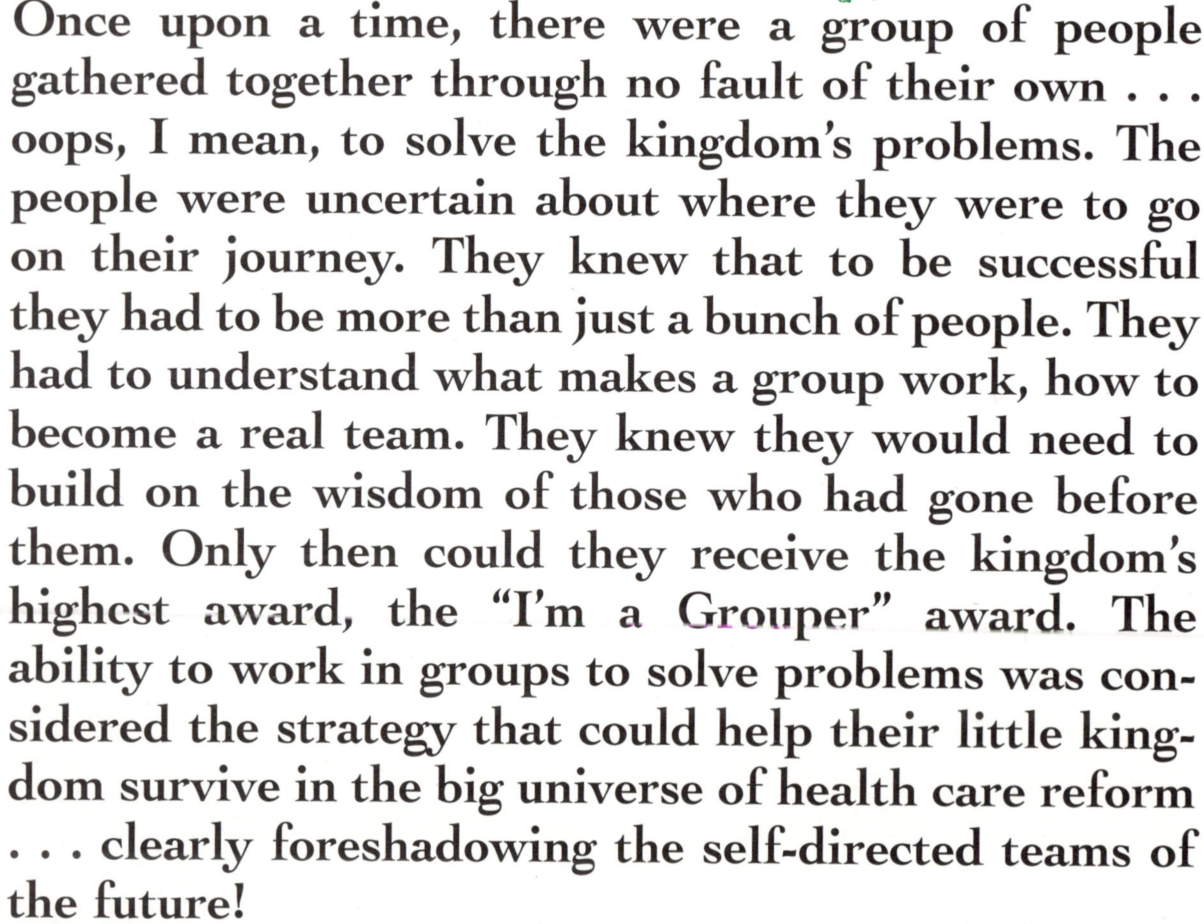

A Fishy Tale

Once upon a time, there were a group of people gathered together through no fault of their own . . . oops, I mean, to solve the kingdom's problems. The people were uncertain about where they were to go on their journey. They knew that to be successful they had to be more than just a bunch of people. They had to understand what makes a group work, how to become a real team. They knew they would need to build on the wisdom of those who had gone before them. Only then could they receive the kingdom's highest award, the "I'm a Grouper" award. The ability to work in groups to solve problems was considered the strategy that could help their little kingdom survive in the big universe of health care reform . . . clearly foreshadowing the self-directed teams of the future!

Can you help this group become a real team by sharing your wisdom from past team experiences?

TO KNOW OR NOT TO KNOW . . . THAT IS THE QUESTION

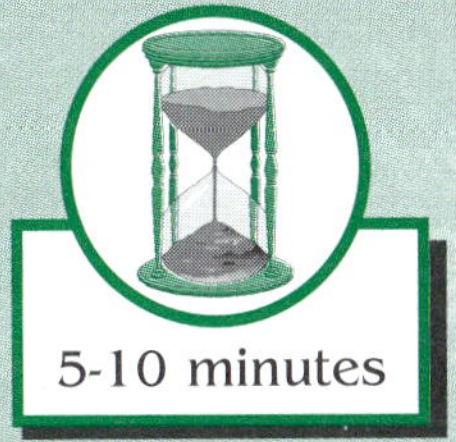

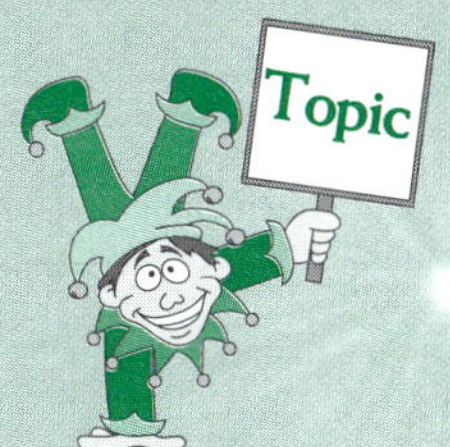

Use to illustrate the importance of identifying resources.

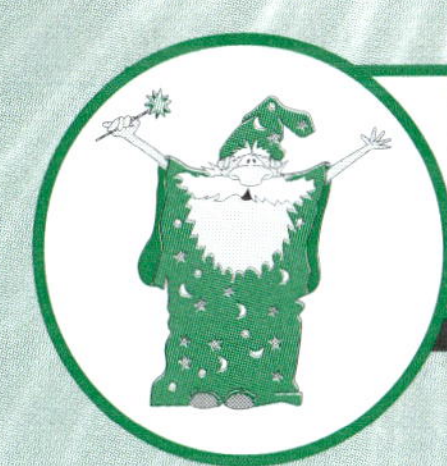

Wizard List Index cards, pens or pencils

Preparation

1. Prepare a list of 3 to 4 questions that require research, or use the following suggestions.
   a. "How can I improve my golf swing?"
   b. "How can I make play dough for my children?"
   c. "How can I learn about the Internet?"
2. Don't identify the answers, but rather how you could find the answers.

Implementation

1. Distribute index cards and pencils.
2. Ask members to write one question to which they would like an answer. Tell them not to supply the answer, but rather how they could find the answer. For example, possible sources are:
   a. Golf pro, friend, video.
   b. Children's craft book, cookbook, home extension service, reference librarian.
   c. Computer wizard friend, sign on to an online service and go for it!, book.
3. Discuss the importance of indentifying the appropriate resource and knowing how to access the information.

Debriefing

It's not important to have all the answers to the questions. What is important is to know where to find the answers.

Magic Touch

Suggest using this exercise in departmental/staff meetings to fully explore available resources for creative problem solving.

Adapted from: Joann Mulqueen

PICK A CARD . . . ANY CARD

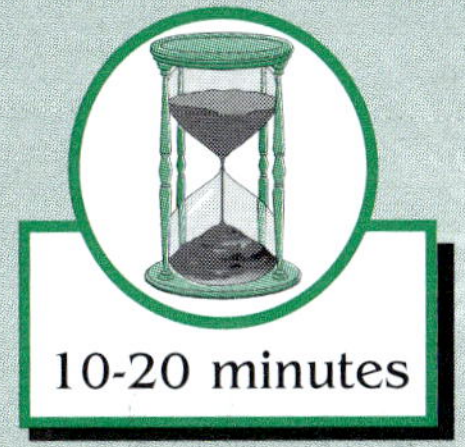

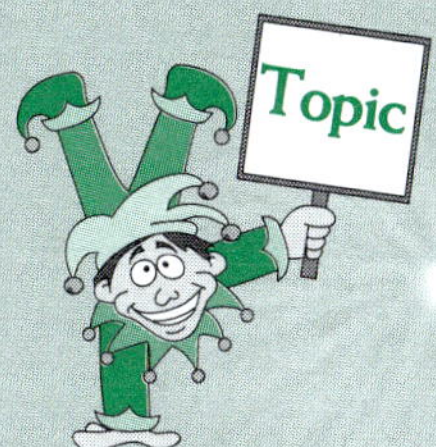

Feedback. Use to form small groups to give feedback about teams.

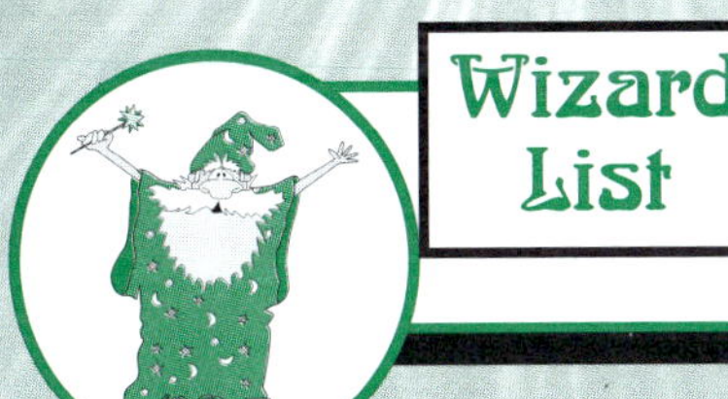

Wizard List A deck of playing cards

Preparation

1. Separate a deck of playing cards into pairs.
2. Select pairs of cards so that each team member, when drawing a card, will be able to find another person with a card with the same number. For example, if you have 8 members, compile 2 aces, 2 twos, 2 threes, and 2 fours.
3. For teams with odd numbers, you will need one card for each team member and one for yourself.

Implementation

1. Put the pairs of cards into a deck and shuffle.
2. Pass the deck, face down, and ask each person to choose one.
3. Ask each member to turn their card over, and find the team member whose card makes a pair with the card selected.
4. (The hardest part is over, honest!) Ask the dyads to discuss their ideas about what is going well with the team and suggest ideas for change.
5. Have participants return the cards for future use.

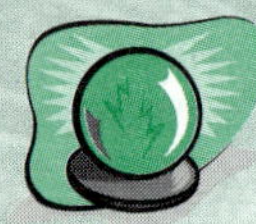

Debriefing

Suggest that it is sometimes easier to talk in small groups before sharing. Ask each group to report what they learned.

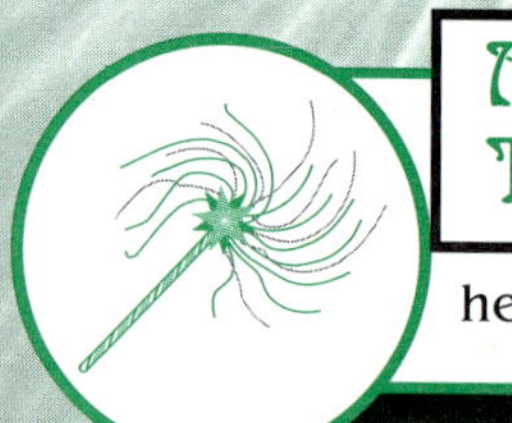

Magic Touch Begin by wearing a top hat and waving the magic wand. "Today we'll focus on the magic of feedback to help our team work more efficiently."

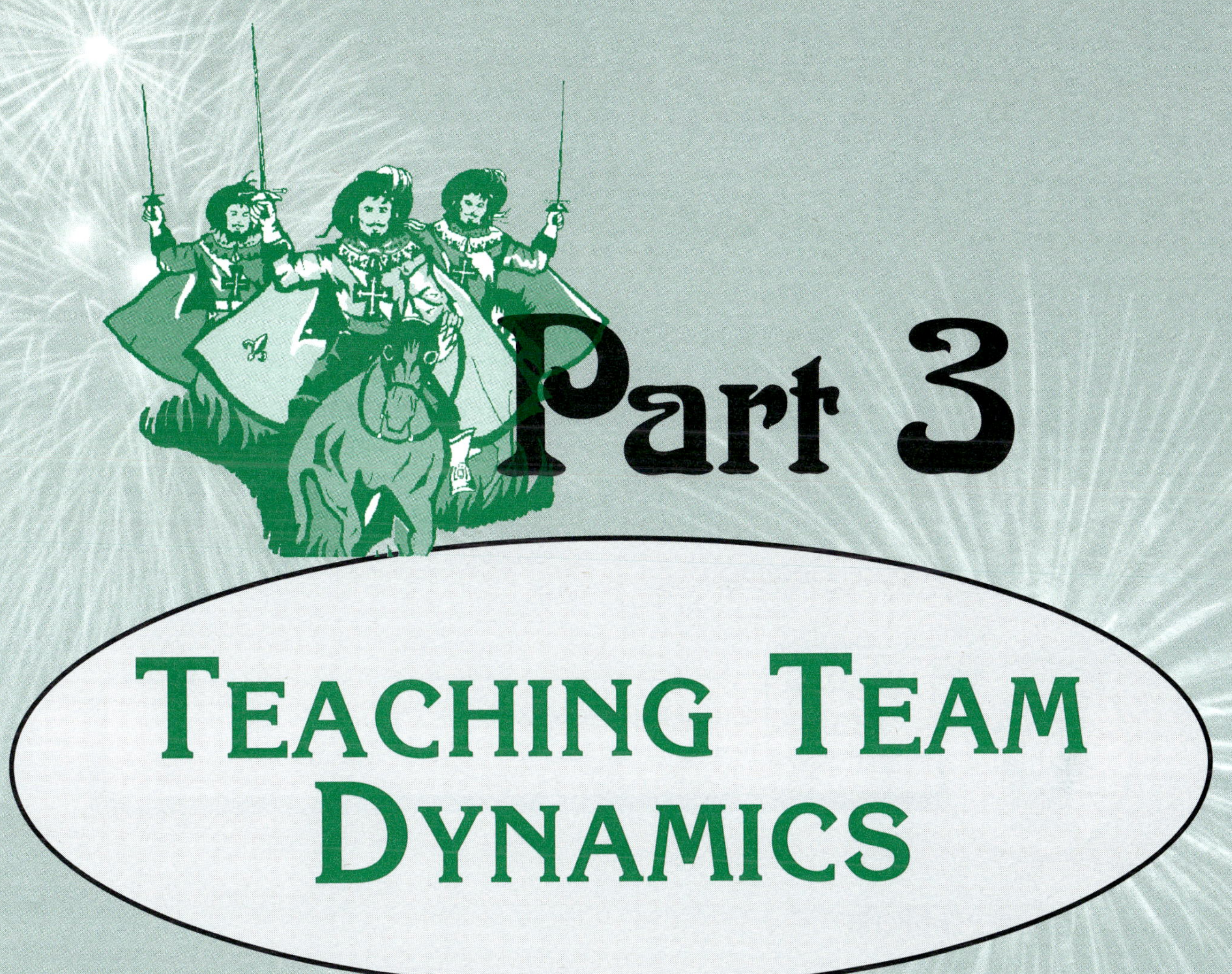

Part 3

Teaching Team Dynamics

People forming a new team arrive with varying degrees of experience with groups, teams, and one another. There is usually some anxiety at the beginning of a new team. Anxiety is defined as a fear of the unknown. Knowledge about teams and how they work can decrease this anxiety and free that energy for the creative work of teams. For example, understanding that total agreement in teams *(groupthink)* may be comfortable but not productive frees people to be honest. It is an eye-opener to understand that *storming* is normal and predictable as team members compete for status and aren't yet sure of the competency of other members. This explains committees that never seem to find a time to reconvene after a stormy meeting. It takes time to build a team. Teaching team dynamics speeds the process. To learn more about team dynamics, see the resources list in this book. I have found Harrington-Mackin's book especially helpful. She identifies four essential behaviors for successful teams (Harrington-Mackin, 1994). In such teams, members:

1. assume responsibility to participate
2. negotiate and build consensus
3. give and receive feedback
4. commit to team goals

The activities that follow can be used in work teams or to accompany team training workshops that are conducted before introducing a formal quality improvement program in a health care organization. These activities reinforce the behaviors essential for team success.

CONGRATULATIONS! YOU'RE ON A TEAM

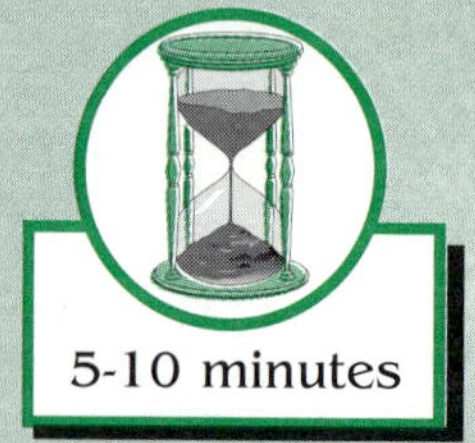

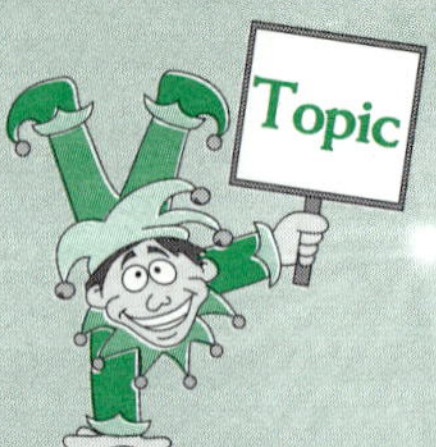

Responsibilities of team membership. Use as an icebreaker to talk about team membership and what it means. Use it for team training or for the first team meeting.

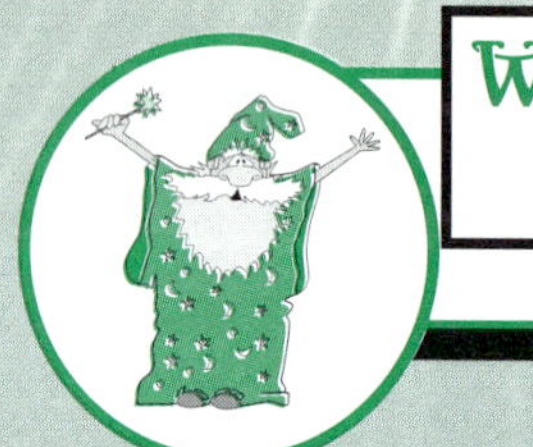

Wizard List

"Congratulations! You're on a Team" pretest, pens or pencils

Preparation

1. Copy "Congratulations! You're on a Team" pretest for each team member.
2. Provide pens or pencils.

Implementation

1. Distribute the "Congratulations! You're on a Team" pretest to each team member.
2. Tell the team that they have one minute to reflect on their experience and ideas about teams and to complete this brief but very important pretest.
3. When all members are finished, ask if the pretest statements are just about right for many committee and team experiences.
4. Ask the team to reflect on each statement and suggest reasons why some team members might see these statements as true.

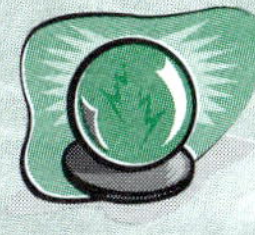

Debriefing

The answer to all five pretest questions is false. Use the following as guidelines to embellish answers if these points are not covered.

- It is not always easy to reach consensus in a team.
- Careful thought needs to go into selection of appropriate team members, with a clear mission statement for a relevant problem.
- It takes effort to inject a little humor and creativity into teams, and it is appreciated.
- Successful teams follow an agenda, hold members accountable for assignments, and maintain a reality check on their work.
- Successful teams need good leadership, active participation, and group facilitation. A plan needs to be made for successful implementation of solutions and a plan to hold the gains of success.

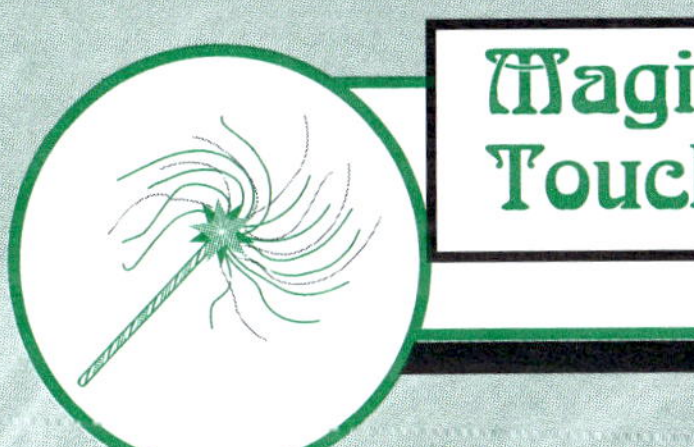

Magic Touch

Use exaggeration and ham it up a bit.

CONGRATULATIONS!

YOU'RE ON A TEAM

Pretest

Take this quick attitude check to see what your experience has been. Answer true or false for each of the following.

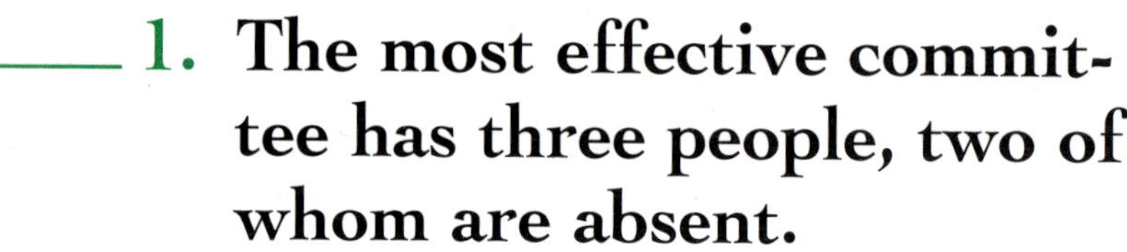

____ 1. The most effective committee has three people, two of whom are absent.

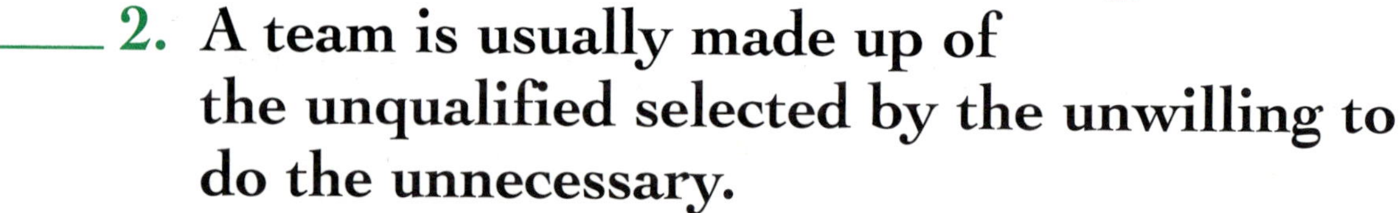

____ 2. A team is usually made up of the unqualified selected by the unwilling to do the unnecessary.

____ 3. Interesting meeting is an oxymoron.

____ 4. A circle is a straight line drawn by a committee.

____ 5. A team is people sitting around talking about things they should be doing.

(Lundy, 1992, p. 108.)

ROLES PEOPLE PLAY

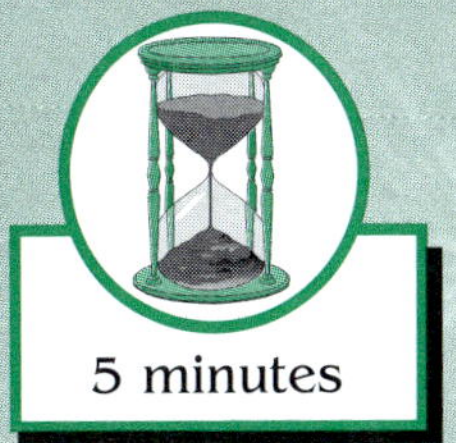

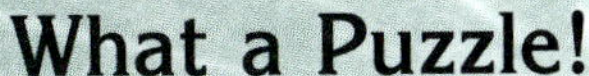

What a Puzzle!

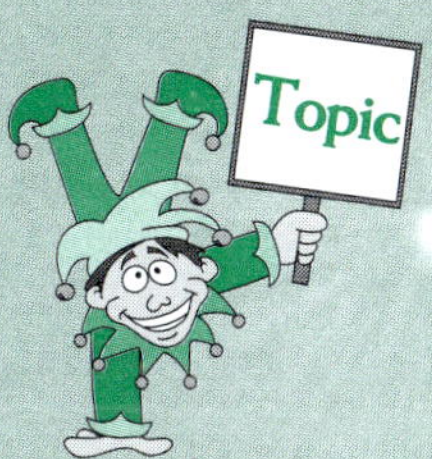

Team member roles. Use to initiate a discussion of group member roles. When teaching team dynamics or when a problematic role behavior impedes group process, introduce this light activity.

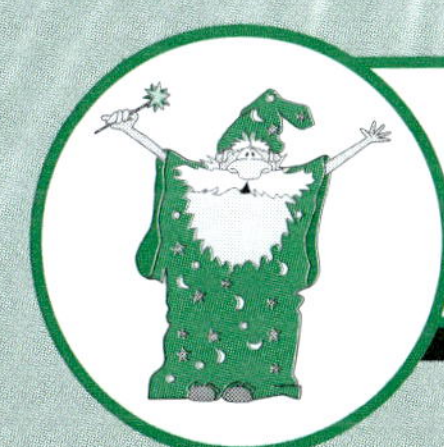

Wizard List

"Roles People Play" crossword puzzle, pens or pencils

Preparation

1. Copy "Roles People Play" for each team member.
2. Provide pens or pencils.

Implementation

1. Distribute "Roles People Play" crossword puzzle to each team member.
2. Ask members if they have ever seen these behaviors in meetings or groups.
3. Ask them to add others they have encountered or studied. Point out that some of these behaviors are in response to the stress of an uncomfortable situation.
4. Ask people to share what they know about their own behavior when in an uncomfortable group setting or a new setting.

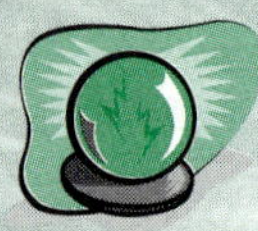

Debriefing

Discuss the use of humor to relieve stress. Some people use humor, for example, to calm themselves and make others more comfortable. This may be very effective or ineffective if overused.

Magic Touch

Variation: Divide the group into pairs to complete the "Roles People Play" crossword puzzle or make a "Roles People Play" crossword puzzle transparency or poster and allow the group to solve the puzzle.

ROLES PEOPLE PLAY

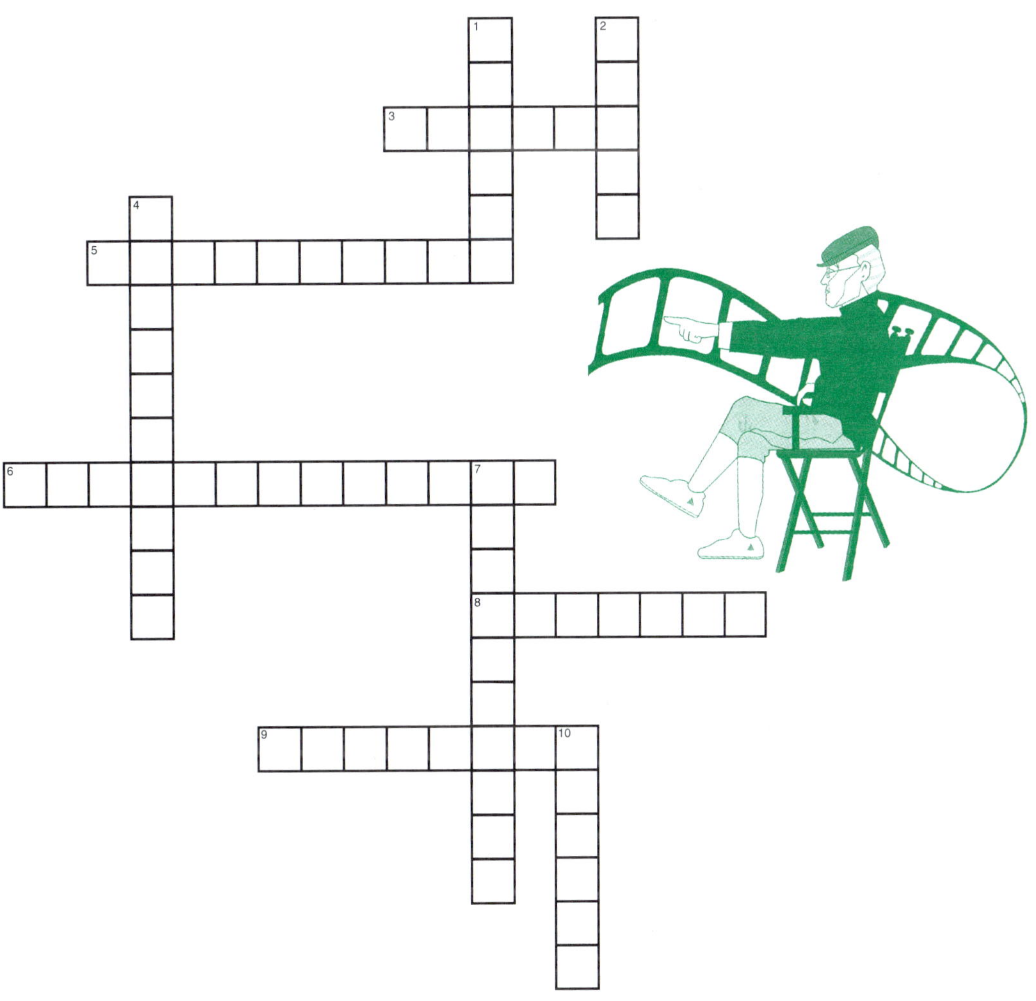

DOWN

1. Does not speak
2. Disinterested
4. Wants power and influence
7. Distrustful, looks for motives in everything people do
10. The "pro," the know-it-all

ACROSS

3. Thinks out loud, monopolizer, chatty
5. Wants to be like everyone else, always agrees
6. Opposite of 2 down, wants to be different
8. Socializes, fools around (male)
9. Opposite of positive

ROLES PEOPLE PLAY

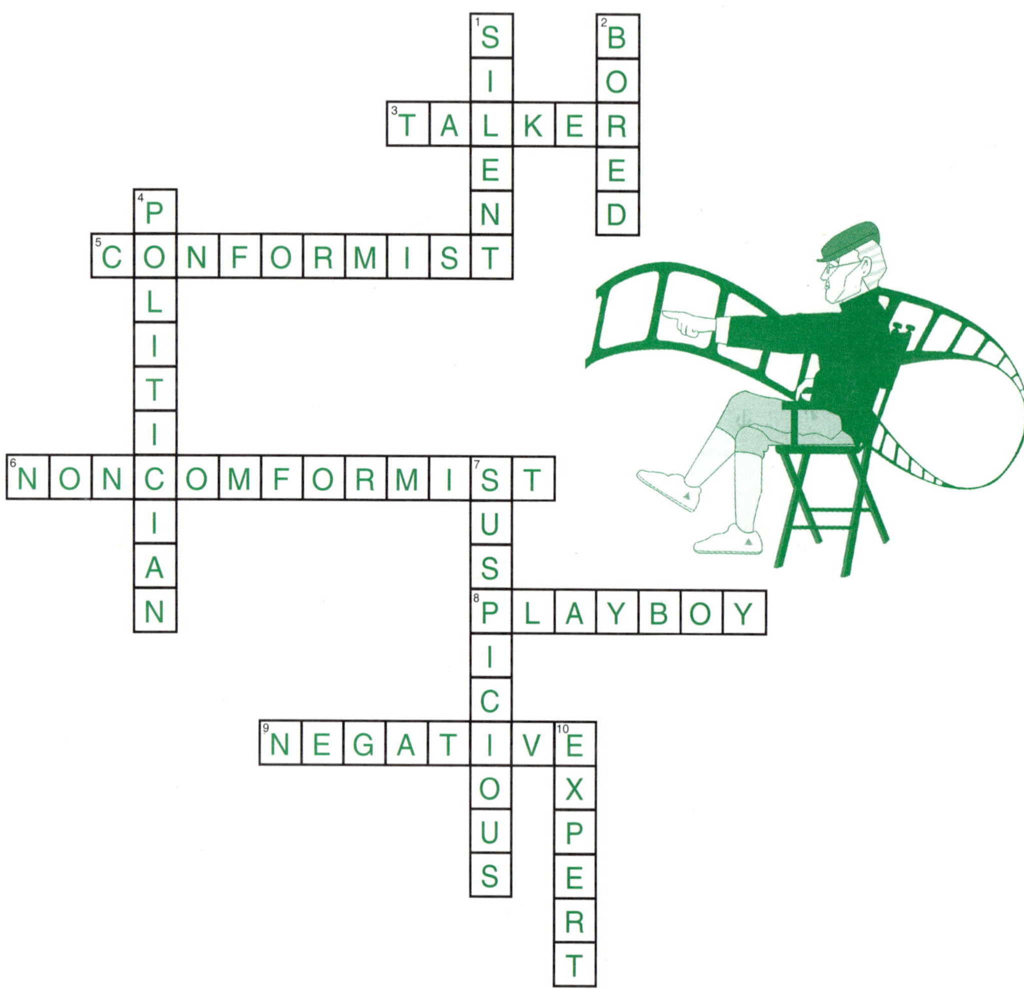

DOWN

1. Silent
2. Bored
4. Politician
7. Suspicious
10. Expert

ACROSS

3. Talker
5. Conformist
6. Nonconformist
8. Playboy
9. Negative

SWEET DIFFERENCES

It Takes All Kinds of Flavors

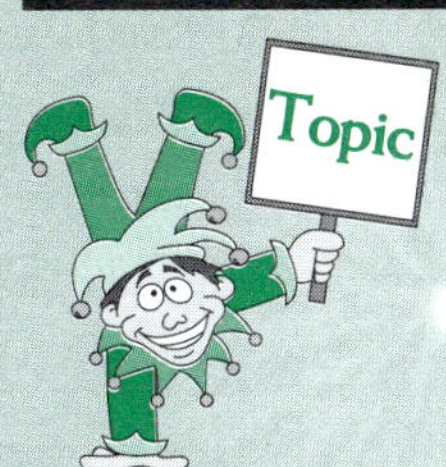

Differences. Use this exercise when your team has a mix of clinical and nonclinical staff, or when teaching a class on team dynamics, or whenever there are different groups mixed and you want to address the issue of differences.

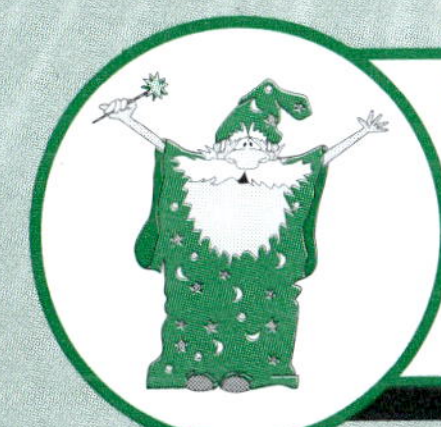

Wizard List

Small plastic sandwich bags, jelly beans (assorted flavors), Jelly Bellies (small gourmet type, assorted flavors)

Preparation

1. Fill small plastic sandwich bags with jelly beans and Jelly Bellies. Keep jelly beans and Jelly Bellies separate. Do not mix. You will need one bag of each for each group within the team.
2. Mark half the bags with "C" for clinical and half the bags with "N" for nonclinical. All of the bags marked with "C" need to contain the same type of candies, for instance, all jelly beans. The goal is for each team member to have at least three to four to taste. More is nice, but time and cost are issues.

Implementation

1. Divide team members into groups. Make sure each group has a variety of backgrounds. (For example, clinical and nonclinical.)
2. Ask that for each group the clinical members distribute the contents of the bag marked "C" among clinical members and

that the nonclinical members distribute the contents of the bag marked "N" among nonclinical members.

3. Distribute blank paper and pen or pencil to each team member.
4. Ask each team member to taste the candies one at a time, pausing after each one to write down the flavor.
5. Ask the clinical staff to communicate with one another about their flavors and make a combined list. Likewise, ask the nonclinical staff to communicate with one another about their flavors.
6. Ask each group to discuss what lessons were learned.
7. Introduce the topic of diversity and discuss how all are different, but all are good.

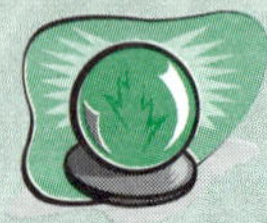

Debriefing

Use these questions:

1. What did you discover when you shared among others of your group with similar work settings?
2. What did you discover when you shared among others of your group with different work settings?
3. Did you enjoy different colors, flavors, and textures?

Points to consider: There were differences in colors, flavors, and textures in the candies, just as there are differences in experiences and skills in health care. To provide quality care, we need to collaborate across departments just as between team members from different specialties and work functions in health care.

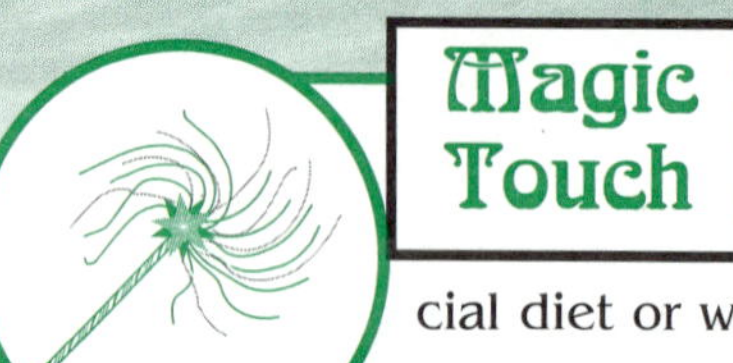

Magic Touch For special needs, have some sugarless candies available. This extra effort allows someone on a special diet or who is a diabetic to participate.

By: June Larrabee, PhD, RN

IS THERE A DOCTOR IN THE HOUSE?

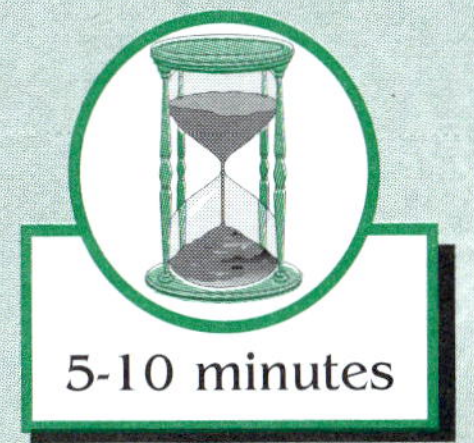

Seuss, That Is

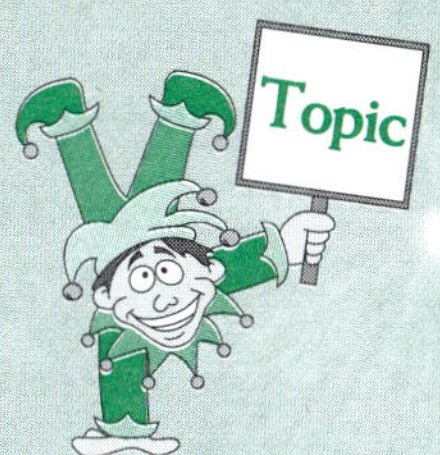

Consensus and implementing change.

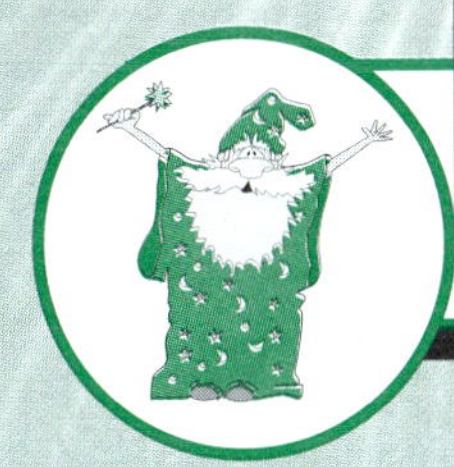

Wizard List

Yertle the Turtle and Other Stories, by Dr. Seuss (New York, 1986, Random House)

Preparation

1. Research children's books for appropriate material to teach a concept.
2. Review suggested listed material "Yertle the Turtle," "Gertrude McFuzzy," "The Big Brag."
3. Choose one or all three to illustrate a concept.

Implementation

1. Explain to the team that you are going to read a story and that they will be asked to identify the moral and apply it to team behaviors and processes.
2. Relate to the team members the following about *Yertle the Turtle.* Yertle the Turtle is king of the pond and craves more power. He climbs on others to build his empire. He is indifferent to the problems he causes for others beneath him. One turtle finally makes a single move that makes all the difference. Illustrated concept: The problem with departments or individuals who lose touch with the needs of the people they are entrusted to lead. Illustrated systems theory: One change can affect the organization; implementing change can sometimes

have larger, farther-reaching ramifications that a team might envision.

3. Relate to the team members the following about *Gertrude McFuzz.* Gertrude McFuzz was a bird who had only one "droopy-droop feather." She was jealous of Lolla-Lee-Lou, whose lovely tail had two feathers. Gertrude goes to great lengths to get more feathers, and gets so many she cannot move. Finally, she returns to her real self and is content with who she is. Illustrated concept: Each team member can offer the most by being himself or herself and honestly expressing views and opinions; it doesn't matter how many more feathers (degress or years of experience) other team members have; each member was chosen for his or her potential to make a unique contribution.
4. Relate to the team members the following about *The Big Brag.* The bear and the rabbit each claim to be the best of all the beasts. One can smell the best, the other can hear the best. A worm teaches them what fools they are to have nothing better to do than sit and argue about who is best. Illustrated concept: The futility of power struggles or how each team member contributes his or her talents; consider how the parts of the body work together: the nose smells, the eyes see; be yourself—when an eye tries to be a nose it doesn't work.

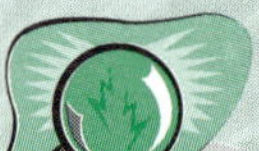

Debriefing

Identify the concept you want to illustrate. Be clear about the purpose of the story. As usual, debriefing is important; if the team did not get the lesson you intended, work with the feedback you get and move it to the point you want to make.

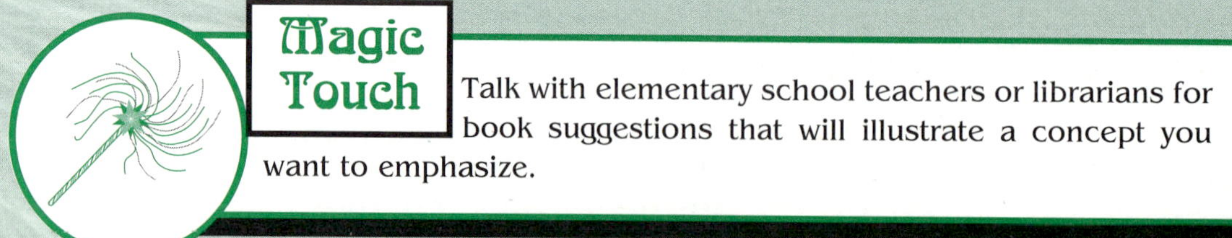

Magic Touch

Talk with elementary school teachers or librarians for book suggestions that will illustrate a concept you want to emphasize.

WE'RE ON A ROLE

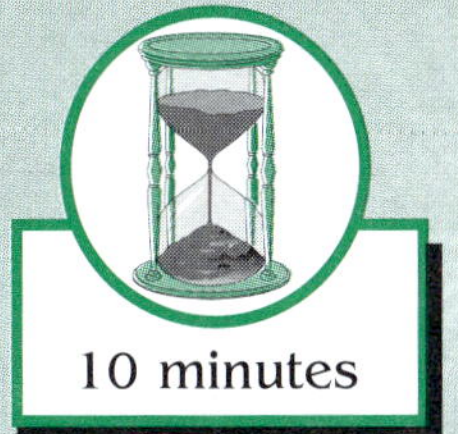

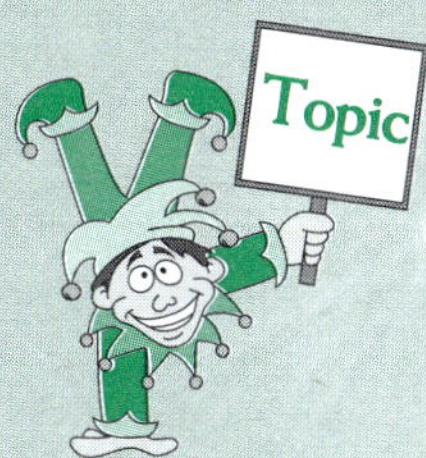

Use to recognize problem behaviors.

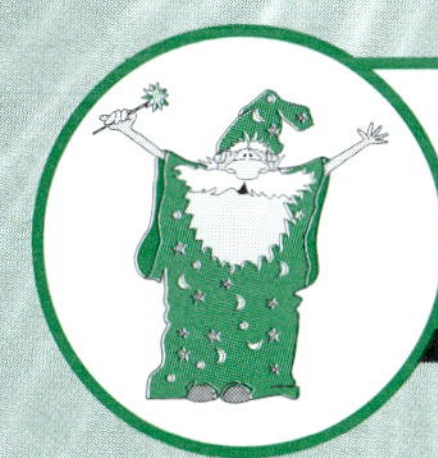

Wizard List

"We're on a Role" labels, construction paper, scissors, scotch tape or paste, paper clips

Preparation

1. Copy "We're on a Role" labels and cut in single strips.
2. Make six headbands from construction paper, 2″ × 28″ strips.
3. Tape or paste one "role label" to each head band.

Implementation

1. Select six volunteers.
2. Take the volunteers outside of the meeting room area and assign a quality improvement project which they will discuss in front of the team, such as holiday celebrations for hospital employees, remodeling plans for the hospital lobby, or a new line of food selections for the hospital cafeteria.
3. Place a role headband on each volunteer. Do not allow the volunteers to see the role on their headband. Use tape or paper clips to make the headbands fit.
4. Instruct the volunteers not to reveal another person's role!
5. Instruct the volunteers to respond and react according to the role or behavior on one another's band.
6. Appoint a group leader to inform the members who were not selected for a role (the audience) that each returning team member will be wearing a headband describing a behavior or a role. Clarify to the audience that the wearer is not aware of what his or her label says.

7. Ask the audience to respond during the dialogue with laughing, sighing, clapping, or other appropriate responses. For example, when the person with the headband *Comedian* talks, they should always laugh, even if the person did not say anything funny.
8. Have the volunteers come back to the main group and sit in chairs in the front of the room in a semicircle facing the audience.
9. Instruct the volunteers to begin working on their quality improvement project. Usually, a leader of the group just emerges and begins the discussion. (Prompt audience participation, if necessary.)
10. Let the group work on their project for 2 to 3 minutes.
11. Stop the activity and ask each volunteer to guess what his or her headband says; then remove and read it.
12. Ask the volunteers to rejoin the group, and initiate a discussion on the exercise. Possible questions are:
    a. What were some of the problems of trying to be yourself under the conditions of role pressure?
    b. How did it feel to be consistently misinterpreted by the group (e.g., to be laughed at when you were trying to be serious, or to be ignored when you were trying to make a point)?
    c. Did you find yourself changing your behavior in reaction to the group's treatment of you (e.g., withdrawing when they ignored you, acting confident when they treated you with respect, giving orders when they deferred to you)?

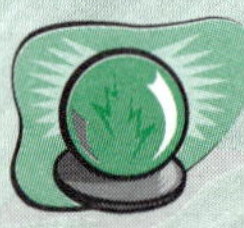

Debriefing

Discuss lessons learned and point out the activity's demonstration of how many different personalities and behaviors come together on a Continuous Quality Improvement (CQI) team and how you have to learn to work and deal with them.

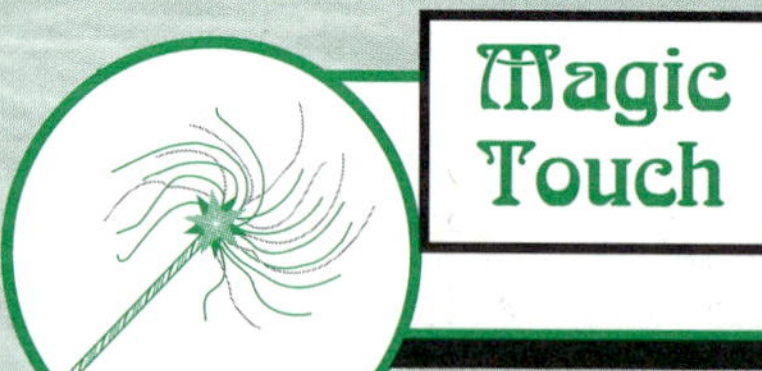

Magic Touch

Interactive exercises make learning fun and can open up quiet members.

By: Judy K. Scott, RN, MSN

WE'RE ON A ROLE

Labels

EXPERT—ask my advice

COMEDIAN—laugh at me

BOSS—obey me

INSIGNIFICANT—ignore me

HELPLESS—support me

IMPORTANT—defer to me

A PICTURE IS WORTH 1000 WORDS

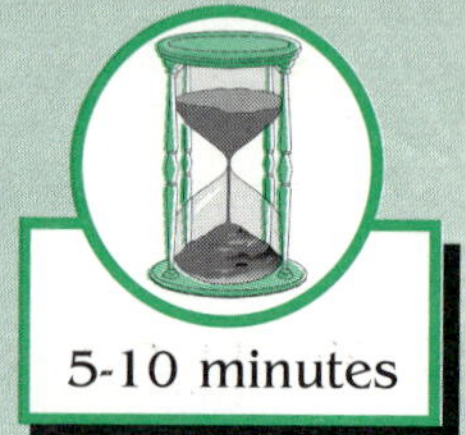

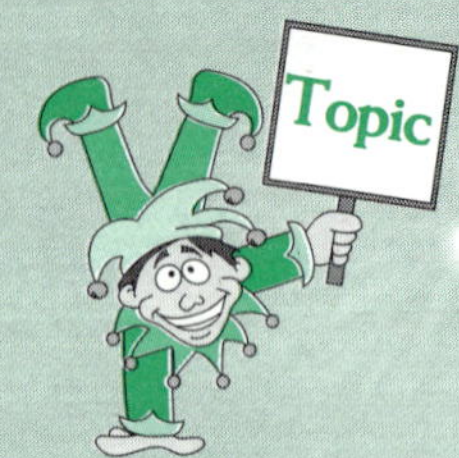

Use to discuss behaviors in groups that can interfere with work.

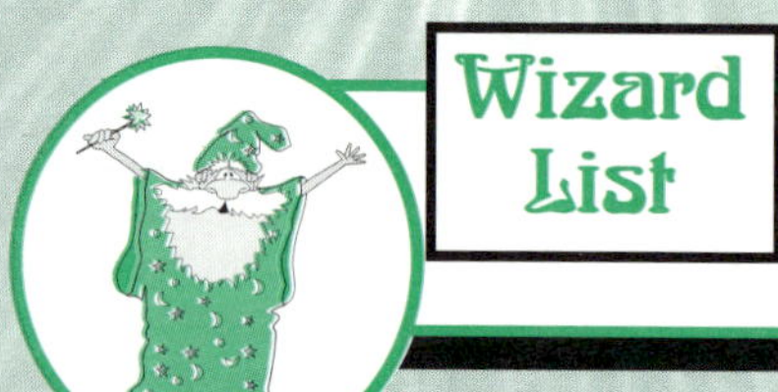

Wizard List

"Who, Me?" cartoon

Preparation

1. Copy "Who, Me?" cartoon for each team member or copy to a transparency.

Implementation

1. Distribute the "Who, Me?" cartoon.
2. Ask the team members to discuss what behaviors come to mind.
3. Invite discussion about experiences with such behaviors.
4. Point out that these may occur when people are anxious. Ask if anyone can see himself or herself in the cartoon.

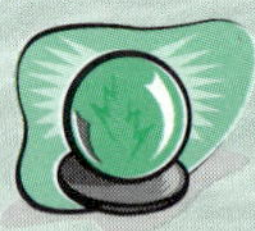

Debriefing

Discuss the following behaviors:

Aggressor Annihilates other group members; destroys other members' self-esteem.

Nonconformer Finds something wrong with almost everything; very negative.

Conformer Agrees with everything.

Recognition seeker Wants to be the shining star; concerned with personal achievements.

Self-confessor Tries to use the group for therapy sessions; shares personal life.

Silent one Does not contribute.

Know-it-all Knows something about everything.

Playboy/Playgirl Lacks interest and involvement; is not committed.

Emotional one Expresses feelings of insecurity to get others' sympathy; has low self-esteem.

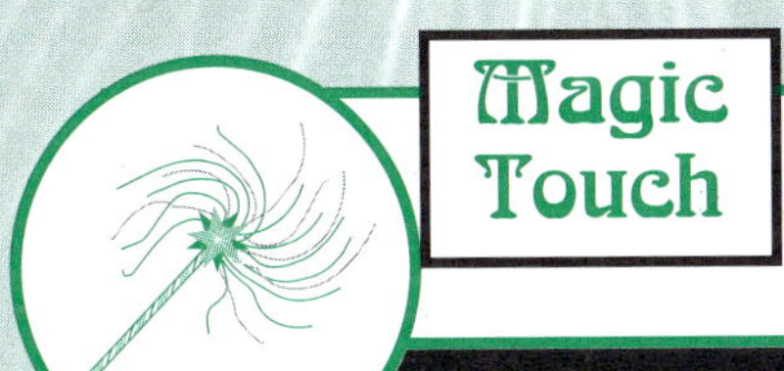

Helping team members recognize negative behaviors encourages positive behavior.

WHO, ME?

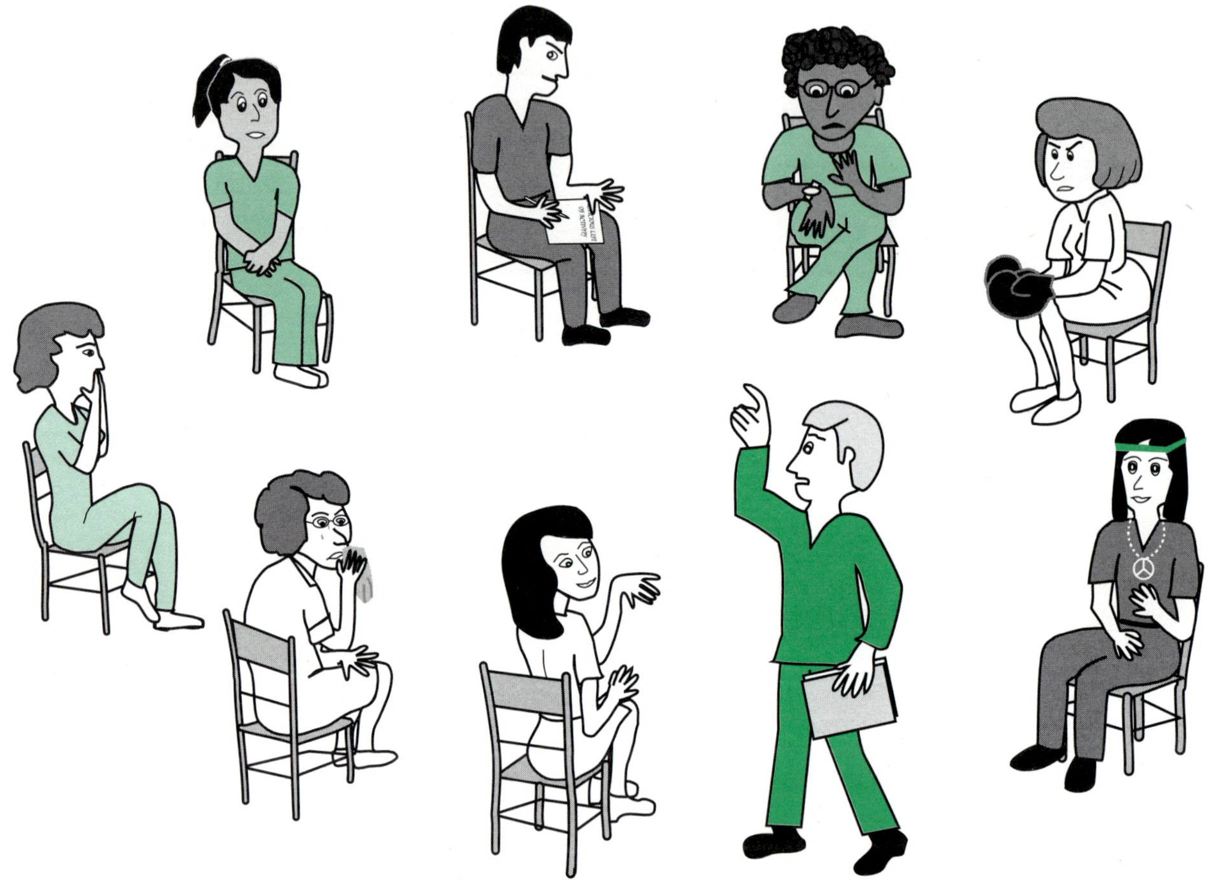

WHO, ME?

Blocker or suspicious one
Conformist
Bored
Aggressive
Silent
Emotional
Playboy/playgirl
Politician or teacher
Nonconformist

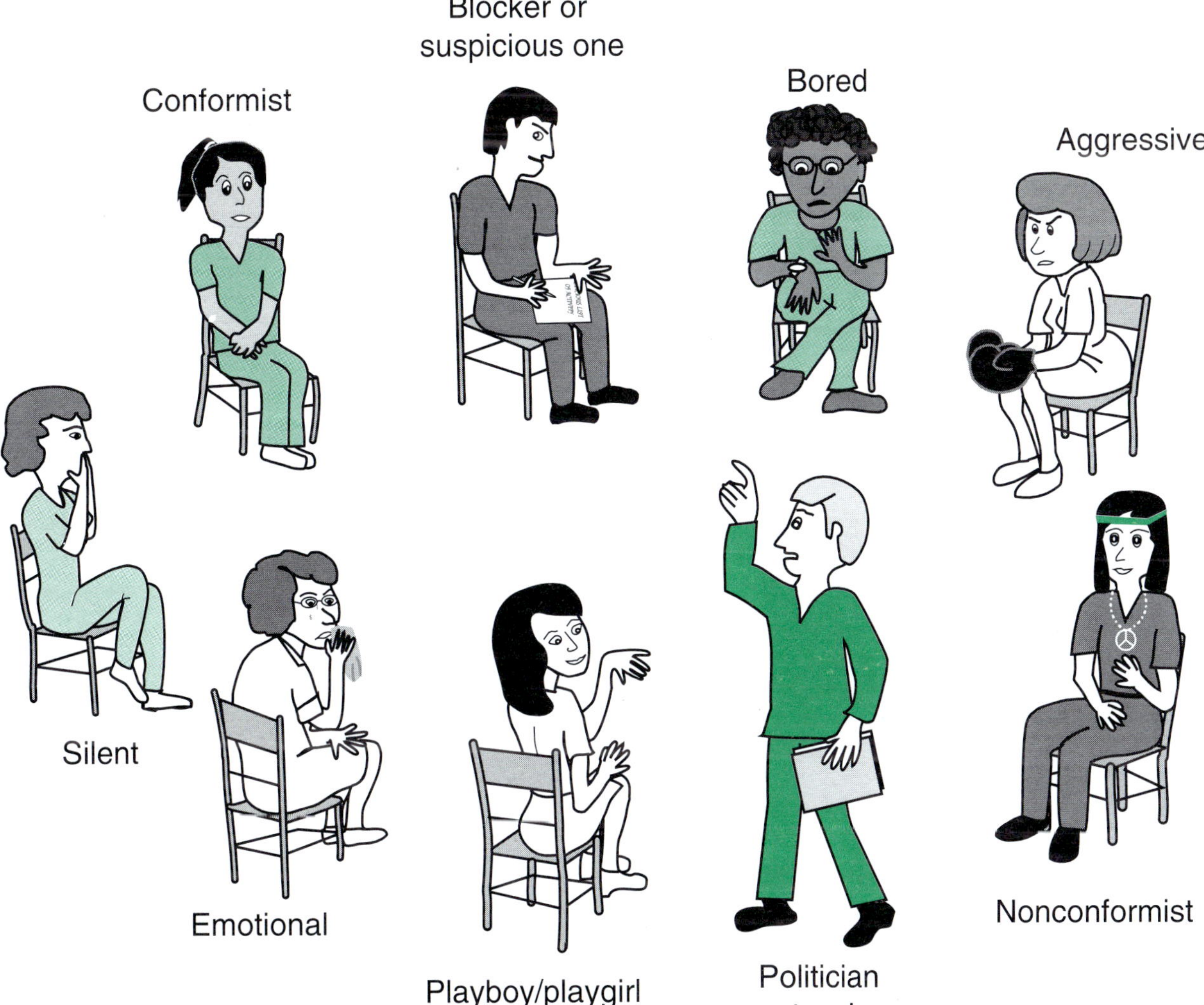

GETTING THE WORK DONE

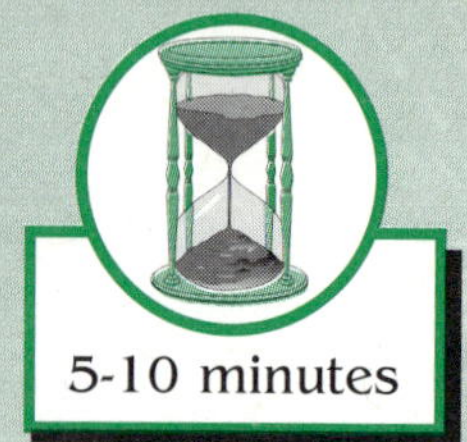

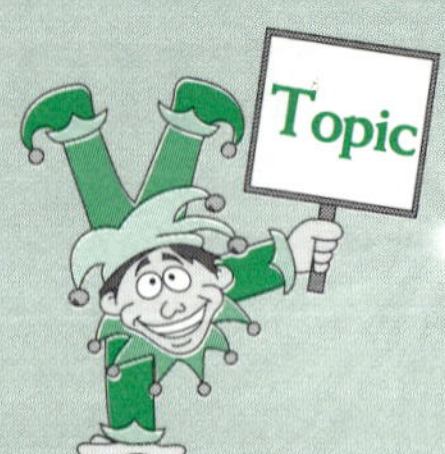

Behavior. Use to distinguish between helpful and problematic facilitator behaviors.

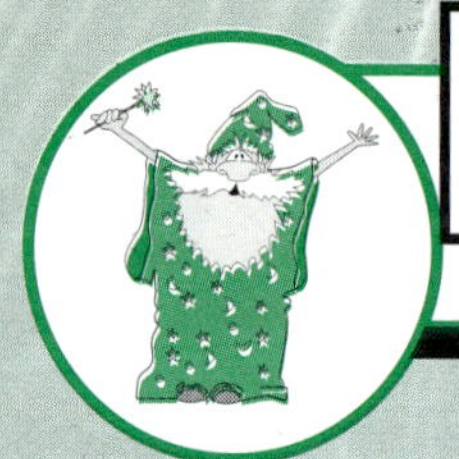

Wizard List "Getting the Work Done" worksheet, pens or pencils

Preparation

1. Copy "Getting the Work Done" worksheet for each team member.
2. Provide pens or pencils.

Implementation

1. Discuss how we know when a group is working well, but we don't always know how to make the meeting process flow. This is the role of a team facilitator. Keep in mind that when there is no appointed facilitator, all team members share this responsibility.
2. Distribute "Getting the Work Done" worksheet and ask the team members to complete the worksheet.

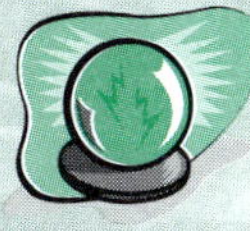

Debriefing

Discuss positive behaviors and mention the facilitator's primary responsibilities:

- **Encourage communication**
- **Use question techniques that encourage communication**
- **Keep the team focused**
- **Foster trust and commitment**
- **Clarify discussions**
- **Keep the team moving forward**

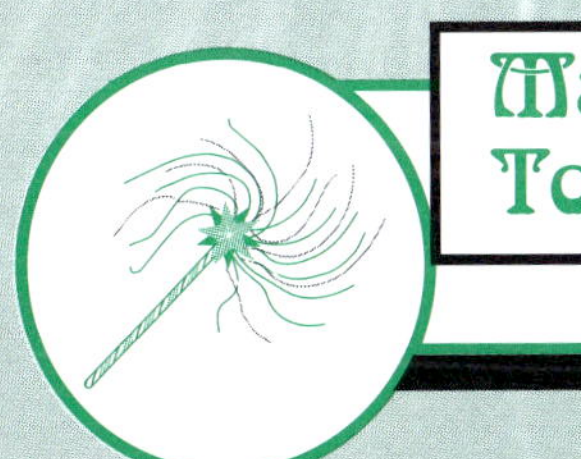

Magic Touch

Make a team member responsibility handout and on it list the responsibilities for each team member role.

GETTING THE WORK DONE

The following is a list of facilitator behaviors. Label positive behaviors with a + and negative behaviors with a −.

____ 1. Allows the team to get off the topic onto tangents.

____ 2. Asks questions to stimulate more careful consideration of an issue.

____ 3. Carefully explains to the team that they have the wrong solution to the problem.

____ 4. Allows thoughtful silences without interruption.

5. Summarizes the work done.

____ 6. Models openness and trust.

____ 7. Ignores some team members and argues with others.

____ 8. Arrives late to meetings and ignores lateness in others.

____ 9. Confronts judgmental comments.

____ 10. Interrupts hostile humor and refocuses the group.

____ 11. Controls the team by dominating the discussion.

____ 12. Listens and maintains open body posture.

____ 13. Pays attention to nonverbal behavior to understand group process.

____ 14. Keeps time.

____ 15. Returns the focus of comments directed to the team.

____ 16. Assumes the role of expert in the group's mission.

____ 17. Does other work on team time.

____ 18. Interrupts a personal attack on a team member.

____ 19. Asks the team why they are letting one person assume responsibility for the work (when that person is monopolizing).

____ 20. Avoids dealing with team problems.

____ 21. Surfaces process issues, such as groupthink.

____ 22. Provides additional information about team dynamics when needed.

____ 23. Encourages the team to clarify questions in data collection.

____ 24. Helps the team decide what data they need, how best to collect it, and how the data will be analyzed.

____ 25. Teaches information about steps of the quality improvement process as needed.

GETTING THE WORK DONE

Answer Key

1. −
2. +
3. −
4. +
5. +
6. +
7. −
8. −
9. +
10. +
11. −
12. +
13. +
14. +
15. +
16. −
17. −
18. +
19. +
20. −
21. +
22. +
23. +
24. +
25. +

HANGPERSON

For the Politically Correct

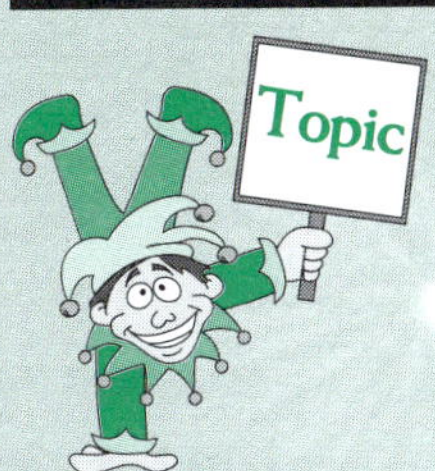

Successful teams. Use to review successful ingredients to teamwork.

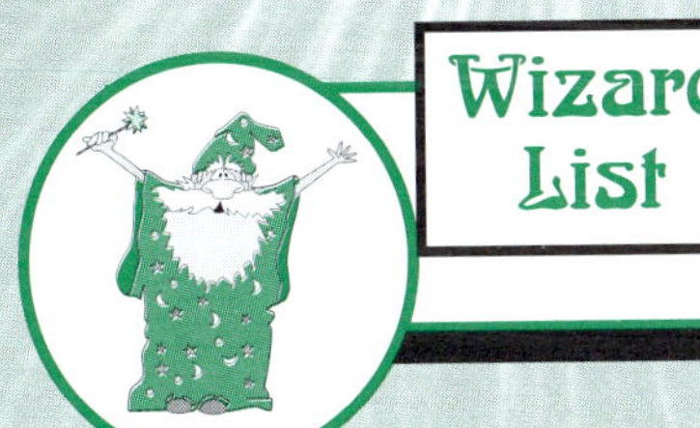

Wizard List "What's in a Team?" word list, pens or pencils

Preparation

1. Print the words from the "What's in a Team?" word list on 3″ × 5″ index cards. Or choose vocabulary from your own team training materials, or have team members think of their own words from team dynamic training sessions.
2. Provide blank sheets of paper and pens or pencils.

Implementation

1. Divide the team members into pairs. It may help to assign numbers, each pair would be numbered 1,2; 1,2 and so on. To start, have all the number 1s be the hangperson.
2. Distribute blank paper and a pen or pencil to each pair.
3. Distribute a deck (5 or 6 cards) of "What's in a Team?" word cards placed face down to each pair.
4. Ask all the number 2s to pick a card and without looking at the card show it to the hangperson (number 1s).
5. Ask all the hangpersons (number 1s) to take the blank paper and draw a scaffold and a noose. (An example appears on the "What's in a Team?" word list page.) At the bottom of the page draw a blank line for every letter in the word that appears on the selected index card. The 2s in each pair state, only to their

partner, a letter he or she thinks might be in the word. If the letter guessed is in the word the hangperson fills in the correct blank on the hangman drawing. If the guessed letter is not in the selected word the hangperson draws a head at the end of the noose. With each incorrect letter that is guessed, another body part is drawn; for example, the neck, two arms (one at a time), two legs (one at a time). If the word is guessed before all the body parts are drawn there is no hanging and pairs change roles. If not, oh well, change roles anyway!

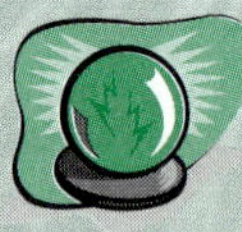

Debriefing

Have team members review the words and ask them to identify how these words relate to team dynamics, and how, when applied, these things speed the process.

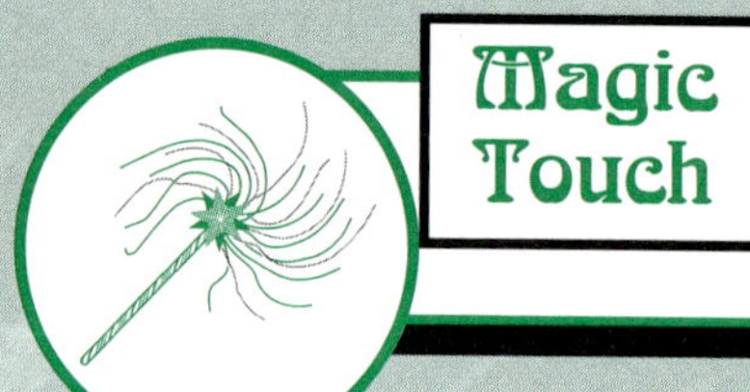

Magic Touch

Laminate your index cards. It's inexpensive, and the cards can be used again and again.

WHAT'S IN A TEAM

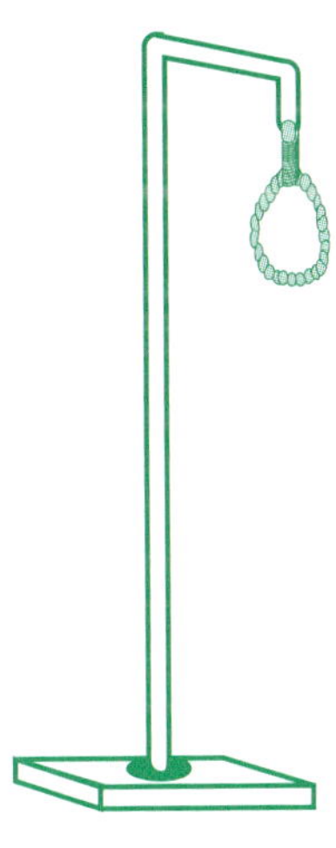

Word List

Trust
Listen
Humor
Support
Open share
Agenda
Honesty
Goal
Mission
Consensus
Feedback
Follow-up
Risk-taking
Prompt

Courtesy
Data
Norm
Storm
Form
Team
Participate
Conflict
Decision
Attitude
Disagree
Negotiate
Communication
Problem-solving

Leader
Morale
Member
Expectation
Customer
Energy
Creativity
Knowledge
Cooperate
Risks
Minutes
Results
Problem
Solution

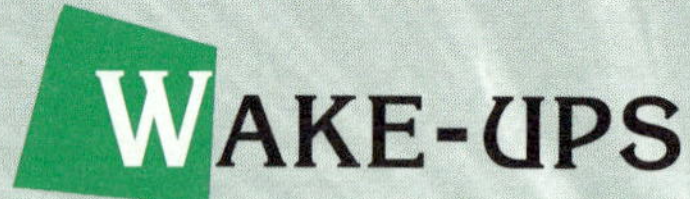

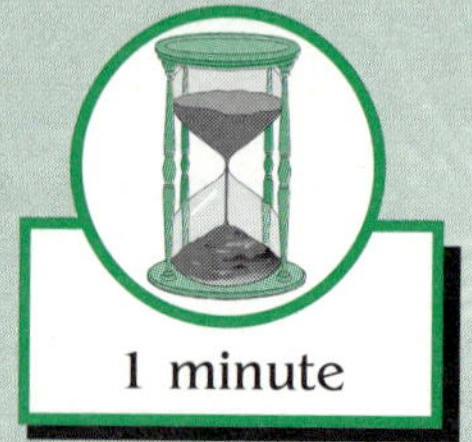

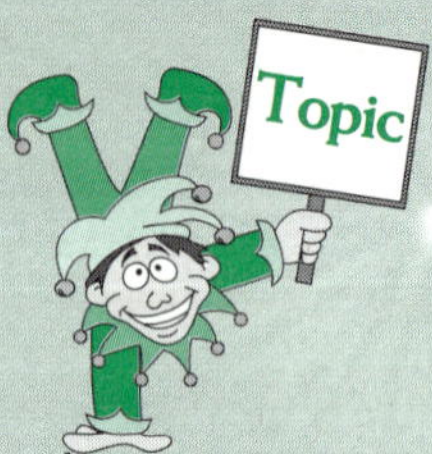

Observation. Use to start a training class, after lunch break, or to start a team meeting.

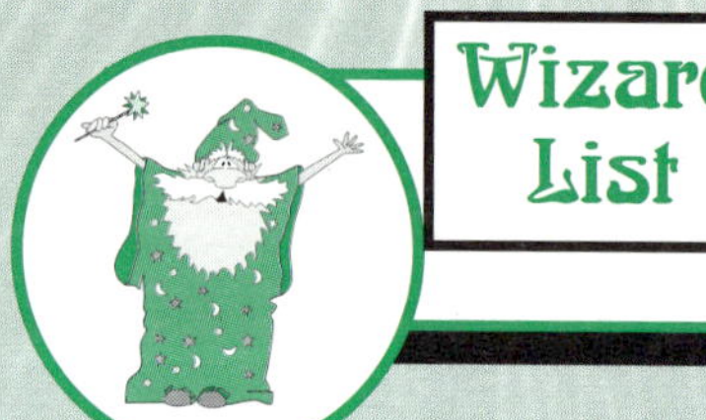

Wizard List "Wake-Ups" list, pens or pencils

Preparation

1. Copy "Wake-Ups" list for each team member.
2. Provide pens or pencils.

Implementation

1. Distribute "Wake Ups" list.
2. Ask team members to complete the "Wake-Ups" list (allow approximately 1 minute).
3. Read the answers aloud to the team.

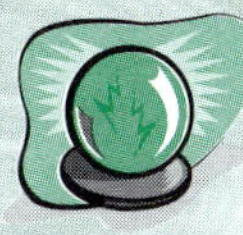

Debriefing

Discuss the importance of careful observation and application of existing knowledge. Parallel the skills used to solve "Wake-Ups" to team dynamics.

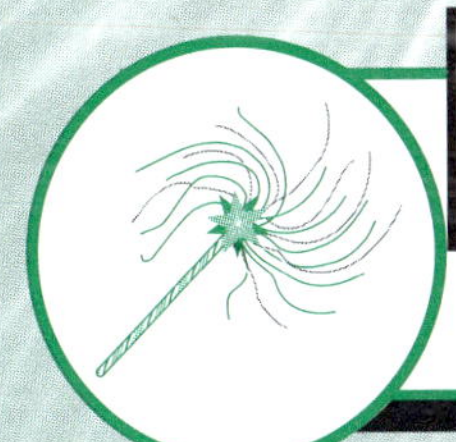

Magic Touch

Variation: To use this exercise as a group activity, copy the "Wake-Ups" list to a flip chart or transparency.

WAKE-UPs

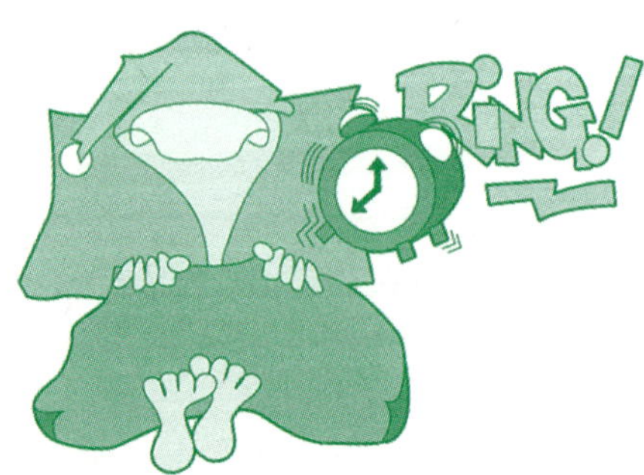

1. Tom and Tammy Teammembers took a vow to treat team members with terrific respect, to take team roles terribly seriously, to treat team data with tremendous seriousness, and to take the time to attend every team meeting. How many *T*'s are there in all? ________
2. Name the Grand Canyon State. ________
3. Name the Peach State. ________
4. Name the Hoosier State. ________
5. Name the Sunflower State. ________
6. Name the Bluegrass State. ________
7. Name the Show Me State. ________
8. Name the Cornhusker State. ________
9. Name the Tarheel State. ________
10. Name the Volunteer State. ________
11. Name the state called Old Dominion. ________
12. Which months have 31 days? ________

____

WAKE-UPs

Answer Key

1. There are no *T*'s in all.
2. Arizona
3. Georgia
4. Indiana
5. Kansas
6. Kentucky
7. Missouri
8. Nebraska
9. North Carolina
10. Tennessee
11. Virginia
12. January, March, May, July, August, October and December. Ask if anyone remembers the childhood verse:

    Thirty days hath September
    April, June, and November.
    All the rest have 31,
    excepting one month alone . . . [February]

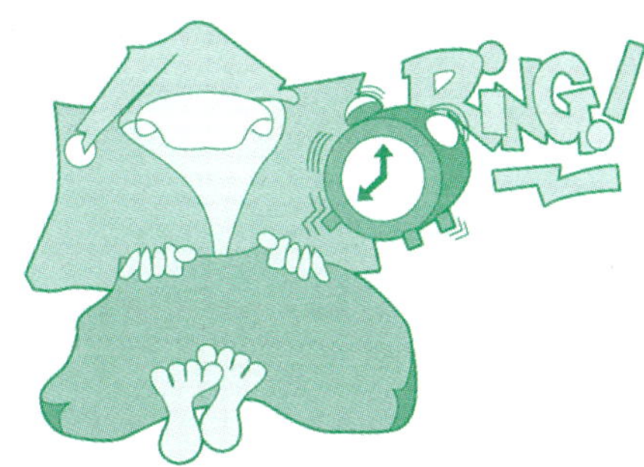

Making Music

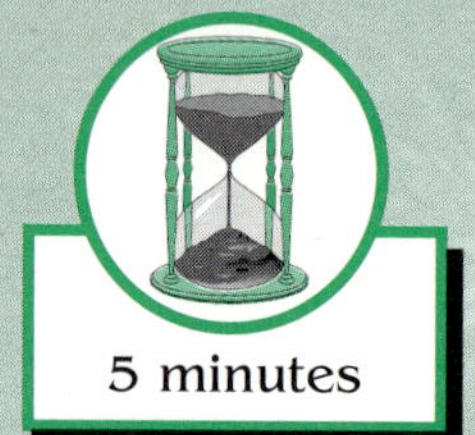

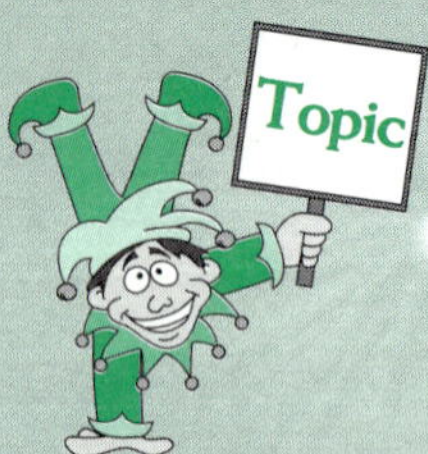

Team training. Use to review essentials for meeting team goals.

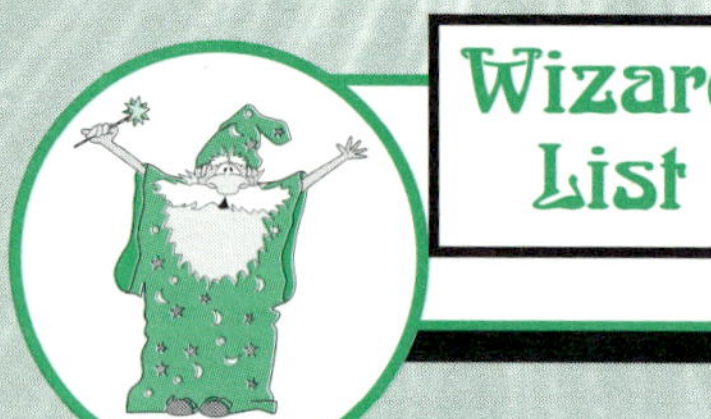

Music, audio equipment, flip chart, markers

Preparation

1. Select orchestra music and appropriate audio equipment.
2. Review Debriefing.

Implementation

1. Play one selection or a short portion of a long composition. (Remember—in training sessions for which a fee is charged, permission must be obtained to play copyrighted music.)
2. Ask the team members what is necessary for an orchestra to play together successfully.
3. Write responses on a flip chart.
4. Ask the group to discuss how these ideas apply to the successful work of a team.

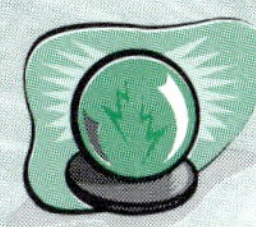

Debriefing

Commonalities might include: common focus or goal; participation by all, but equally, so one person does not stand out in a way to take away from the work of the whole; trust in the leader and one another; a score or agenda from which to work; practice and commitment to timely rehearsals; perseverance; solos when one special skill is needed.

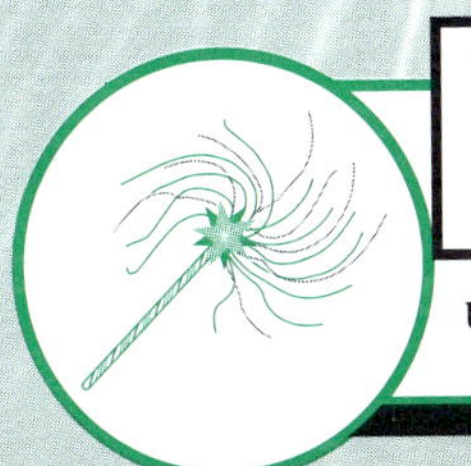

Magic Touch

Each comes to the orchestra with a talent that compliments those of the others to make a greater product than could be made alone.

RECIPE FOR SUCCESS

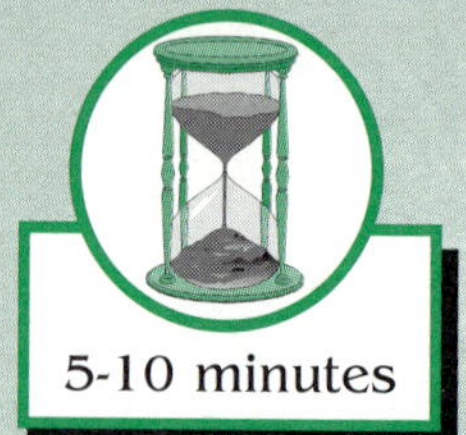

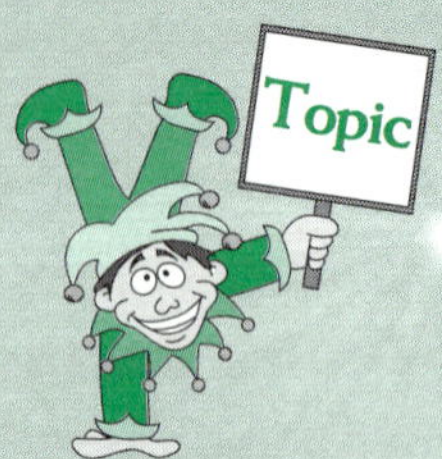

Use to discover what ideas team members have about teamwork.

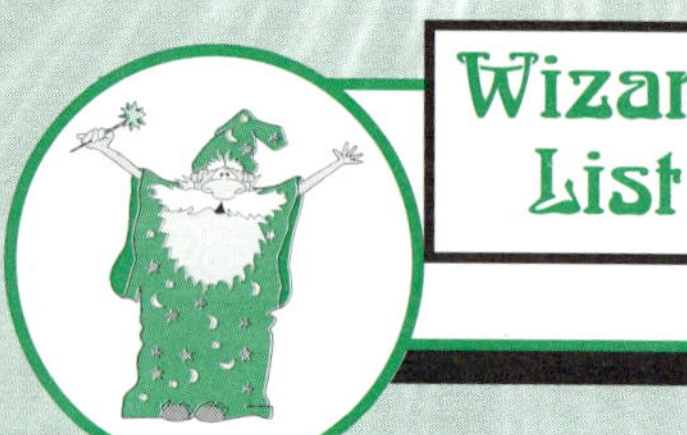

Wizard List

Index cards, pens or pencils, flip chart, chef's hat, apron, other cooking paraphernalia, a mixing bowl

Preparation

1. Assemble supplies.
2. Label a flip chart page "Recipe for a Successful Team."

Implementation

1. Display your gear with flourish—have fun with this.
2. Discuss how important the right ingredients are for a successful dish.
3. Distribute an index card and a pen or pencil to each team member.
4. Ask them to consider what they think are essential ingredients for a successful team and write the ingredients on the index card.
5. Pass the mixing bowl around to collect all the index cards.
6. Ask for a volunteer to read the cards.
7. Record the results on a flip chart labeled "Recipe for a Successful Team."

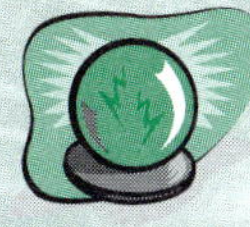

Debriefing

Tie the results to concepts you want to stress. For example, preparation, managing conflict, time management, reaching consensus, assignment completion, note taking (recording), agenda.

Magic Touch

Collect results from groups with which you work and compile these to share with other teams. People like to hear what others have contributed. And have fun with the recipe theme—bring refreshments and provide the recipe. Make cookies or get a volunteer to do so and provide that recipe. Collect free recipes from the grocery store and distribute them.

QUALITY IMPROVEMENT LIVE!

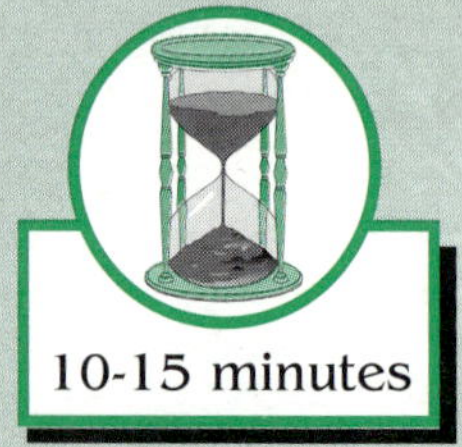

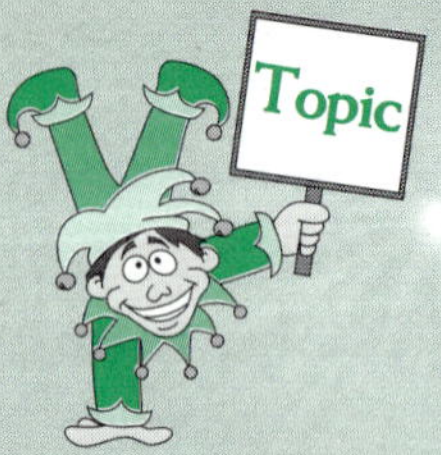

Use to demonstrate results of quality improvement teams.

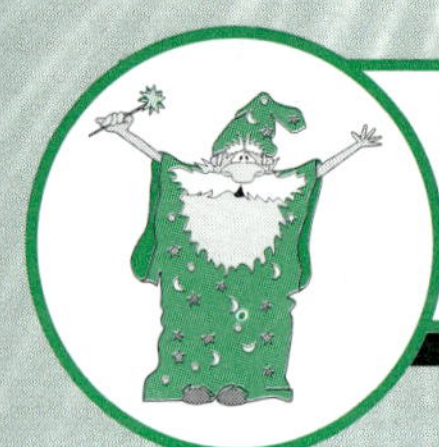

Wizard List

An experienced quality improvement team, storyboard

Preparation

1. Select, invite, and schedule an experienced quality improvement team to make a storyboard presentation of the steps they took to problem solve.
2. Give the presenters a time limit and explain what you would like them to include. An outline might be helpful.

Implementation

1. Explain a storyboard if anyone in your group is unfamiliar with this type of demonstration.
2. Introduce the experienced team.
3. Ask for questions.

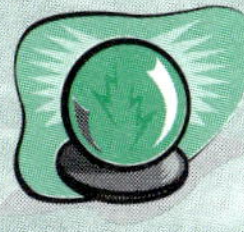

Debriefing

Make a list of the points you want to emphasize and be prepared to apply applicable information if the question-and-answer session does not highlight these points.

Magic Touch

Shared team experiences and visual demonstrations (storyboard) help team members pull the content of a team training session together.

Rules for Success

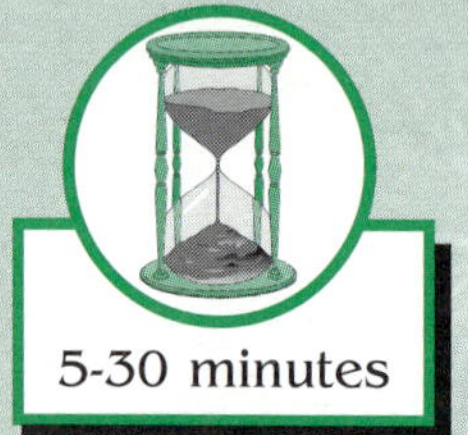

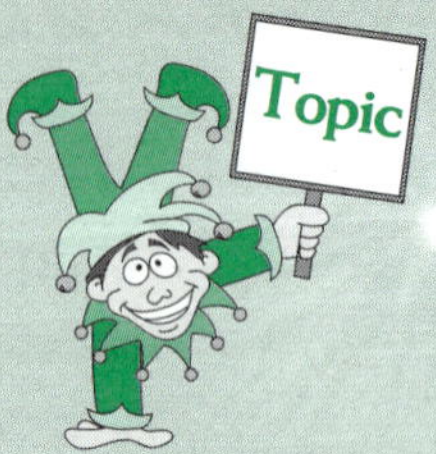

Ground rules. Use to develop team norms.

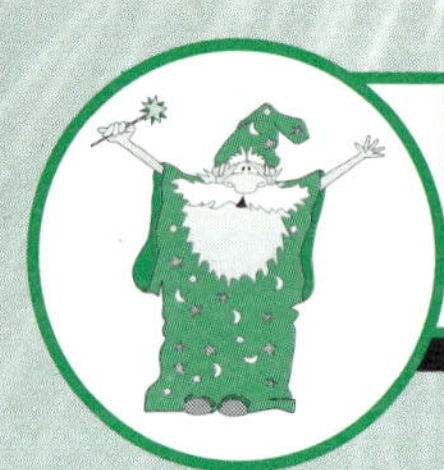

Wizard List

"Rules for Success," flip chart, marker, masking tape

Preparation

1. Copy "Rules for Success" for each team member.

Implementation

1. Explain that the purpose of establishing team rules is to make sure everyone can fully participate in the team and to honor members' time.
2. Distribute "Rules for Success" poem and allow a few minutes for review. You may also read "Rules for Success" aloud.
3. Ask members to work together to formulate ground rules for working together.
4. Consider the points in "Rules for Success," and brainstorm about what the group sees as important and what they are willing to abide.
5. List all suggestions on the flip chart.
6. Work together to reach a consensus on an acceptable list.
7. Write the final selection on a clean flip chart sheet and tape the sheet to the wall for future reference.

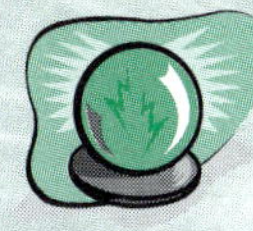

Debriefing

Rules such as participation and starting on time set the expectations, or the norms, for how the team will work together.

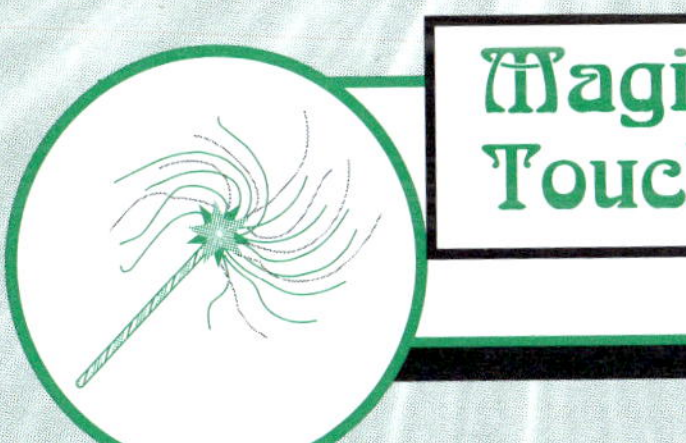

Past experiences with groups or teams lay the foundation for setting up the team for success.

RULES FOR SUCCESS

Start on time
And end that way, too.
Show up for the meeting,
Yes, that means you!

Someone is leader.
Someone takes minutes.
Providing an agenda
Reinforces these tenets.

A facilitator can help
Keep the team on task.
If someone doesn't speak,
One can just ask.

We share the work
And our own good humor.
Teams can work,
Or at least that's the rumor.

YES, WE'LL FORM, STORM, NORM, AND PERFORM

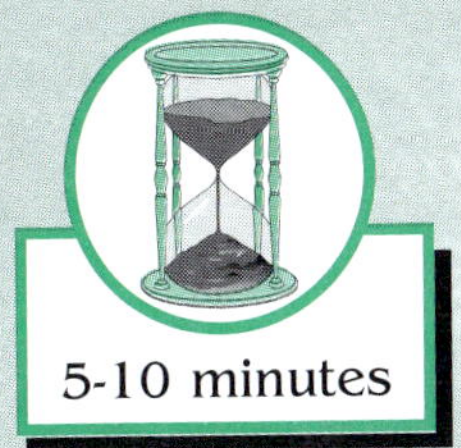

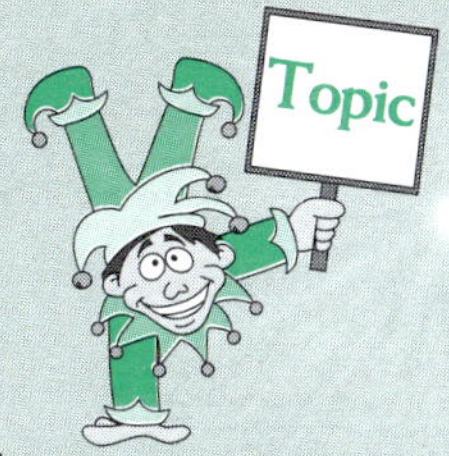

Use to teach team stages.

Wizard List "Form, Storm, Norm, Perform" transparency master, "Yes, We'll Form, Storm, Norm, and Perform" overview, "Yes, We'll Form, Storm, Norm, and Perform" pretest/posttest, pens or pencils, flip chart (optional)

Preparation

1. Make "Form, Storm, Norm, Perform" transparency or write "Form, Storm, Norm, Perform" on a flip chart.
2. Review "Yes, We'll Form, Storm, Norm, and Perform" overview.
3. Copy the "Yes, We'll Form, Storm, Norm, and Perform" pretest/posttest for each team member.

Implementation

1. Display the "Form, Storm, Norm, and Perform" transparency or flip chart.
2. Talk about how helpful it is to understand the dynamics of the development of a team, both for this current experience and to understand the behaviors in other work or community groups.
3. Explain that some members already may have been exposed to this and have remembered or forgotten the forming, storming, norming, and performing stages. It is new to others, so to bring all to the same place you will present a brief overview in a few minutes.

4. Distribute the pretest/posttest, explaining this is for the individual's own use to help guide learning.
5. Deliver the content and ask the members to answer the questions again.
6. Review the "Yes, We'll Form, Storm, Norm, and Perform" answers.

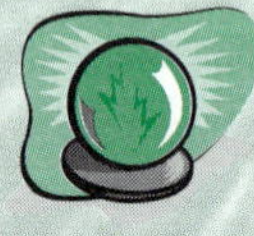

Debriefing

The correct answers are as follows: 1. d, 2. a, 3. c, 4. b.

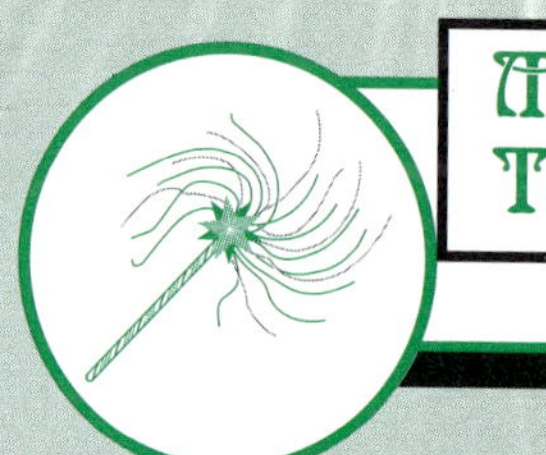

Magic Touch

Knowing what to expect helps team members to react in a positive way.

FORM

STORM

NORM

PERFORM

YES, WE'LL FORM, STORM, NORM, AND PERFORM

Overview

Four stages occur in the development of a group. Although there is no set time for these stages, and it may seem that members move back and forth among the stages, it is helpful to be aware of the information to help you figure out what is going on! The stages are forming, storming, norming, and performing. Think about individual development, and consider how the stages compare: Forming is like childhood. Storming is like adolescence! (If the group really does its stuff, it may look like it too!) Norming is like young adulthood. Performing is like adulthood.

In *Forming,* people are polite yet impersonal, testing the water, unsure about their commitment. The team is figuring out team goals and beginning to get a clear idea about the work to be done. People are testing out group relationships to see how the work will get done.

In *Storming,* overt or covert conflict may be evident, people may be hostile, engage in power struggles, be apathetic, and not do great work! People are resisting the process of teamwork. People resist cohesion and collaboration and do not have a commitment to the team.

In *Norming,* the group is getting organized, figuring out necessary rules and norms to get the work done, confronting problems and issues in a constructive way, and giving feedback. People clarify goals of the team, define the tasks and procedures for the work to be done. People move into cohesion and collaboration, and they demonstrate commitment.

In *Performing,* the work is getting done. People are open, can collaborate, are flexible and productive. People begin to do quality work, respect and support one another, motivate others by group achievement, and become flexible in their roles.

(Hamilton and Kieter, 1986.)

YES, WE'LL FORM, STORM, NORM, AND PERFORM

Pretest/Posttest

Match the following descriptions with the four phases of group development.

____ 1. Forming
____ 2. Storming
____ 3. Norming
____ 4. Performing

a. Resistance and conflict are expected now. There is little or no evidence of group cohesion or team commitment.

b. The work gets done. Team members feel good about their achievements and are flexible in their roles to meet team goals.

c. Team members clarify group goals and figure out the rules necessary to get the work done.

d. Team members are polite, begin to identify group goals, and test relationships.

TEACH WITH A TEAM THEME

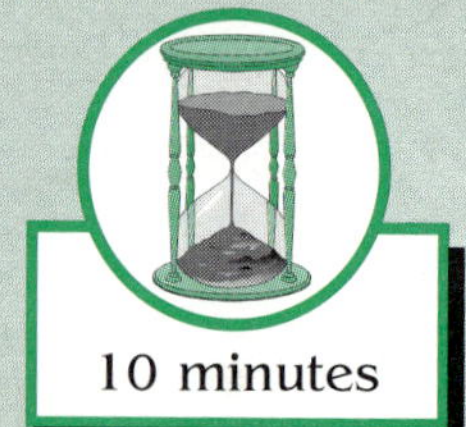

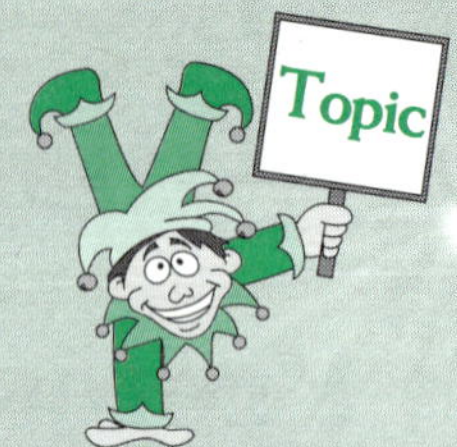

Stories. Use a story to teach a theme.

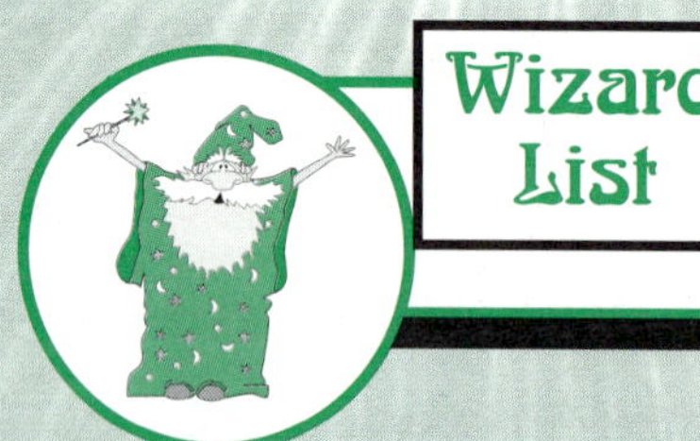

"Quality in the Kingdom" story

Preparation

1. Copy "Quality in the Kingdom" for each team member.
2. Review "Quality in the Kingdom."

Implementation

1. Distribute "Quality in the Kingdom" to all members.
2. Read "Quality in the Kingdom" aloud as the members review their copy.
3. Ask the team members to identify the moral.
4. Discuss comments.

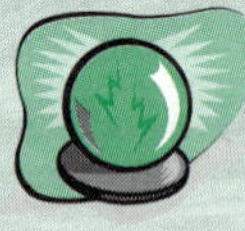

Debriefing

The moral of the story . . . executives and managers cannot disown quality and expect to have a "quality department." Quality is a culture, a way of doing business, a way of meeting customer needs that is deliberately constructed. It is *not* simply a set of procedures.

Magic Touch

Use this story and modify it to fit your own terminology to teach quality concepts.

You might want to use children's coloring books to illustrate a story, or draw your own illustrations in storyboard format. Think about how you could use "The Three Little Pigs," "Jack and the Beanstalk," "Little Red Riding Hood," but be careful about copyright infringement.

To serve as a theme reminder, use a rubber stamp that depicts the team theme on team memos.

Modified from: Kathleen Shutrump, RNC, CNA

QUALITY IN THE KINGDOM

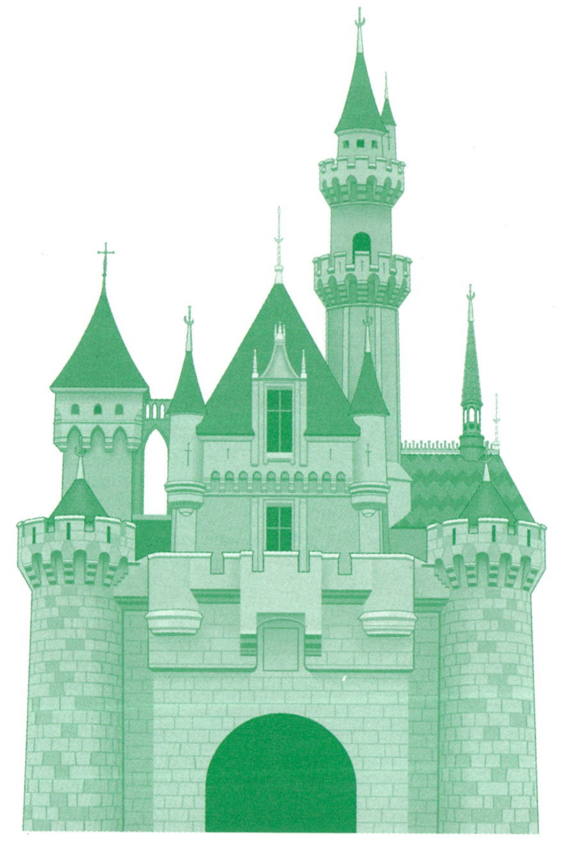

Having gone about living happily ever after in their kingdom, the Prince and Snow White fine-tuned their management skills and implemented their own program, "Quality in the Kingdom," throughout their land. Older now and needing a power name, and since his land was not called the princedom, the prince changed his name to *King Demming* to spread the news of quality education. (Okay, so he could probably time-travel, too, and so admired the Demming philosophy that he and Snow White used it to manage the kingdom.)

Now the king, being the quality-conscious nobleman he was, when called upon, left the Kingdom for a stint as a quality consultant to spread his philosophy of how to build a quality culture. He agreed to this project and had no fear for Snow's safety because she and her friends were well grounded in the principles of quality management. He reminded her before he left, "There is no process so good or so perfect that it cannot be improved. You can always make things better in the Kingdom, Snow. We believe in never-ending improvement, which in later years will come to be called Continual Improvement." [Time-travel again, or fairy-tale license.] "What we used to do is not wrong, it's just that in today's world, it is just 'not right.' "

Snow managed quite well until the *Witch-of-Everything-Is-OK-as-It-Is* ventured into the kingdom. "Listen, sweetie . . . Why do you want to work so hard to improve? Look around you. This place is Okay. Nobody needs to work harder to make things different or better. Who says different is better? What is wrong with the way things are?"

But luckily, Snow knew better, and she escaped into the *Forest of Opportunity,* where she met up with four friends, *Will, Belief, Doing,* and

Wherewithal. They reminded her that change is not easy and is resisted by many; they reinforced what she already knew. They explained to Snow how an organization begins to change.

Will said that nothing can happen until people want to change. *Belief* reminded her that just wanting to change is not enough; people must believe that change is possible. *Wherewithal* emphasized that even when people want to change and believe they can, they need the tools to make it possible. These tools are training, support, and "buy-in." *Doing* spoke last to Snow. "My part is the easiest. Once the first three things have been accomplished, all that remains is for everyone to get involved and do whatever it takes."

As Snow went farther into the *Forest of Opportunity,* she met her friends, the *Seven Dwarfs,* who had formed their own team to improve their mining operation. You may know them from your own organization. They are:

Willingness—"Sure we can do that; how can I help?"
Organization—The organization person, the bean counter.
Bad Attitude—Attitudes are contagious . . . is yours worth catching?
No-buy-in—Does not share the vision or goals of the group.
Hesitation—"I don't know if we will get the results we expect."
Procrastination—"I'm awfully busy now. Let's wait until next week, month, quarter, fiscal year . . . ."
and *Distraction*—Represents how easily we can be distracted from the mission of the team.

Snow, however, recognized that her friends each had his own point of view, and she worked with them to facilitate the team. The journey of teamwork is not smooth, however, and the *Witch-of-Everything-Is-OK-as-It-Is* again reared her ugly head, saying, "Don't work so hard." "Who are you trying to impress?" "Why are you trying to change?" "Aren't we happy here?" "We don't need change." "We don't want to change." "Just take a bite of my shiny red apple . . . ." You know the story. Snow bit and fell into the *Deep Sleep of the Status Quo.*

Who can save her? The prince, now *King Demming,* returned and kissed her to awaken her with the Kiss of Commitment. She awakened from the *Deep Sleep of the Status Quo* and they eventually had a lovely child named *Productivity.* They lived happily ever after and the Kingdom *continually improved forever.*

A LETTER HOME

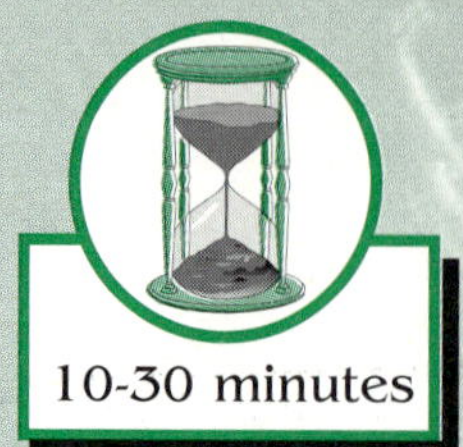

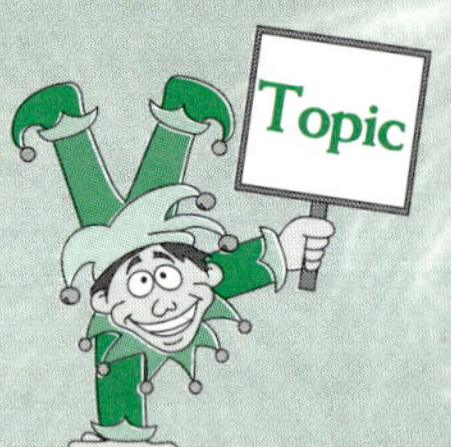

Icebreaker. Use to get acquainted. Appropriate for a half day or full day of training.

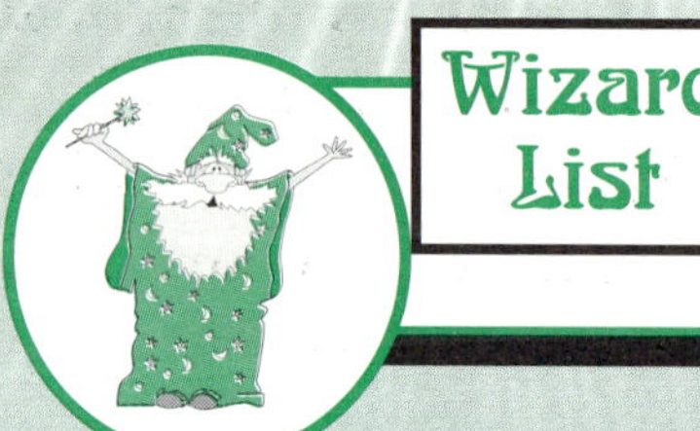

Wizard List

Paper, pens or pencils

Preparation

1. Provide a blank sheet of paper for each team member.
2. Provide pens or pencils for each team member.

Implementation

1. Distribute writing materials.
2. Ask each group member to reflect on what he or she will be doing 20 years in the future. (Gauge the number of years you select by the age of the team members. With older members, try 5 to 10 years.)
3. Ask each person to write a letter back to the group after 20 years. Explain what he or she is doing, describe the location, and so forth. Add that the letter will be shared with the group.
4. Have members read their letters to the group.

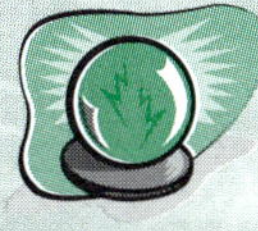

Debriefing

Ask the group if they learned anything about anyone that they did not know. Sharing these letters can give insights into personal interests, aspirations, goals, and so forth. Also it may be fun just to participate in an extravagant fantasy.

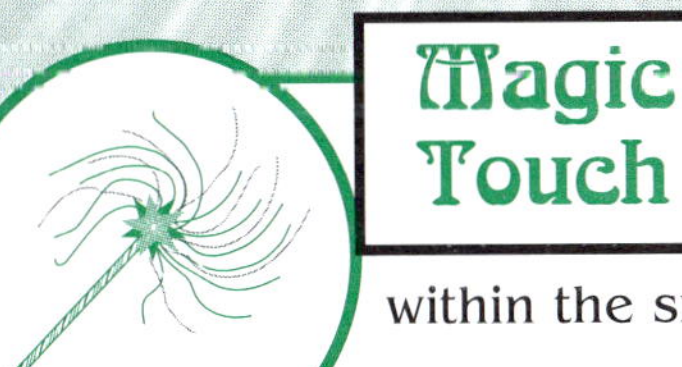

Magic Touch

Variation: For large groups, to save time, divide team members into small groups and share the letters within the small group.

By: Jaye Lynn Hall

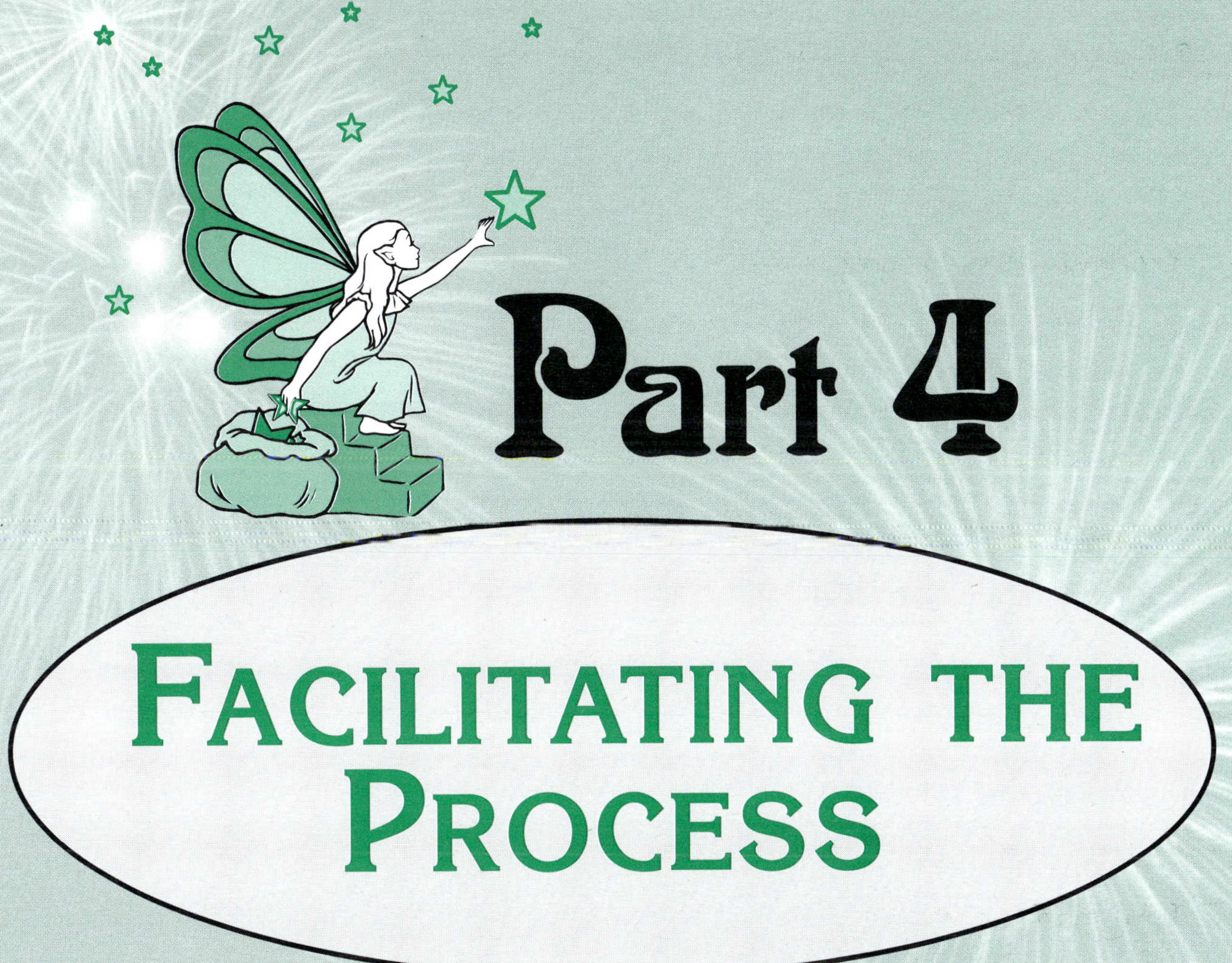

Part 4

Facilitating the Process

Facilitation in teams is the process of initiating teams and smoothing the process of the work. Facilitator training draws on information about team dynamics and offers skills for effective interventions in challenging situations within groups. Schwartz's book, *The Skilled Facilitator: Practical Wisdom for Developing Effective Groups,* is an excellent guide with detailed information for facilitators. See the Resource list.

Brief exercises can focus members' attention to communication issues that can impede or stimulate productive teamwork. This section contains activities to help you start the team, meet the challenges, and check the team's progress.

Remember to ask directly for team feedback, and let these exercises lighten your journey of team facilitation.

I DON'T DO MORNINGS!

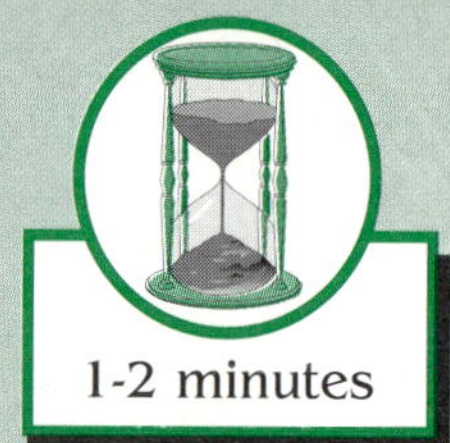

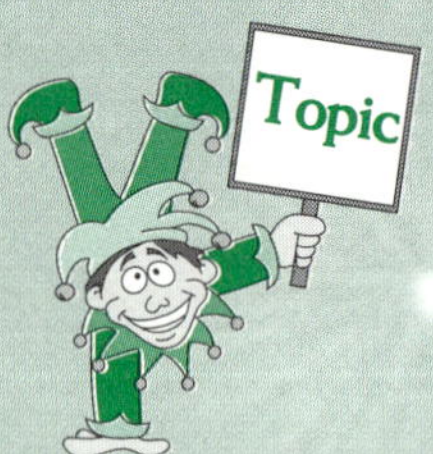

Use in the forming stage as a light way to choose meeting time.

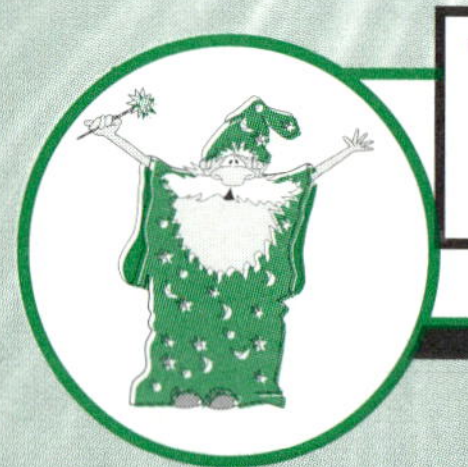

Wizard List No supplies needed

Preparation

None needed.

Implementation

1. Ask for a show of hands of who is a morning person and who is an evening person.
2. Select a recorder to record times.
3. Ask the morning team members what time they wake up in the morning and ask the evening team members what time they go to bed at night.
4. Invite the group to learn more about one another's peak energy times by lining up in order from the person who is the earliest "morning person" to the latest "night person."

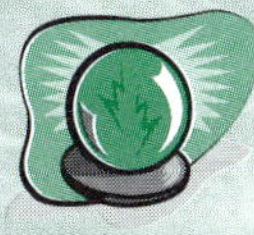

Debriefing

Point out that this exercise illustrates just one way in which team members can work together even though they are different. We all have to stretch a bit out of our comfort zone to survive!

Magic Touch

Use the Implementation procedures to begin a negotiation of team meeting times and to set the stage for members honoring one another's differences.

By: Judy Trawick, RN, BSN

NAME THAT TEAM

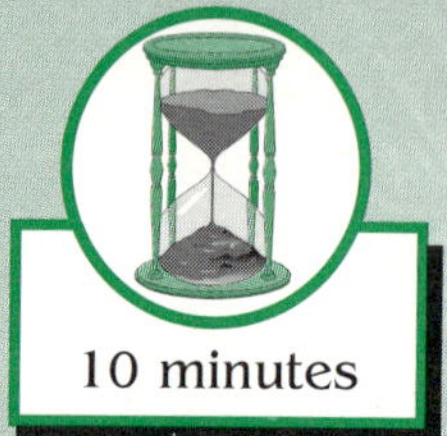

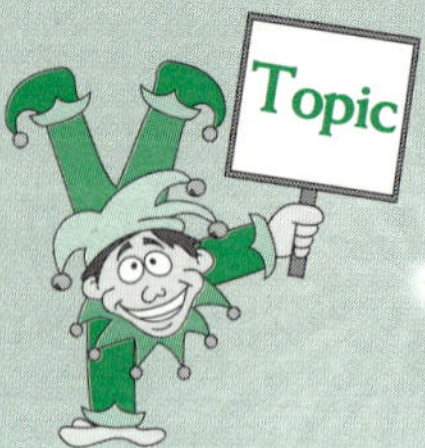

Use in the forming stage to choose a team name.

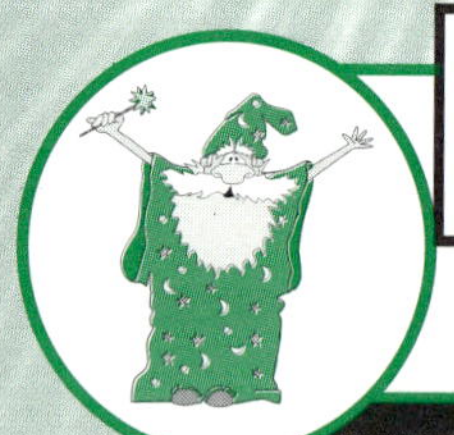

Wizard List

"We Named that Team," "In the News: Gold Miners Hard at Work," "In the News: Beauty and the Beast," flip chart, marker, prizes (optional)

Preparation

Make copies of "We Named that Team," "In the News: Gold Miners Hard at Work," and "In the News: Beauty and the Beast" for each team member.

Implementation

1. Suggest that the team come up with a catchy team name to identify their team.
2. Distribute "We Named that Team" and "In the News" articles to each team member and allow a few minutes for review.
3. Ask for other examples team members may have heard.
4. Ask for team name suggestions and record responses on the flip chart.
5. Vote to reach a consensus on a team name. If you cannot come up with a name for the team, ask team members to think about it and bring their suggestions to the next meeting. Explain that the team will vote on a name at the next meeting.
6. Give a prize to the team member whose name wins and/or to each team member that submits an idea!

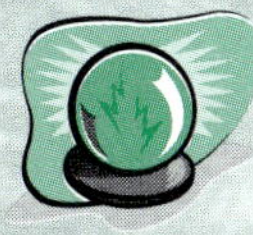

Debriefing

A team name can contribute to team identity and cohesiveness. It helps when the team does presentations about progress in order to catch the attention of administrators and other employees whose help and resources are needed to implement the team solutions.

Magic Touch

Have items imprinted with the team name, such as a coffee mug, to give to the team members and use the team name on all paperwork. Highlight team progress in the organization's newsletter. (See In the News.)

WE NAMED THAT TEAM

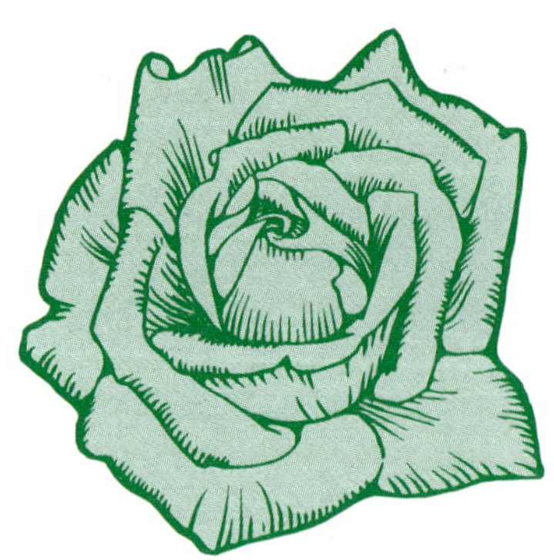

What's in a name?

The Gold Miners—a dietary department team to increase customer satisfaction (see the newsletter excerpt, "In the News")
T.J. Walkers—care path for total joints
The Wellness Kings—reducing the dollars spent on healthcare claims for our employees
S.T.A.R.S. (Stroke Treatment and Recovery Steps)—care path for strokes
A.S.A.P. (Ambulatory Surgery Assessment & Processing)—improving the flow of patients scheduled for ambulatory surgery
Pump-n-Parkit—ensuring IV pumps are cleaned between patient use
Path-o-Gems—timing of prophylactic IV antibiotics before surgery
Eliminators—reduce the completion days of medical records
Sump Pumps—care path for congestive heart failure
Homeward Bound—coordinate the discharge planning process for OB patients
Dominoes—improve purchasing and the accounts payable process regarding paper flow
The Impossible Dream—discontinue the long-standing practice of physicians who write post-op orders to "resume home medications" without specifically naming what medications the patient had been on
On the Road Again—improve discharge planning on medical oncology unit
Beauty and the Beast—improve the process of patient diet instruction (see the newsletter excerpt "In the News")

By: Judy K. Scott, RN, MSN

IN THE NEWS

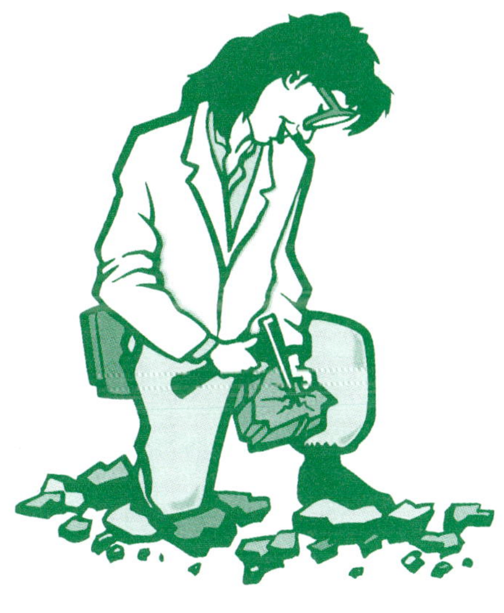

Gold Miners Hard at Work

by Mary Ewalt

Dietary CQI team members are hard at work "sharpening their pick axes and shining their miner's lamps" for the work ahead. Part of our strategic plan in the dietary department is to increase the satisfaction of physicians and other customers. We selected the Outpatient Diet Instruction Process as a topic for our CQI efforts for 1994. We call our team "The Gold Miners" because this is a golden opportunity to improve this important process. In flowcharting and fish bone diagrams, we discovered that patient referrals and communication from the physicians' staff to our department were occasionally untimely, and patients were sometimes lost as they tried to find our Outpatient Diet Clinic. As we worked through PLAN and DO, we have revised the outpatient nutritional counseling protocol and provided inservice to the clinic staff. Letters have been sent to physicians. Additional inservice for the office staff will be planned as indicated in our CHECK and ACT team functions. We intend to "keep digging for that gold!"

IN THE NEWS

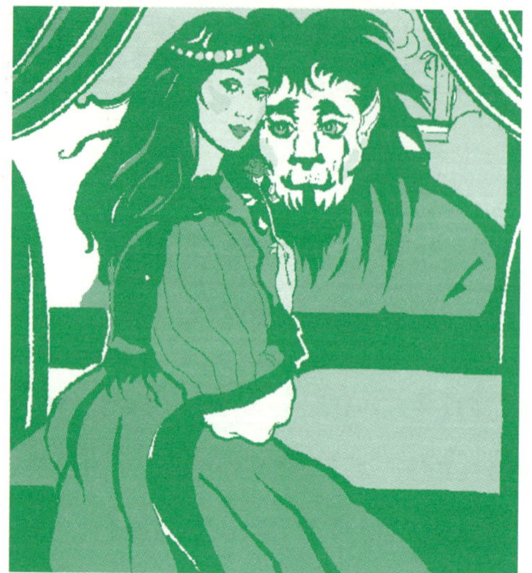

Beauty and the Beast

by Mary Ewalt

This dietary CQI team stresses the beauty of good nutrition and turns the beast of poor food habits into the handsome prince of health food choices through patient education. We want to improve the process of patient education and diet instruction. We have gathered data regarding how many patients receive a menu from which to select. We found that many patients are in for such a short time that we often do not even provide a meal. We also found many patients receive only a clear liquid diet during their stay. When we ask them to evaluate our efficiency, courtesy, and diet instructions, they have nothing to evaluate. We want to provide some nutritional information for each patient we serve.

We are planning to provide the pyramid food guide for each patient on a general diet. We will try this for two months, and evaluate our progress. If we find that we have improved patient satisfaction in this area, we plan to expand our efforts to other diets and continue the effort to reach all patients with nutritional education.

THE TEAM PLEDGE

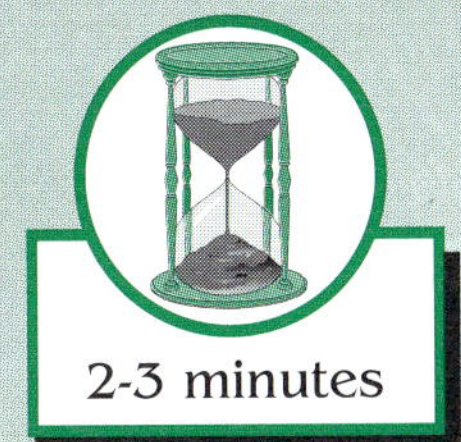

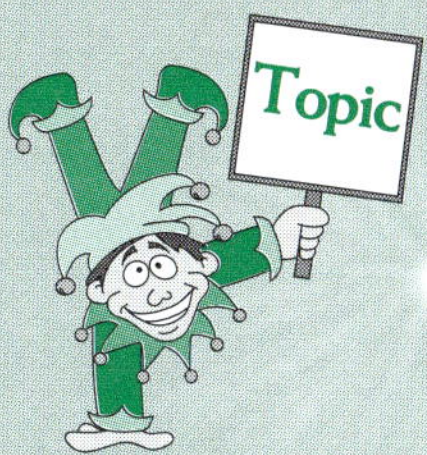

Team Spirit. Use in the forming stage or to lighten up!

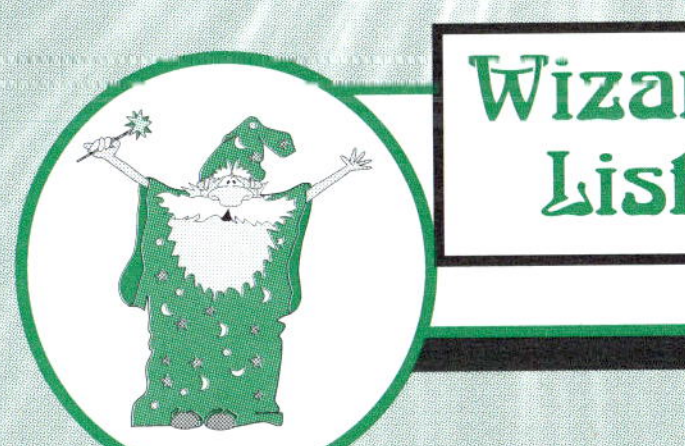

Wizard List

"The Team Pledge"

Preparation

1. Copy "The Team Pledge" for each team member.
2. Obtain a clown nose (optional).

Implementation

1. Ask team members if they think they are ready to take the team pledge.
2. Distribute copies of "The Team Pledge."
3. Explain that when one hospital defined behaviors to demonstrate team spirit, these are some of the objectives they devised.
4. Ask the team to reflect and comment on their willingness to take the pledge!

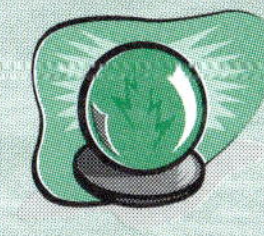

Debriefing

Comment that we often talk about team spirit but don't define it. When times are tough, remind the team of the pledge and request a show of hands of people who will promise to keep their sense of humor. Wear a clown nose if desired in order to make the point. Consider distributing noses so each person can put one on when a bit of humor is needed.

Magic Touch

Have the team write its own pledge. Add the pledge to the storyboard or use it to add a light touch to a team presentation of team findings.

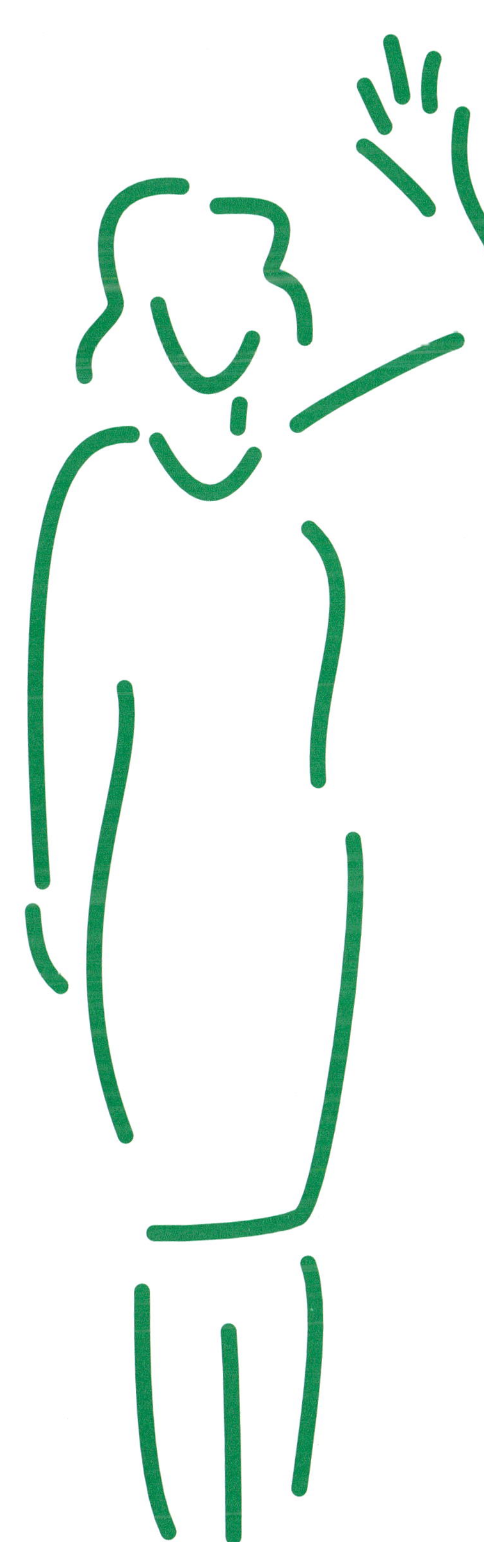

THE TEAM PLEDGE

We promise to:

Promote team spirit through genuine respect for one another and consistent willingness to cooperate, and by exhibiting a positive attitude and a sense of humor as measured by observation and feedback.

Recognize and acknowledge each team member's unique contribution by offering encouragement, support, and appreciation as measured by observation.

PROPPED UP FOR SUCCESS

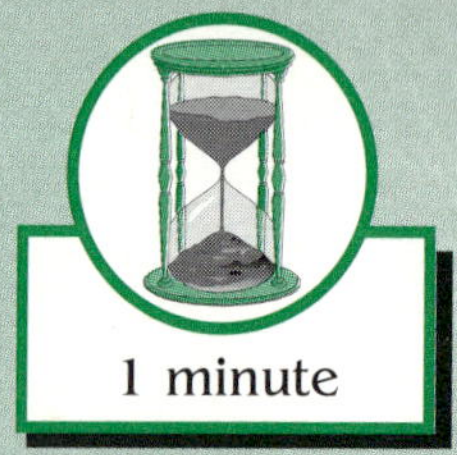

Toys That Teach

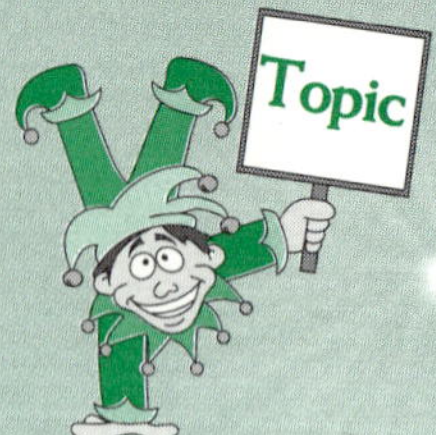

Use to illustrate a concept, a stage of team development, a process issue, etc.

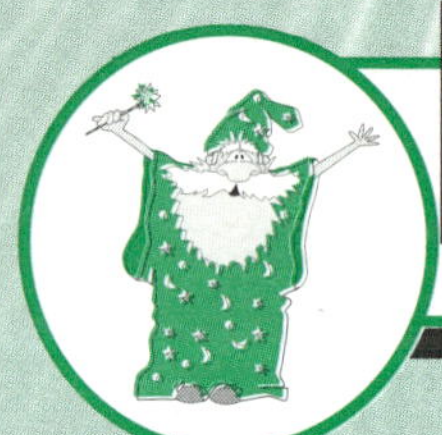

Wizard List

"Getting to the Heart of the Matter," "We're Right on Target," assorted props

Preparation

1. Review "Getting to the Heart of the Matter."
2. Collect the props appropriate for your meeting.
3. Make a copy of "We're Right on Target." (See Item 9 of "Getting to the Heart of the Matter.")

Implementation

1. Display the selected item and explain the connection to the point you are making. Refer to "Getting to the Heart of the Matter" for Concept Connectors.
2. Reinforce an important concept you are illustrating with a toy or other item that can be associated with the concept. Distribute the item to the team.

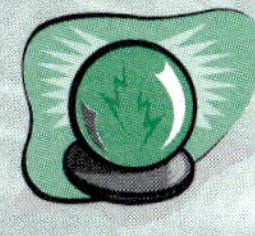

Debriefing

For example, for brainstorming display a light bulb, a common symbol for creativity. Distribute light bulb-shaped erasers. Tell participants to display them as a reminder that we are all capable of great ideas.

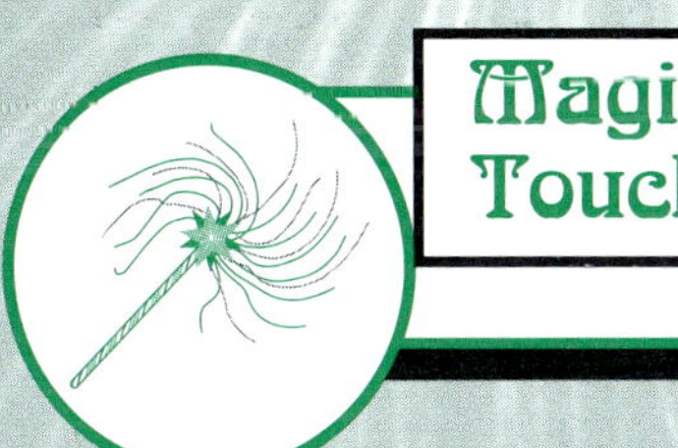

Magic Touch

Create your own list of Concept Connectors.

GETTING TO THE HEART OF THE MATTER

Item	Use	Concept Connector
1. A heart-haped item or red paper heart.	When you are stuck in data analysis or in the storming phase, or when the team seems to lose its focus.	"The patient is the heart of the matter."
2. A light bulb eraser.	When introducing problem-solving tools	"Bright ideas."
3. A huge eraser found in novelty stores, a huge pencil (clown prop), or any eraser.	When the team has made a mistake or has worked through a time of conflict.	"It's time to start fresh. That's why erasers were made."
4. A variety of hats.	When turf issues arise or different disciplines have trouble seeing other perspectives.	"Here we have to wear a variety of hats." or "Today I am wearing the hat of the group facilitator in order to introduce a process issue." It may be helpful to designate one hat as a facilitator's hat when other team members want to introduce a nonagenda process issue.
5. Pictures, such as a bull with horns.	When the team hesitates to make a decision.	"Okay, it's time to take the bull by the horns."
6. Electric, extension, or large industrial-strength cord, or a battery recharger.	When there is group apathy and more energy is needed.	"There's plenty of power in this group to get the work done. How can we plug into it? What do you need to get started?" Or, "Looks like we need a recharge to get going again." (Serve high-powered refreshments—dub them "high-powered" with a sign.)

Item	Use	Concept Connector
7. Fuses.	When there is a power struggle or conflict (storming).	"We need a lot of power to get our work done and it needs to be evenly distributed or we'll blow a fuse."
8. Scotch tape, stapler, brads, string, ribbon, white glue.	When the group resists cohesion and commitment (storming phase).	"Remember the phases of team development? Looks like we're at just the right place—storming. It takes more than these [hold up items] for us to form a team that can stick together and have cohesion. We need to discuss our normal responses in this phase—conflict, hostility, power struggles, and apathy."
9. An illustrated target (use "We're Right on Target!" to make a transparency or poster).	Whenever the team is functioning in a way that illustrates the stages of team development, and you want to point it out to facilitate the process.	"It is a marvelous thing to hear that you are okay and doing the right thing." Use this frequently and make it part of the group lore. "We're right on target!" Then, add the appropriate words, such as, "We are forming, storming, norming, performing, struggling with consensus, grappling with the design of a data collection tool," etc.
10. A Slinky spring toy, or any flexible object such as piece of connector tubing (used to vent a clothes drier).	When the team is doing a good job, being flexible, or needs more flexibility. (Role flexibility is a characteristic of the stage of performing.)	"We could use a little more of this just now." Or, "Look at us, we are just as flexible as this."

WE'RE RIGHT

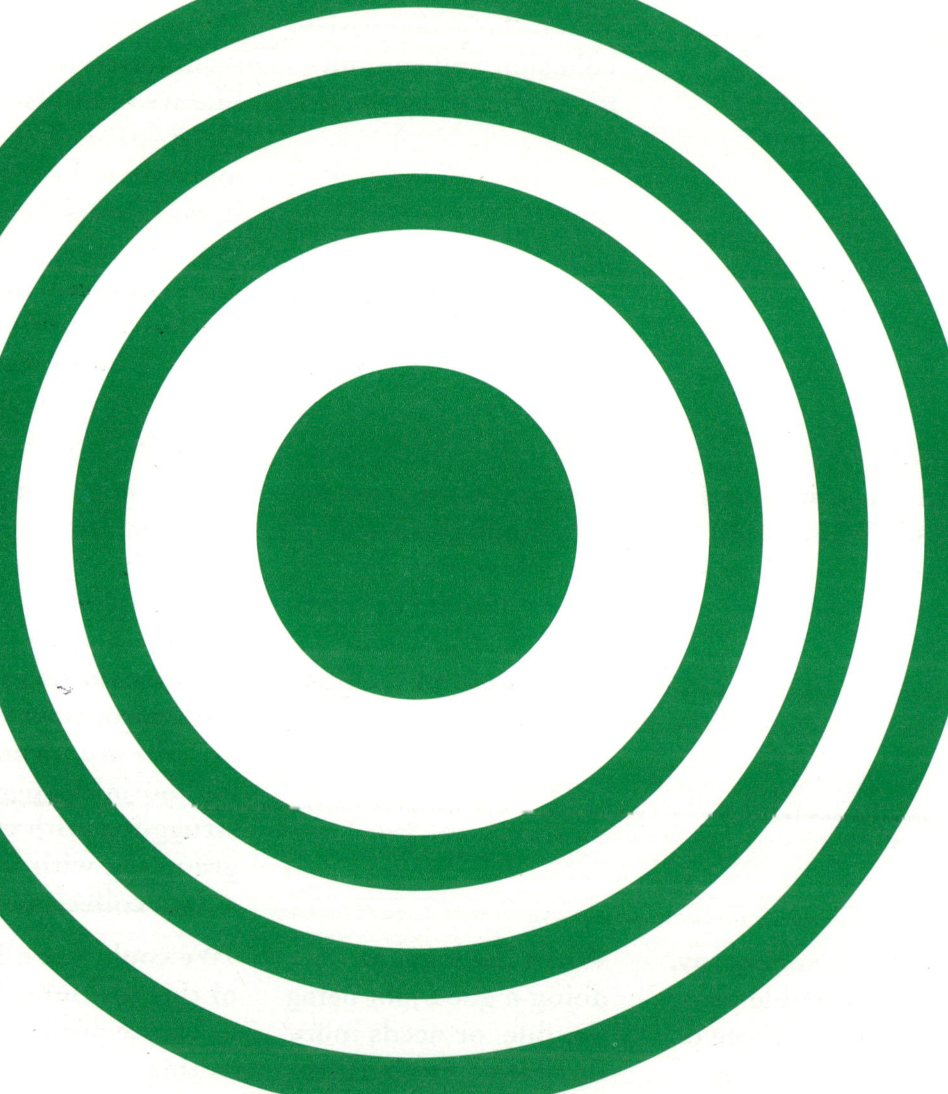

ON TARGET!

ONE STEP AT A TIME

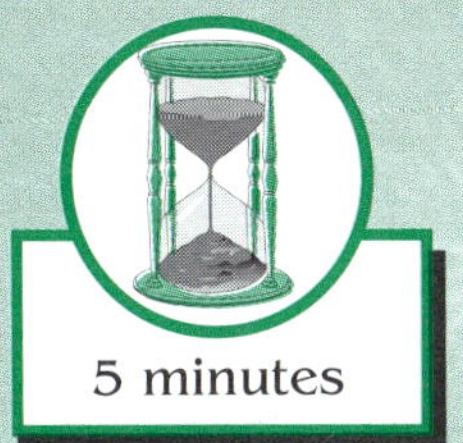

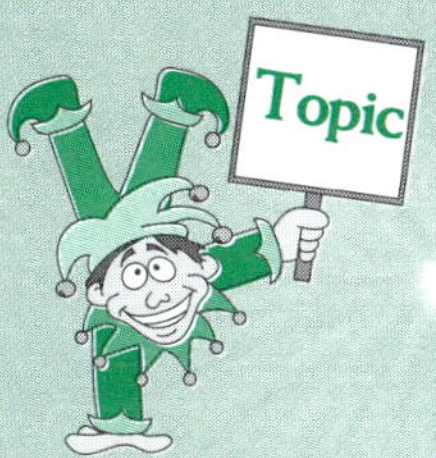

Use when members want to skip steps in the problem-solving process, or think they know answers without supporting data.

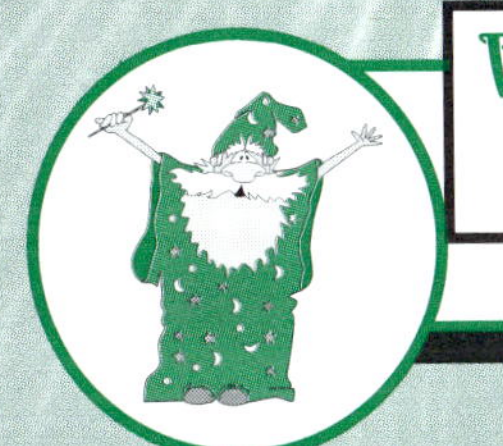

Wizard List

"How To Paint a Room" signs, thumbtacks or tape, flip chart

Preparation

1. Make one copy of each "How To Paint a Room" sign.
2. Provide thumbtacks or tape to post signs on a flat surface or flip chart.

Implementation

1. Explain that sometimes we jump right into problem solving without taking all the necessary steps.
2. Ask if anyone has ever painted a room. Ask what is the first thing they really want to do. The answer will probably be *"Paint!"*
3. Explain that you have signs that list the steps required for painting a room, and you need the team to put the signs in order so the painting is completed in an organized manner.
4. Ask for a volunteer to hang the steps according to the team's decision on their order.

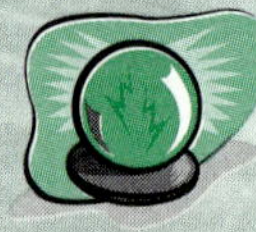

Debriefing

Conduct a light-hearted comparison of the hazards of painting without first protecting the floor and furniture and compare it to jumping to quick solutions to chronic problems.

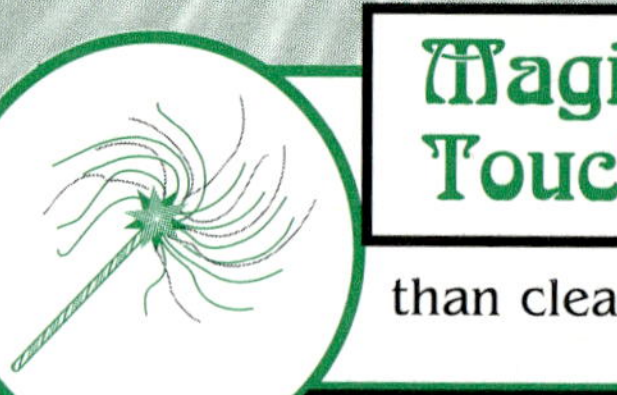

Magic Touch

In addition, remember that a plan must be flexible. It's easier to spend the time up front collecting data than cleaning up the mess afterwards.

From: Julia W. Balzer, One Step at a Time. *Quality Connections*, August 1994.

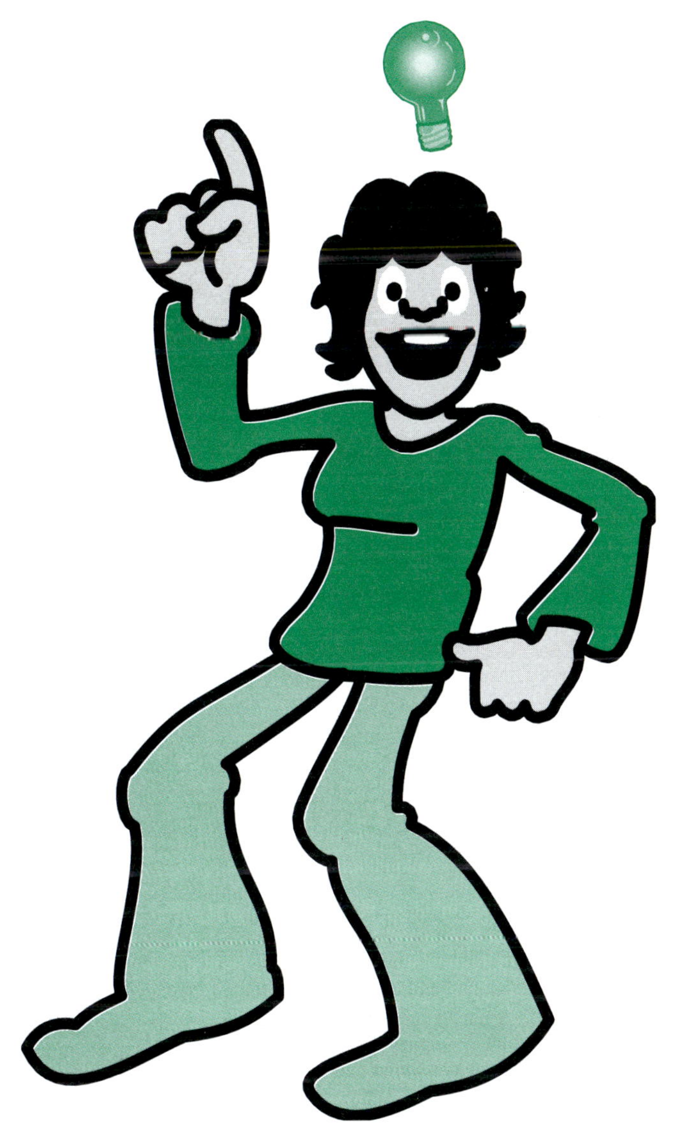

DECIDE TO PAINT

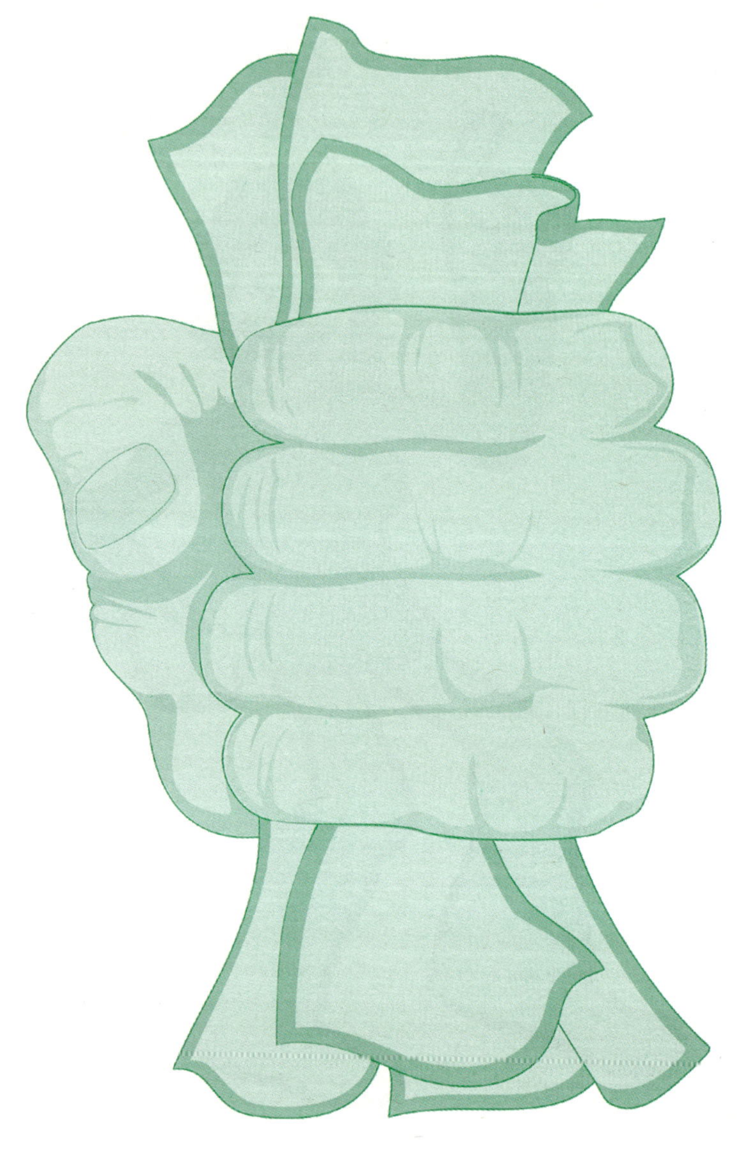

BUDGET THE MONEY

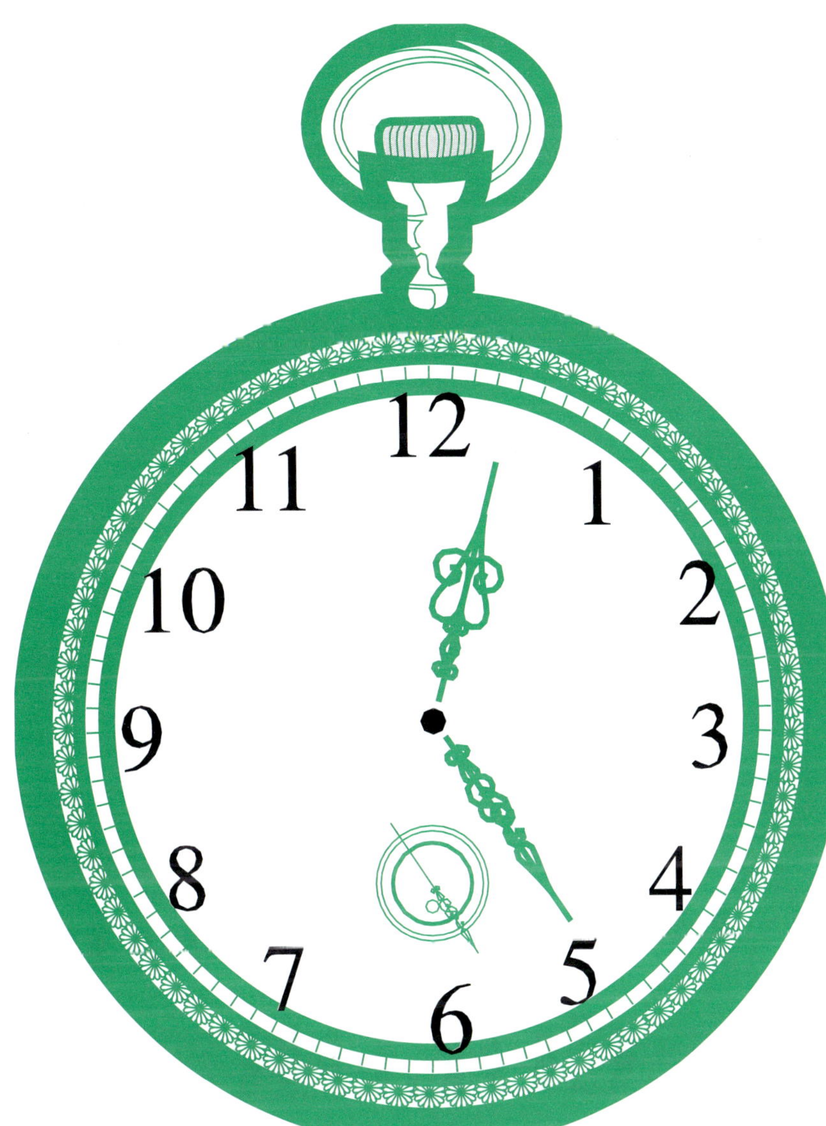

ARRANGE A TIME

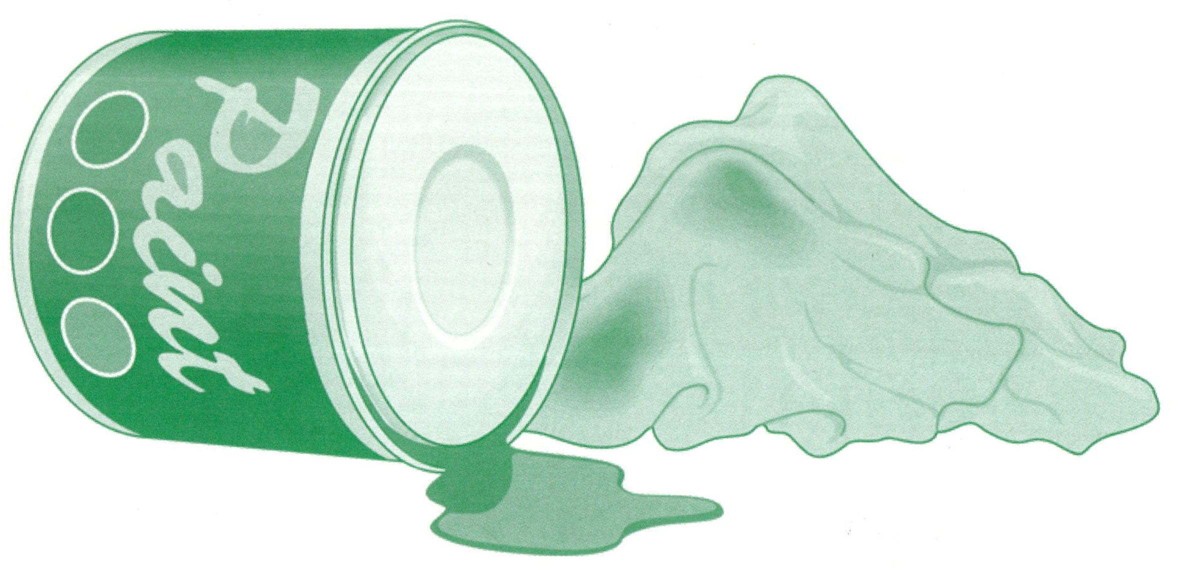

CHOOSE THE COLOR

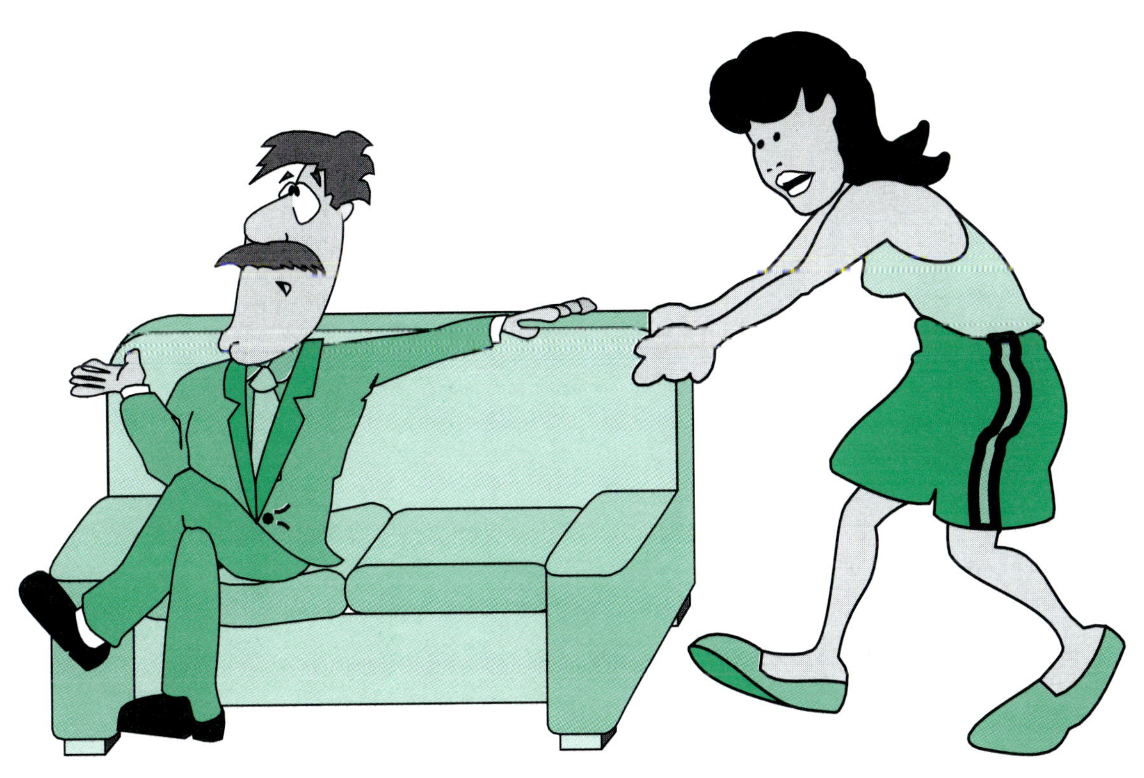

MOVE THE FURNITURE OUT OF THE WAY

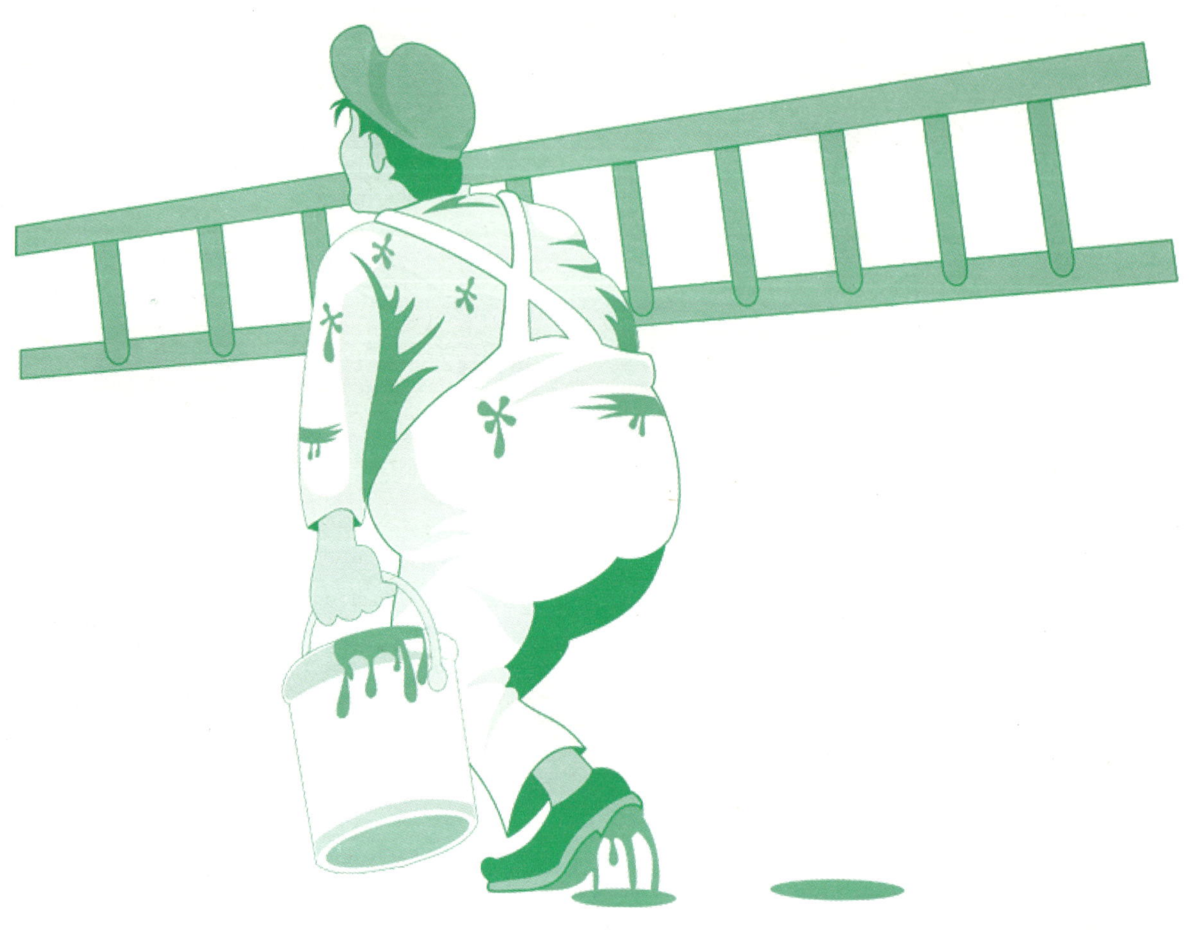

ASSEMBLE THE TOOLS

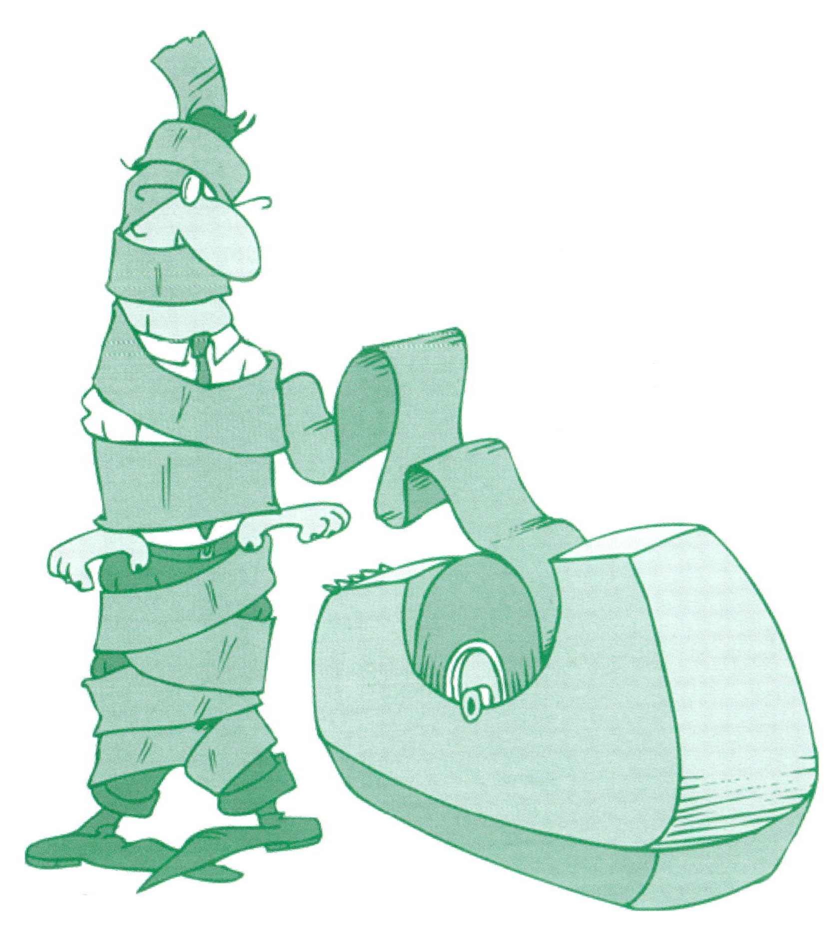

TAPE THE WINDOWS AND WOODWORK

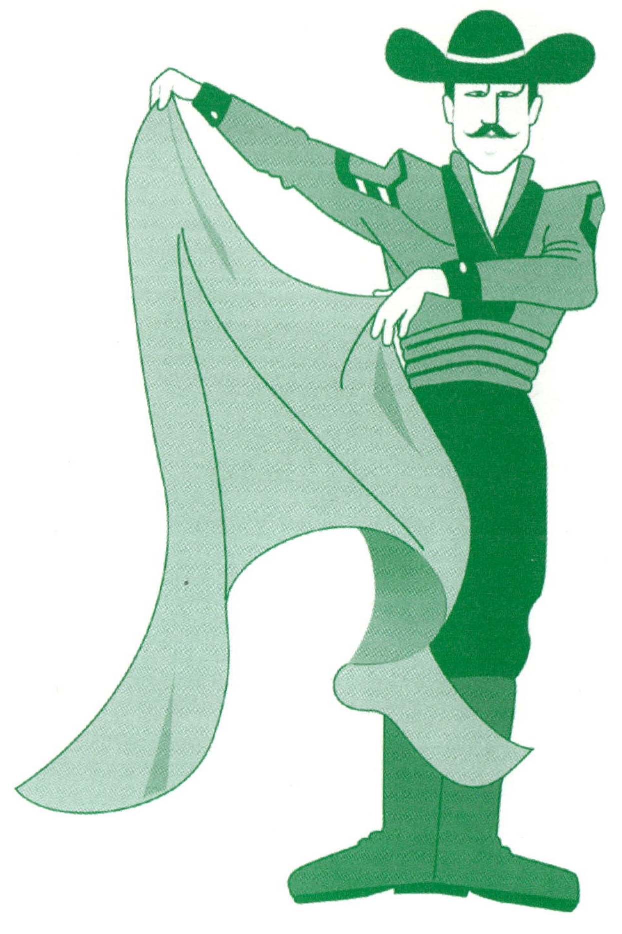

COVER THE FURNITURE AND FLOOR WITH DROP CLOTHS

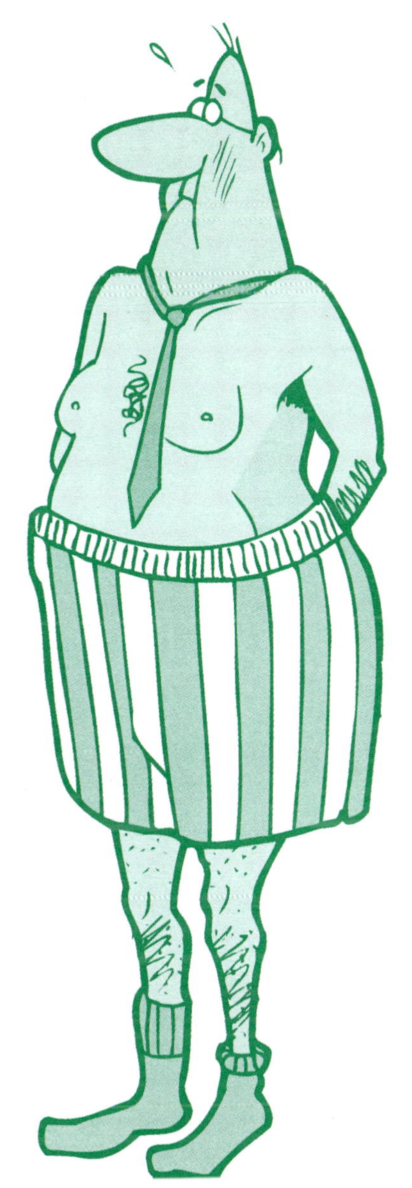

PUT ON OLD CLOTHES

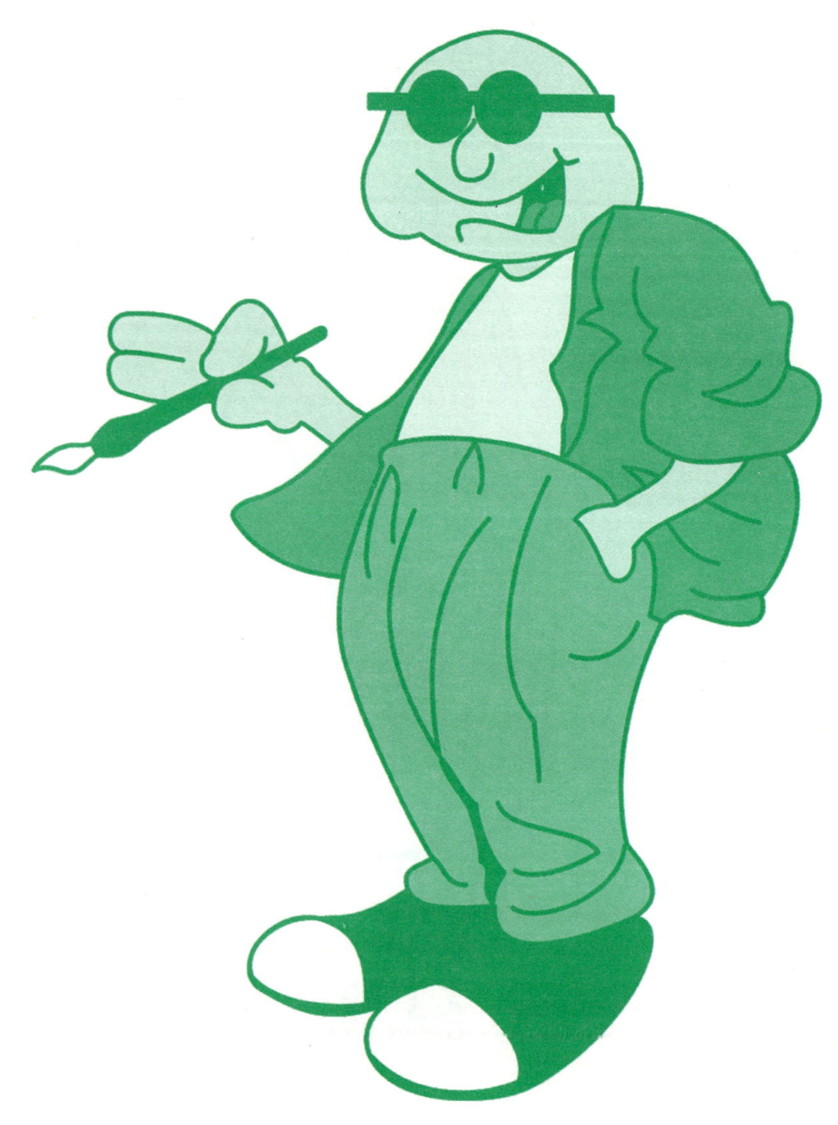

EDGE

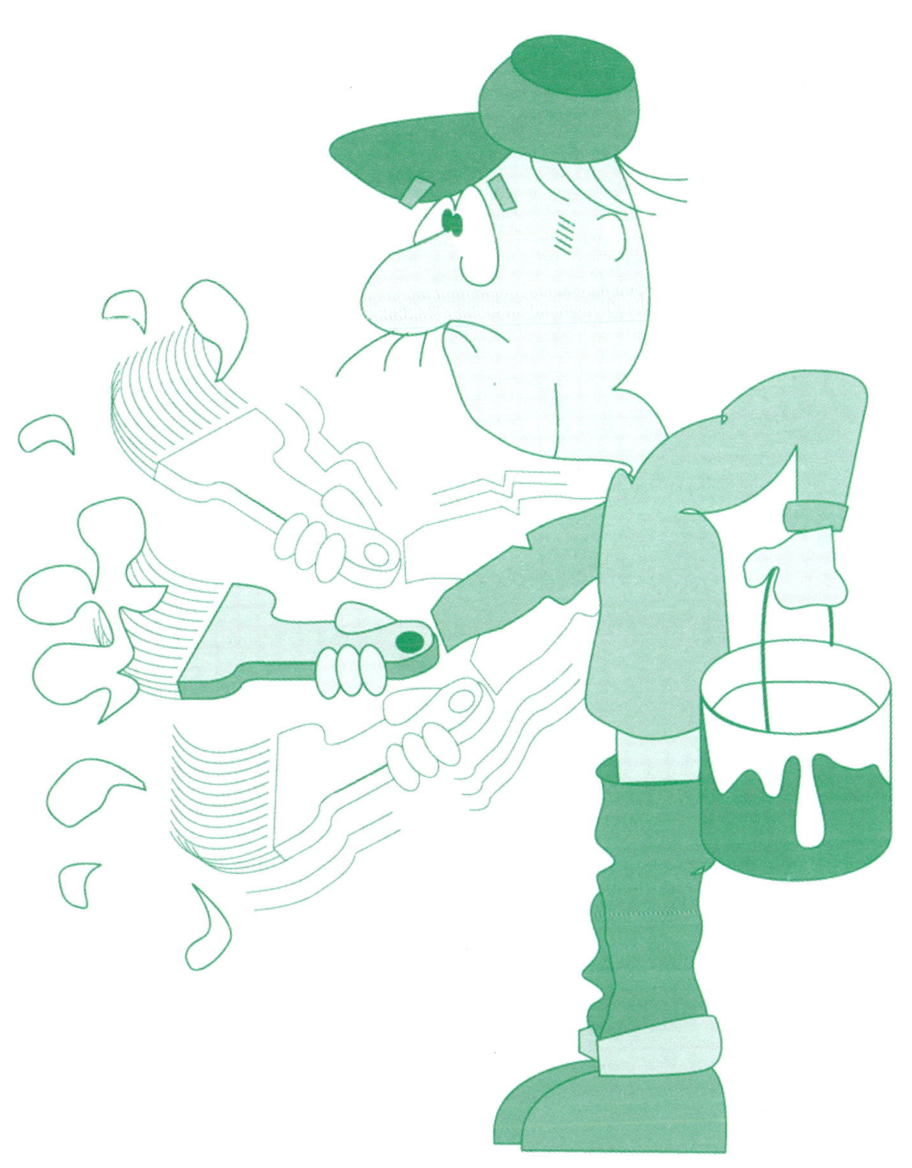

PAINT

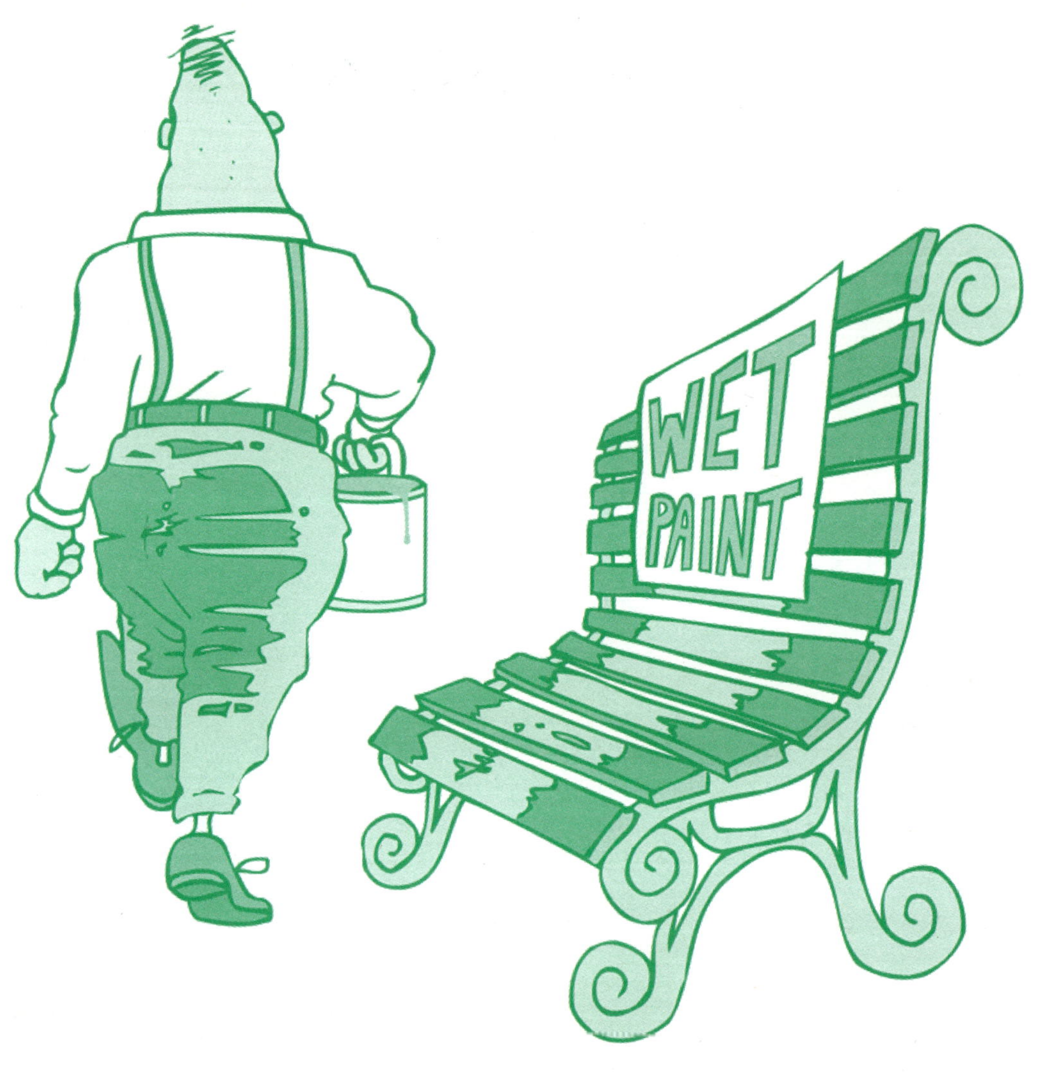

LET THE PAINT DRY

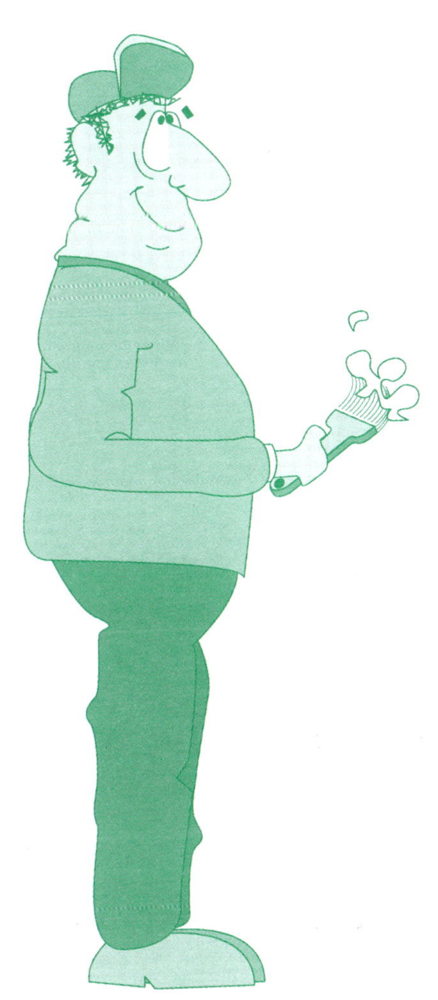

PAINT A SECOND COAT, IF NECESSARY

HOW TO PAINT A ROOM

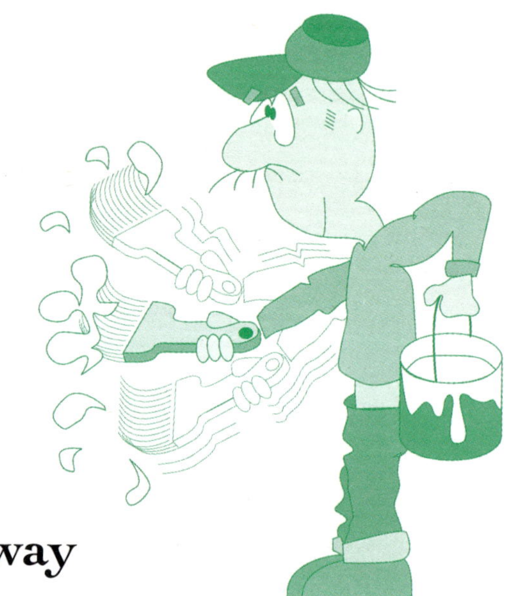

Answer Key

Decide to paint

Budget the money

Arrange a time

Choose the color

Move the furniture out of the way

Assemble the tools

Tape the windows and woodwork

Cover the furniture and floor with drop cloths

Put on old clothes

Edge

Paint

Let the paint dry

Paint a second coat, if necessary

MINING THE GOLD

Do You Talk to Think or Think to Talk?

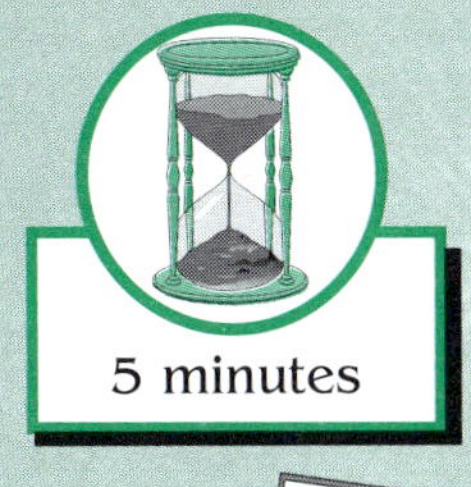

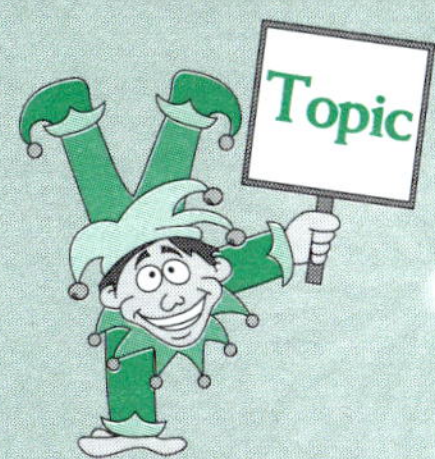

Encouragement of equal participation. Use when some team members are contributing more than others and the quieter team members do not seem to have space in the discussion to add their ideas.

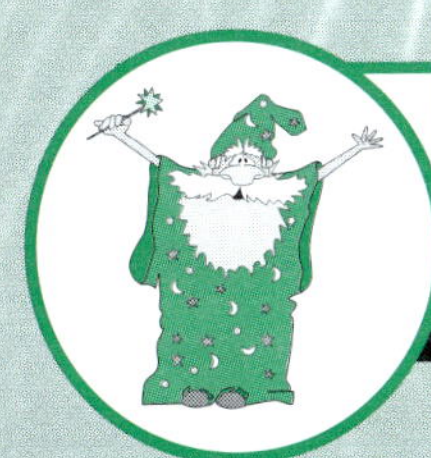

Wizard List

"Mining the Gold," rock and gold paint or chocolate coins wrapped in gold foil

Preparation

1. Spray a rock gold or purchase chocolate coins wrapped in gold foil. If you decide on the chocolate gold coins, these can be shared with the team.
2. Review the "Mining for Gold" Guidelines.
3. Explain (and discuss) that some people talk to think while others think to talk.

Implementation

1. Show the "piece of gold" or the gold coins. Suggest to the team that team members all have valuable information to share, but that, just like gold ore, sometimes it must be mined. It takes skill to do this. Some can share more easily because they think out loud. Others choose to listen and process information before they share their thoughts.

2. Explain that a little information about differences in how people think may be helpful and can provide strategies for the team in mining their own gold.
3. Use the guidelines to briefly teach the differences.

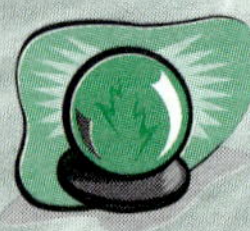

Debriefing

Discuss with team members whether this makes sense and how they can use this information here.

Magic Touch Reintroduce the gold rock or keep one of the gold coin candies to show later if those who talk to think don't allow time for those who think to talk!

MINING THE GOLD

Do You Talk to Think or Think to Talk?

GUIDELINES

DESCRIPTIONS

Talk to think! Some people think out loud and get their energy from fast-paced conversations with quick exchanges of partially formed ideas. They get excited about their ideas and do their best work with time to talk it through. These people aren't afraid to toss out an idea to see how it lands. This does not mean that they necessarily believe what they say.

Think to talk! Some people prefer to mull over their ideas before sharing them. They use fewer, measured words and prefer not to share until their ideas are well thought through. They are less likely to respond quickly to a question because they want to give their best answer.

PITFALLS

If team members are not aware of these different styles for thinking and sharing ideas, the people who talk to think may carry the load and not get help from those who think to talk.

The talkers resent the lack of participation of the quieter members or, perhaps, never even notice. The thinkers believe their opinions are not wanted and stop trying.

STRATEGIES

To honor these differences and mine the team gold, the talkers can practice their listening skills, understanding that silence may be needed for processing and that it does not necessarily mean consensus; they can consciously slow down and ask only one question at a time, allowing time for a response. The thinkers can understand and allow the talkers time to process aloud; they can ask for a moment to think and take the initiative to make sure they are heard. With this knowledge, the team can recognize violations of one another's styles and use the "mining the gold" reference to add a light touch to facilitate the best work of the team.

This information refers to personality preferences called Extraversion (talks to think) and Introversion (thinks to talk). The Myers-Briggs Type Indicator is a personality inventory that helps people learn more about their own preferences in communication and problem solving.

(Kroeger and Thuesen, 1988.)

GETTING TO THE BIG PICTURE

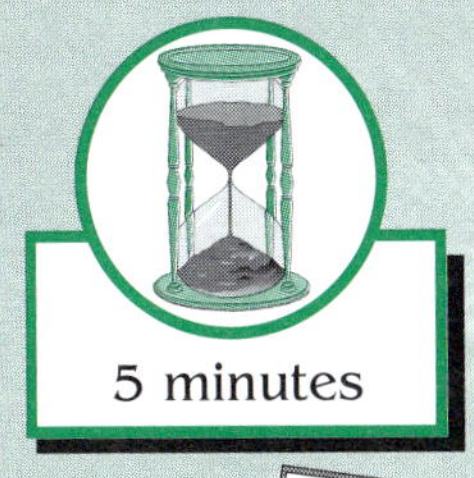

Or, Don't Bother Me with the Facts!

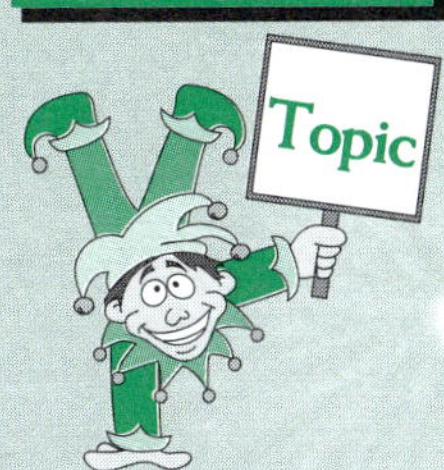

Problem Solving. Use when some members are dealing with details and others want to move more quickly.

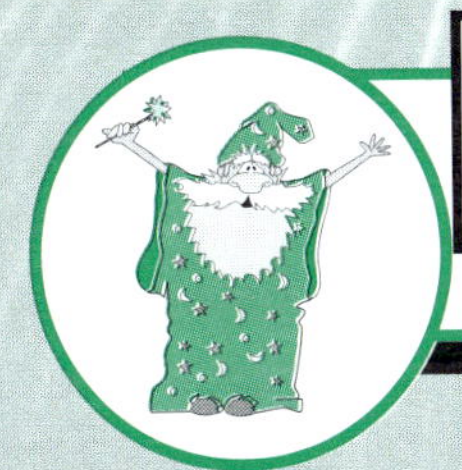

Wizard List

"Getting To the Big Picture" Guidelines, jigsaw puzzle in its original box

Preparation

1. Obtain a jigsaw puzzle in its original box.
2. Review "Getting to the Big Picture" Guidelines.

Implementation

1. Show the puzzle box lid. Point to the picture. Explain that this is the goal, to make the puzzle pieces fit together.
2. Open the box and spill some of the pieces onto a table.
3. Explain that individuals problem-solve in different ways.
4. Use the "Getting To the Big Picture" Guidelines to teach about these differences.

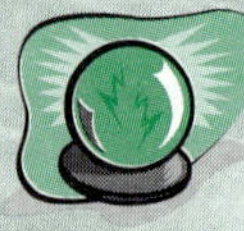

Debriefing

Discuss the advantages and disadvantages of the different ways in which people problem-solve.

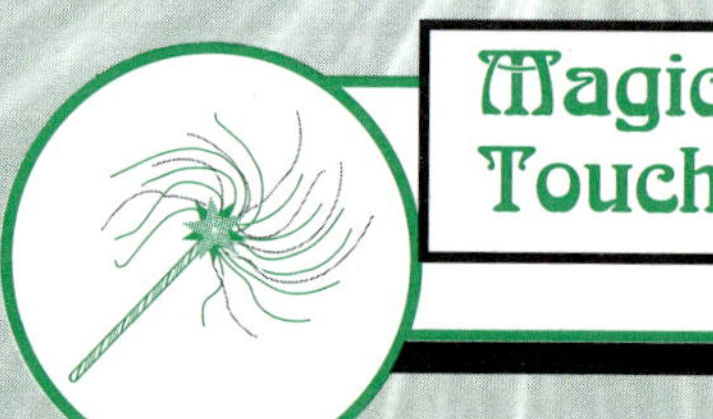

Magic Touch

Repeat an analogy to the team if the same problem arises.

GETTING TO THE BIG PICTURE GUIDELINES

DESCRIPTIONS

Sees the big picture! Some people look for the end product and anticipate it. They may skip steps on the way to the end, thinking A . . . oh, yes, D. They solve problems by depending on their intuition to get to the right answer.

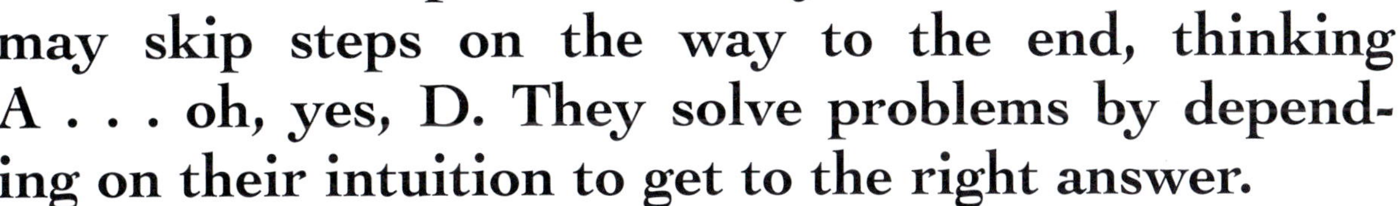

Collects data! Some people want to know how many, how big, when, what, where, and who. They think A . . . B . . . C . . . , and oh, of course, D. They solve problems by collecting all the facts.

PITFALLS

Big picture people may present what seem like unrealistic, fantastic ideas. They may jump to conclusions and make decisions without careful consideration of all the practicalities of implementing their ideas. Data collectors may have trouble making a decision because they can never get all the data they would like.

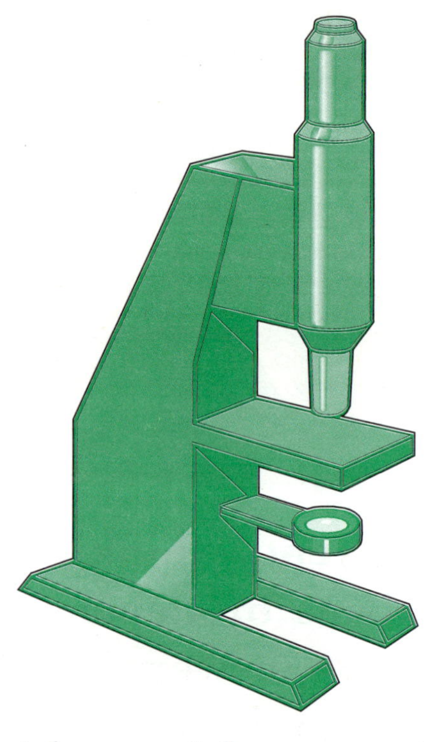

STRATEGIES

To honor these differences and complete the puzzle, big picture people can listen to the detail people to avoid making hasty decisions. They can be more patient with the necessary process of attention to details. They can focus on the current issues to be solved before a solution can be implemented. Data collectors can give the others time to express their ideas without rapid dismissal, so the creativity may be harnessed. They can understand that all the little pieces fit together to make the big picture.

This information refers to personality preferences called Intuition (the big picture person who uses intuition for problem solving) and Sensing (the detail person who collects facts to solve problems). The Myers-Briggs Type Indicator is a personality inventory that helps people learn more about their own preferences in communication and problem solving.

(Kroeger and Thuesen, 1988.)

CATCH A FALLING TEAM

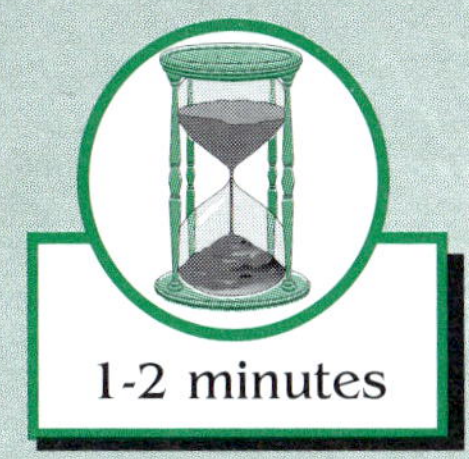

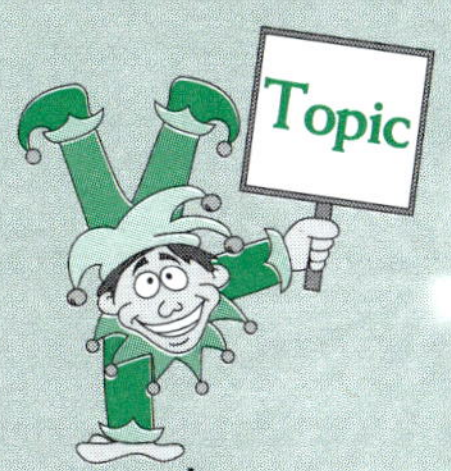

Roadblocks. Use in the storming phase, when the team is stuck, when the mission needs clarifying, or when conflict needs to be surfaced.

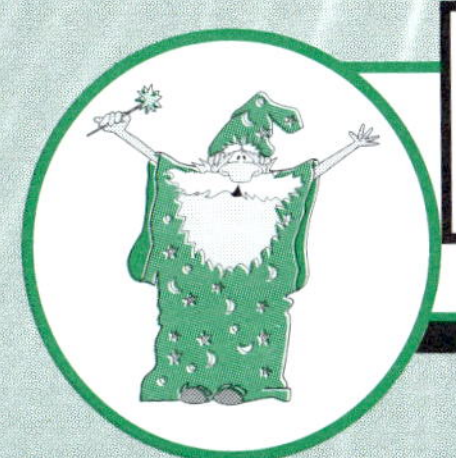

Wizard List

"Catch a Falling Team"

Preparation

1. Make copies of "Catch a Falling Team" for each team member.
2. Make sure someone on the team knows the melody to "Catch a Falling Star," sung by Perry Como.

Implementation

1. Invite the team to play for just a moment. Ask if they would be willing to have a bit of fun singing a silly, but significant, song.
2. Distribute "Catch a Falling Team" and have someone lead the singing to the tune of "Catch a Falling Star."

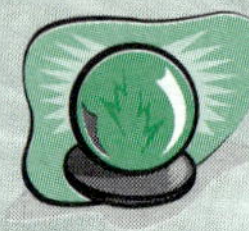

Debriefing

Ask if anyone sees the relevance of the lyrics. Initiate a discussion about what is not currently working for the team or how team members' behavior signify the team's phase of storming.

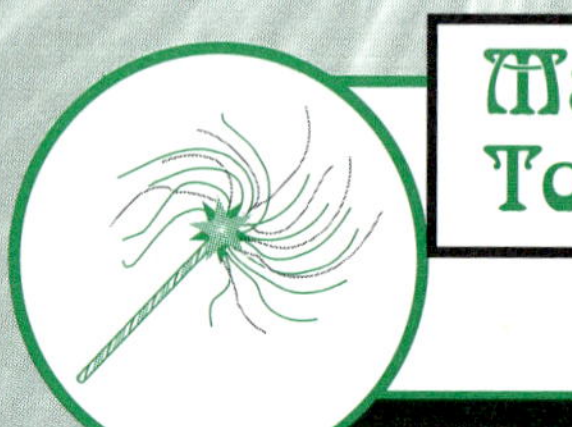

Magic Touch

Discuss how the things that are not working on the team can be changed to make the team process work.

CATCH A FALLING TEAM

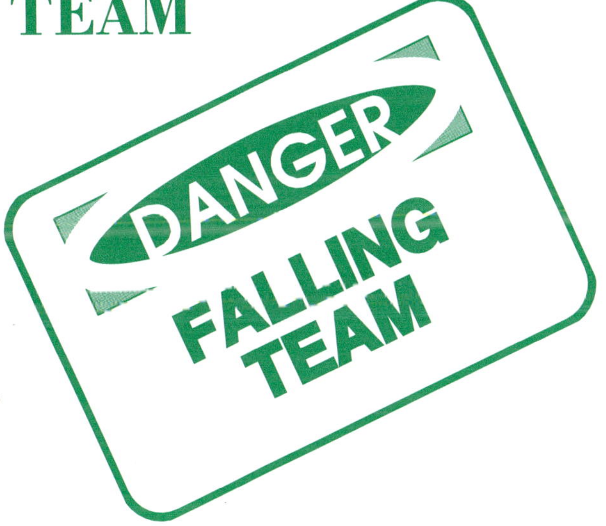

Catch a falling team
And put it on your docket,
Examine how it works today.
Ask the members just what
They think's not working.
Do it now and don't delay.

For surfacing conflict and
Rethinking your mission
Might just save the day.
You might as well
Work on all your problems,
Because they won't just go away.

Catch a falling team
And put it on your docket
Examine how it works today.
Ask the members just what
They think's not working.
Do it now and don't delay.

ON A LONG VOYAGE IN SPACE

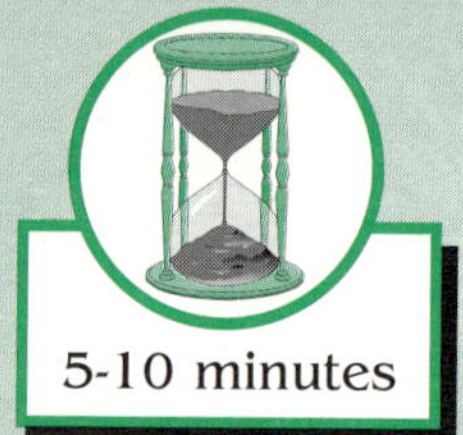

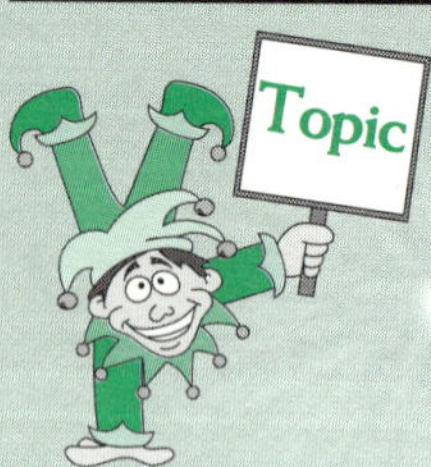

Teamwork. Use to generate discussion about team cohesiveness.

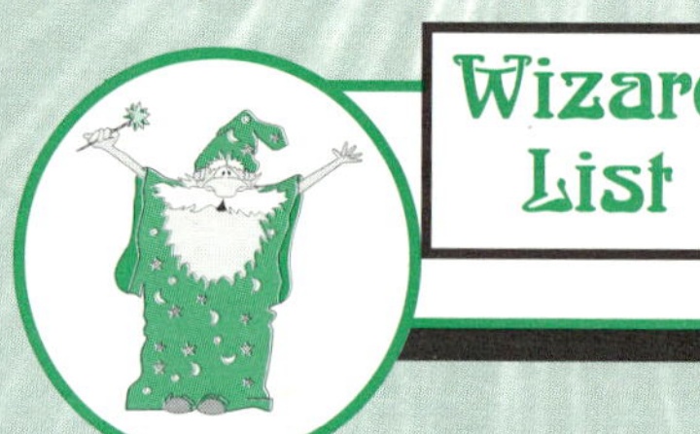

Wizard List "Lessons Learned from the World of Science Fiction"

Preparation

1. Make copies of "Lessons Learned from the World of Science Fiction" for each team member.

Implementation

1. Ask if any team members are Star Trek fans or if they know people who are.
2. Mention that there is an unofficial book about life lessons from Star Trek that applies to the team process.
3. Distribute copies of "Lessons Learned from the World of Science Fiction."
4. Generate discussion about how the team sees itself using the lessons learned from the world of science fiction.

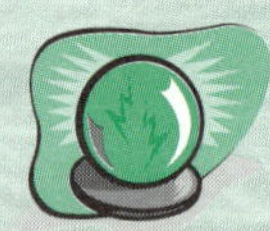

Debriefing

Not all of these can apply to every team. Certainly, few leaders or members can be as secure and open as the fictional, futuristic characters in a science fiction series. Yet, when we consider the mass popularity of these heroes, perhaps, we would all aspire to build such teams, and we can reflect on how we might move in that direction.

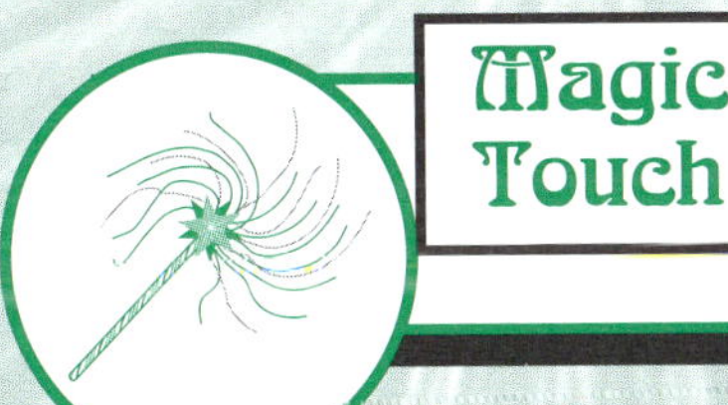

Magic Touch

For added enthusiasm, bring Star Trek toys or memorabilia. Serve snacks on space-related paper goods.

LESSONS LEARNED FROM THE WORLD OF SCIENCE FICTION

The Star Trek characters used teamwork to survive in space. In the unofficial book, *Boldy Live as You've Never Lived Before,* the authors identify four types of heroes on the team— leader, warrior, relater, and analyst. As all team members use their talents proudly and to the fullest, they achieve an interdependence that is admired. Here are seven secrets to good teamwork. How do we measure up?

1. Crew members accept themselves as they are.
2. Crew members have confidence in themselves and their abilities without apology.
3. Crew members are able to trust one another completely.
4. Crew members trust the captain's judgment implicitly.
5. Crew members value being a great team more than being great individuals.
6. Crew members forgive one another for their mistakes. The past is "space dust!"
7. The crew plays together, mourns together, and seeks help from one another.

Now substitute the word "team" for "crew" and what do you think?

(Raben and Hiyaguha, 1995.)

THE SUGGESTION BOX

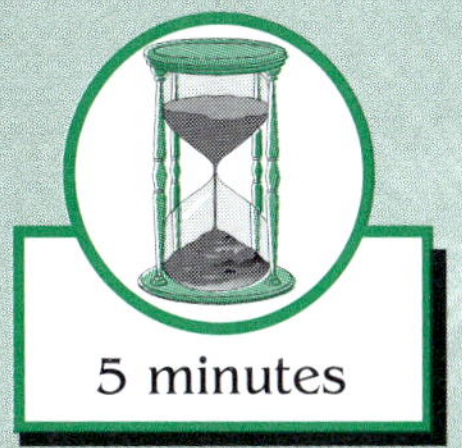

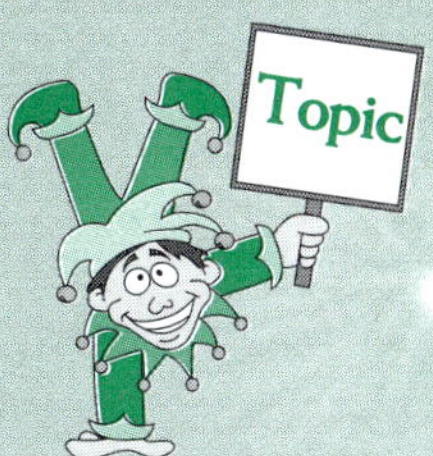

Anonymous feedback. Use when it is difficult to get verbal feedback about the team.

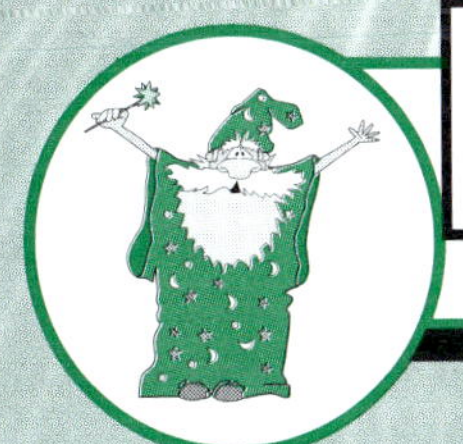

Wizard List

Shoe box, wrapping paper, tape, marker, index cards or small pieces of paper, pens or pencils

Preparation

1. Cover a shoe box with wrapping paper and label it *Suggestion Box.* Wrap box and lid separately to open easily.
2. In the lid of the shoe box, cut a hole big enough to insert slips of paper.
3. Bring the supplies listed to a group meeting.

Implementation

1. Distribute the index cards or small pieces of paper and pens or pencils to each team member.
2. Request that each team member write one suggestion to improve team meetings. These suggestions might pertain to adherence to group rules, participation, or other group issues. Positive comments about the group are acceptable!
3. Have the team members place their suggestions in the Suggestion Box.
4. Explain that these will be reviewed by the facilitator/leader and shared at the next meeting.

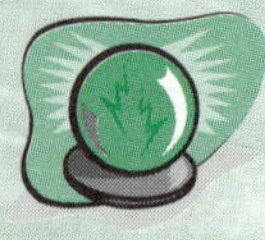

Debriefing

Explain that the participants' feedback about the work of the group allows for positive changes that can contribute to the success of the group. Explain that this activity honors some team members' lack of comfort with sharing.

Magic Touch

Have the team members vote to prioritize the team's suggestions in order of most important to least important in order to see what suggestions would benefit the team the most.

FORTUNE COOKIE WISDOM

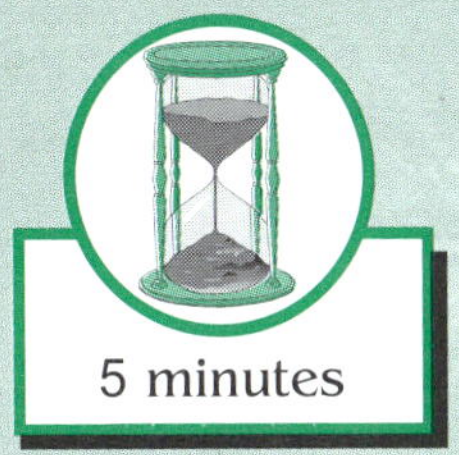

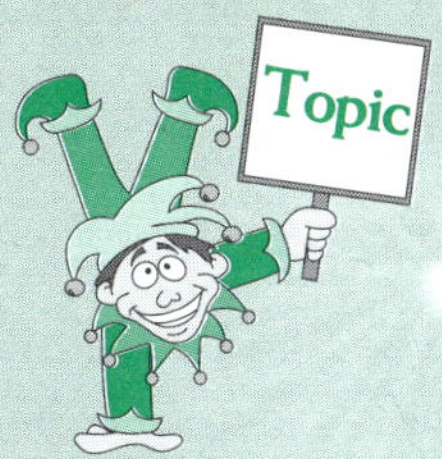

Anonymous feedback. Use this as a regular exercise to review progress.

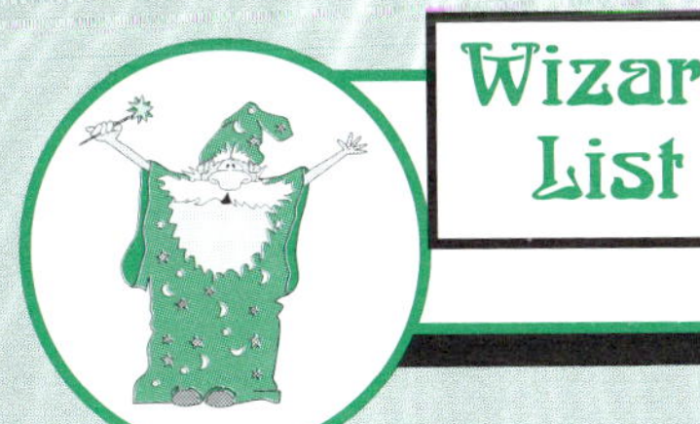

Wizard List

Fortune cookies, flip chart, marker, paper, pens or pencils, small container to collect papers

Preparation

1. Purchase fortune cookies, which are available at Chinese restaurants or in the oriental food section in the grocery store.
2. Prepare flip chart and markers.
3. Cut narrow strips of paper (fortune-cookie size).
4. Provide pens and pencils for each team member.

Implementation

1. Suggest to the team that they have just opened a unique consulting business. As consultants, they examine the activities and functioning of teams and write fortunes, like those in fortune cookies, with bits of wisdom (anonymous observations) customized for this team.
2. Distribute pens and narrow strips of paper. Ask each team member to write his or her bit of wisdom for the team at this time. What is going well? What needs work? What predictions would you make for team success?
3. Ask the team members to fold up their team fortunes, then collect them in a container.

4. Ask for a volunteer to read the team fortunes aloud. Write the team fortunes on a flip chart.
5. Discuss the observations.

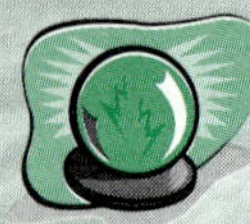

Debriefing

We need to be able to make observations and suggestions for team improvement. Sometimes a creative way makes it easier and opens important areas for discussion.

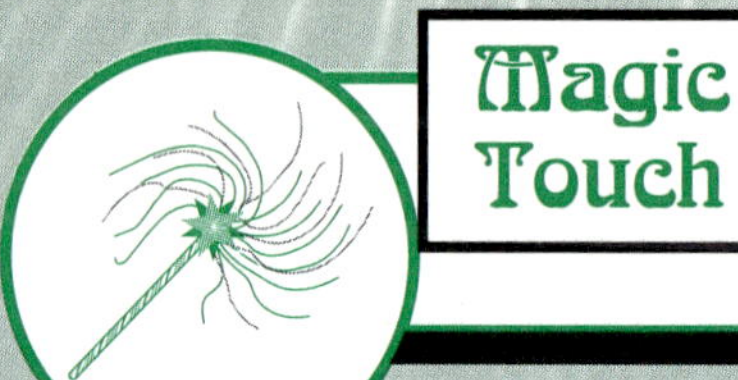

Reward with fortune cookies. Share your fortunes just for fun.

THE FOUR SEASONS OF A TEAM'S LIFE

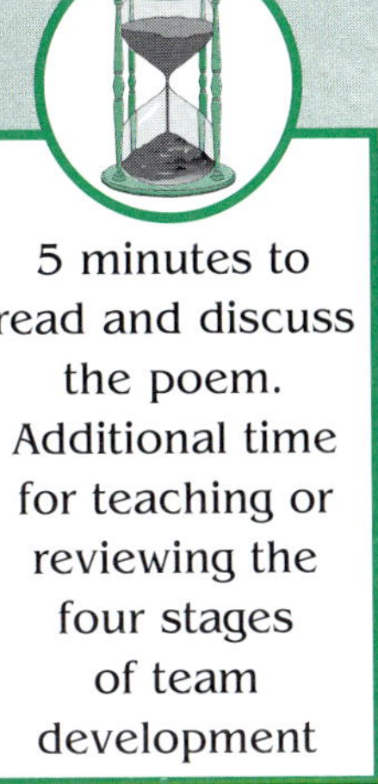

5 minutes to read and discuss the poem. Additional time for teaching or reviewing the four stages of team development

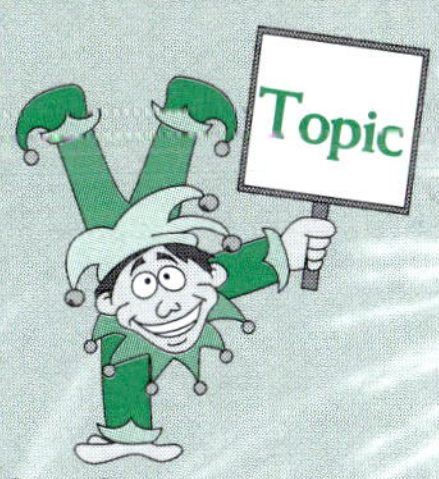

Knowing where you are. Use this exercise to help identify the team stage.

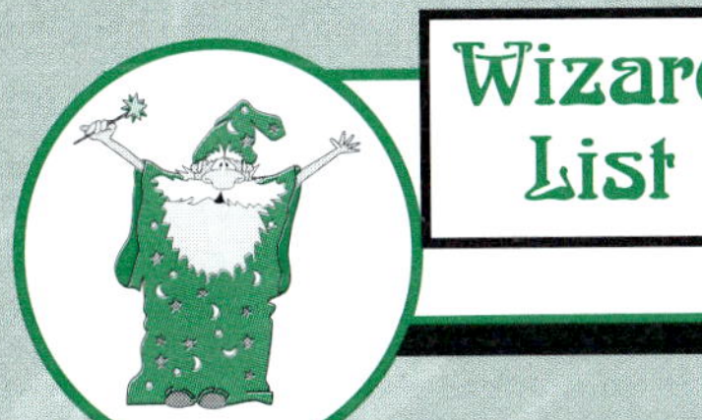

Wizard List

"The Four Seasons of a Team's Life"

Preparation

1. Prepare a short lecture on the four stages of team development: forming, storming, norming, and performing. (Or see the activity "Yes, We'll Form, Storm, Norm, and Perform," page 139.)
2. Copy "The Four Seasons of a Team's Life" for each team member.

Implementation

1. Give the short lecture, if desired.
2. Distribute copies of "The Four Seasons of a Team's Life" and read it aloud.

3. Options:
   - Use the poem to complement the lecture or use it alone to review.
   - Use the poem to add comic relief during the different stages of the life of the team.
4. Ask team members to comment on which parts of the poem relate to each of the four stages. See the Key, which corresponds the parts of the poem to each stage.

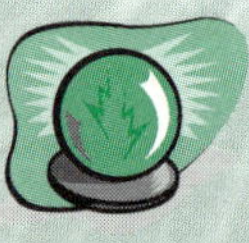

Debriefing

Discuss the importance of understanding team dynamics to the success of the team. All the stages are normal, but they are not always clear-cut. Committees and other groups often disband during the storming phase due to the discomfort caused by conflict. It is important to recognize and expect team issues, such as the need to build trust, the need to have ground rules, the healthy function of recognizing and surfacing conflict and opposing points of view, and the importance of team cohesion when implementing solutions and holding the gains made by new procedures or changes.

"The Four Seasons of a Team's Life" Content Connection Key

Stage one:	Forming, stanzas 1–2
Stage two:	Storming, stanzas 3–6
Stage three:	Norming, stanzas 7–12
Stage four:	Performing, stanzas 13–16

Magic Touch Engage other team members in adding stanzas to the team poem or writing their own poem to reflect the team's dynamics. Try it yourself; it's fun, and expertise at poetry is clearly not needed!

THE FOUR SEASONS OF A TEAM'S LIFE

by Julia Balzer Riley

1
Together we are,
Like it or not.
In for the long haul,
Work hard or not!

2
A bunch of people
For a team do gather.
Working alone is
What they would rather.

3
Feathers ruffled
As we do our dance.
Can we work together
Or just take a stance?

4
Whose degree is bigger?
Who has been here longer?
Will you make your peace
Or be a war monger?

5
Put your toe in the water,
It isn't too cold.
There's work here for all.
Come on and be bold.

6
Nothing to gain
By fighting the tide.
Join in. Be a team.
Come along for the ride.

7
Share your knowledge,
Ideas, and dismay.
The water is fine here.
Come on in; let's play.

8
We'll have to have rules, though.
On time to begin.
Work hard and steady,
And on time we can end.

9
Everyone speaks
When there's something to say.
Quiet one stretching;
Extraverts held at bay.

10
When an assignment is given,
Or taken at will,
Do it on time
Or the team stands still.

11
Conflict managed
By speaking your peace.
Open and frank,
Not anger released.

12
Speak up in the room,
Right in the meeting,
Not after you leave,
When colleagues you're greeting.

13
Consensus is reached,
But not always easily.
Commit to group goals,
Not shallow and breezily.

14
When time comes to implement
Tough team decisions,
A united voice
Prevents useless division.

15
Commitment from members
Goes a long way,
So problem resolution
Does not go astray.

16
Holding the gain
Is not as hard as it sounds
When from all team members
Great support does abound.

WHEN YOU'RE HAPPY AND YOU KNOW IT

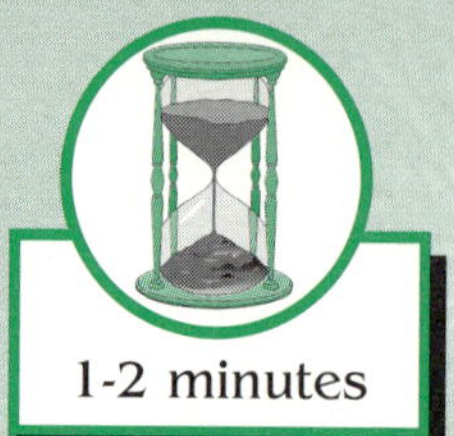

. . . Oh, Give It a Try!

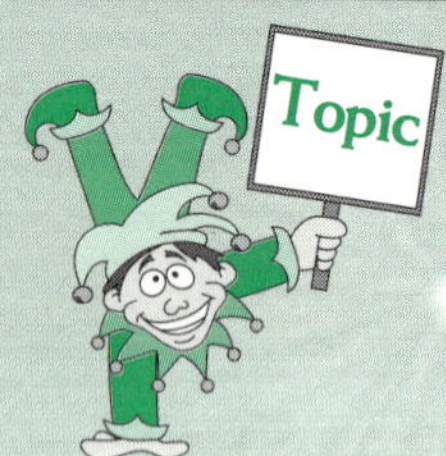

Moods. Use a song for a pick-me-up.

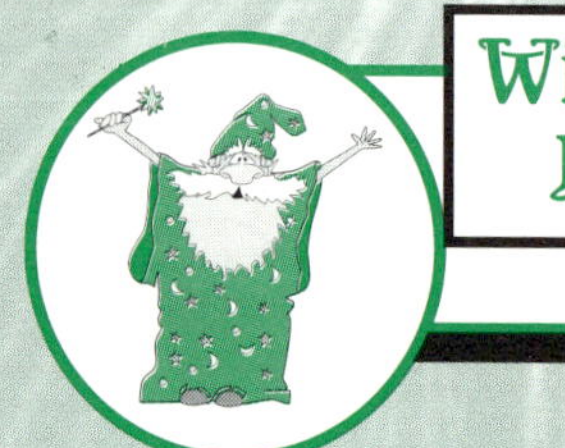

Wizard List "When You're Happy" lyrics, flip chart and marker (optional)

Preparation

1. Copy "When You're Happy" for each team member.
2. Review melody. If you don't know the melody to the song, find someone who does!

Implementation

1. Distribute "When You're Happy" or write the lyrics on a flip chart.
2. Lead the team in song.

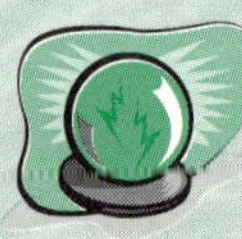

Debriefing

Poking fun of our varying moods and attitudes through the group process helps us laugh at ourselves and then get back to the team's work.

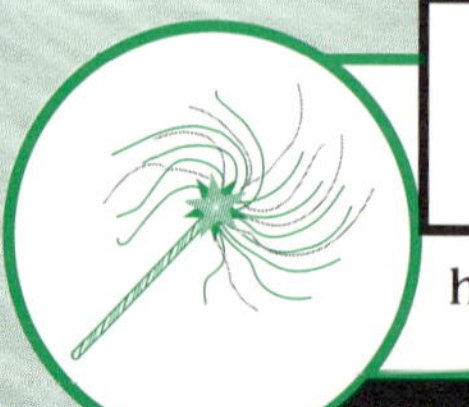

Magic Touch Variation: Substitute the word *grumpy* or other moods as needed. Humor and music work hand in hand to lighten moods.

WHEN YOU'RE HAPPY

When you're happy and you know it

Clap your hands (clap, clap).

When you're happy and you know it

Clap your hands (clap, clap).

When you're happy and you know it

And you really want to show it,

When you're happy and you know it

Clap your hands (clap, clap).

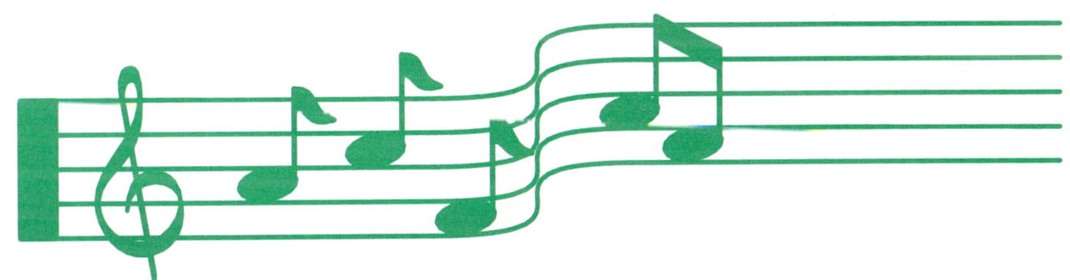

When you're happy . . . stomp your feet! etc.

When you're happy . . . tap your head! etc.

When you're happy . . . touch the ground! etc.

When you're happy . . . turn around! etc.

—Author unknown, lyrics passed on by moms and nursery school teachers

ROAD MAP FOR SUCCESS

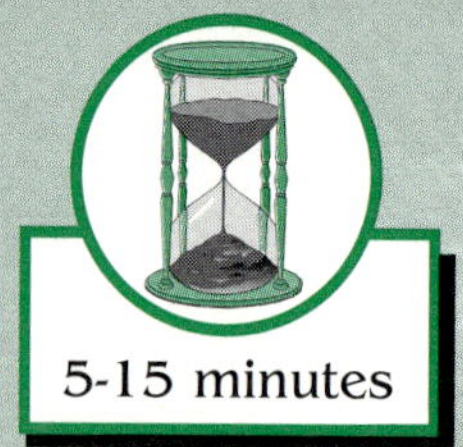

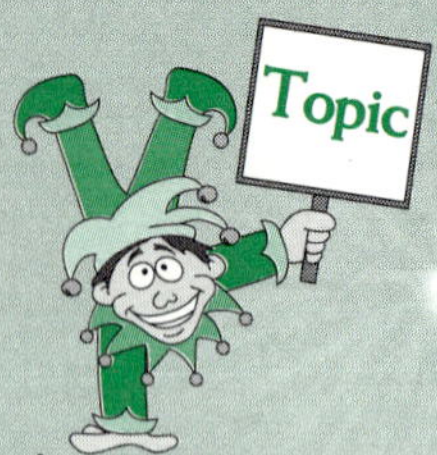

Team progress. Use to refocus on team mission or when there are roadblocks to team progress.

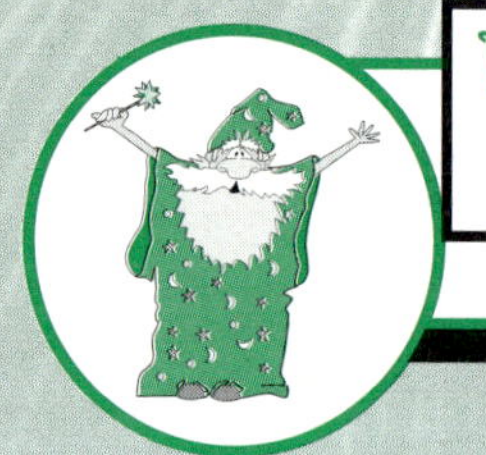

Wizard List

"Road Map for Success Guide," several road maps, flip chart, markers

Preparation

1. Review "Road Map for Success Guide" and make a copy for yourself.
2. Collect maps to be used as handouts (team members can share, if necessary).
3. Make sure flip chart is available.

Implementation

1. Ask for a volunteer to write responses on the flip chart.
2. Ask how many people use road maps.
3. Pass out the road maps and ask people to discuss what information can be found on a road map.
4. Ask what additional information is needed to make a trip successful. Record this information on the flip chart.

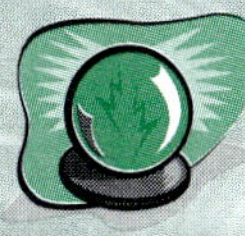

Debriefing

This activity uses the analogy of maps to discuss what is needed for a successful team journey.

1. Ask the group how they would compare what it takes to be successful on a trip with what it takes to be successful on the journey of a team.
2. Ask them to identify potential roadblocks and add any you see with the team.
3. Keep your copy of "Road Map for Success Guide" handy, so you can facilitate the discussion.

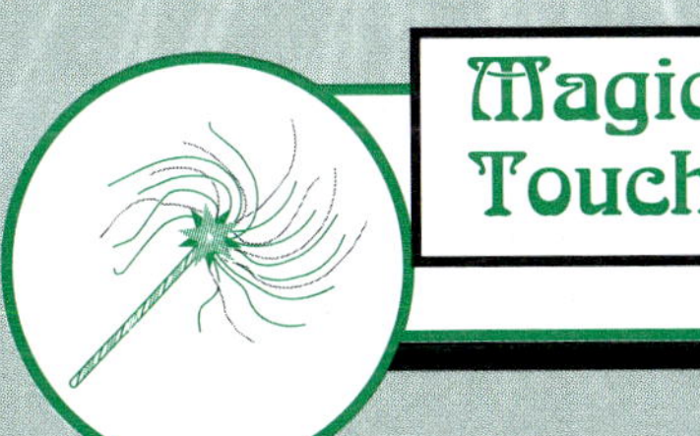

Magic Touch

Obtain maps from mountain and beach resort areas and ask about favorite vacation spots.

ROAD MAP FOR SUCCESS GUIDE

What information is found on the map?

1. City names
2. City locations
3. Mileage
4. Points of interest
5. A legend to explain the symbols and distances on the map
6. Delineations of quality of road
7. Planned, but not yet finished, sections of road (if current)
8. Advertisements for hotels, restaurants (optional)
9. Quadrants of a map to break it down, and references to these in an index
10. Other optional features

What additional information is necessary for a successful trip?

1. Weather
2. Detours
3. Outlet malls, golf shops, etc., that may lengthen the time of the trip!
4. Tourist attractions or other distractors
5. Strategies to keep travellers from being grumpy

What comparisons can be made between a car trip and the team journey?

1. Must identify destination—Mission of team
2. Must estimate how long it will take—Time constraints of team

3. Legend of map—Steps in the problem-solving process, such as steps of the quality improvement framework being used
4. Map is source of information if you know how to read it—What are the team's resources?

Identify potential or current roadblocks.

1. Weather—What is the organizational culture or current climate that impacts possible solutions and their implementation?
2. How current is the map?—Is the problem still timely?
3. Are the travellers grumpy, or do they need food, water, bathroom breaks, amusing games and toys?—Does your team take time out to energize, break bread together, have fun?
4. Time for trip—Do you begin and end meetings on time?
5. Map—Do you follow an agenda?

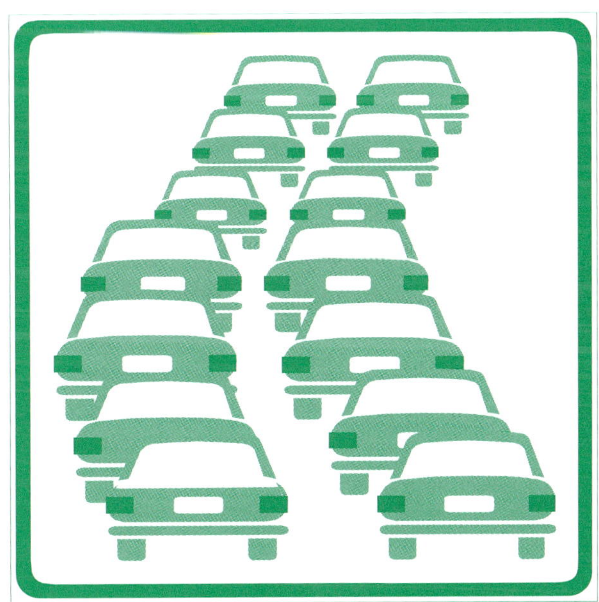

Part 5

Using Problem-Solving Tools

Quality Improvement (QI) or Continuous Quality Improvement (CQI) teams have introduced into health care the tools and techniques for problem solving that have usually been seen in other industries. These problem-solving tools and techniques may seem intimidating at first, but as one administrator quipped, "It's not rocket science!" Although he is right, the use of these tools do require an in-depth understanding, which can be found in your own organization's quality improvement training materials. For an overview of tools and different approaches to quality improvement, see Patricia Schroeder's book, *Improving Quality and Performance* (St. Louis, 1994, Mosby), and Eleanor Green and Jacqueline Katz's book, *Managing Quality* (St. Louis, 1994, Mosby).

This section of the book offers creative and humorous ways to introduce and work with problem-solving tools in teams. A quick definition of the quality improvement process is "data-driven problem solving." Helping teams to look at processes for improvement and collecting data in a systematic way can be a struggle because it is time-consuming. We may think we know solutions, and we may jump to conclusions without examination of the processes. These activities grew out of attempts to lighten the journey, to add a bit of humor or creativity in order to clear both the air and our heads and to get back to work. When all else fails, write a funny song or poem. Read on!

BRAINSTORMING

A Practical Packing Tool

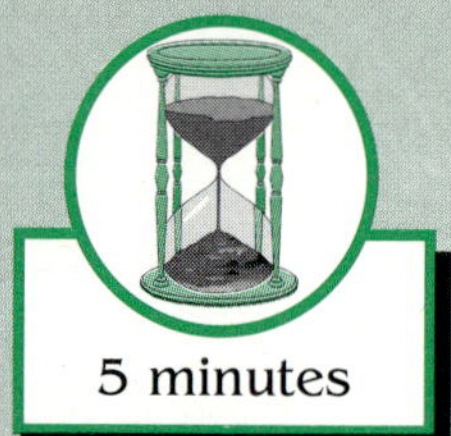

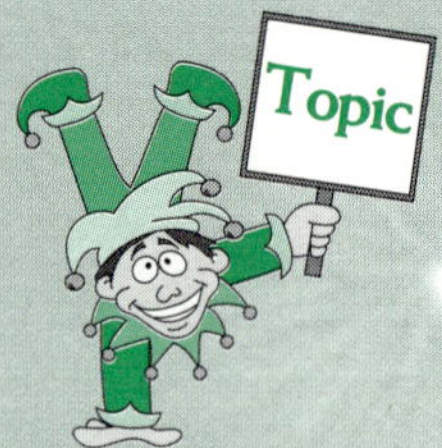

Use to introduce or teach the tool of brainstorming, to warm up a team before brainstorming, or to show benefits of planning when implementing solutions.

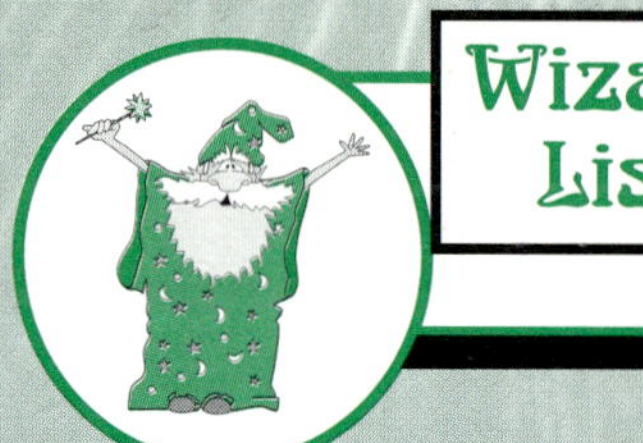

Wizard List "Brainstorming Rules," flip chart, marker

Preparation

1. Copy "Brainstorming Rules" for each team member.
2. Provide flip chart and marker.

Implementation

1. Distribute "Brainstorming Rules."
2. Review "Brainstorming Rules" with the team.
3. Ask for a volunteer to record ideas. Remember, the recorder does not contribute ideas.
4. Ask how many people have occasion to travel by air. If a good number do, use the example of packing bags for air travel. If not, use the example of packing for a vacation by car.
5. Ask the team to brainstorm all the items needed to pack for the trip.
6. Identify one team member as a starting point. That member calls out his or her idea, and the recorder writes the idea (comment) on the flip chart. Then the next member responds, and so on. The goal is to call out ideas as quickly as possible. If

someone does not have a response, he or she should say "pass," and the next member takes a turn.

7. Ask if anyone has ever forgotten an item on a trip. What were the consequences?

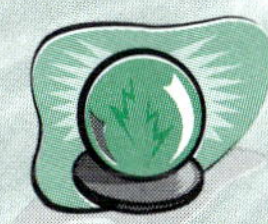

Debriefing

Point out the comprehensive list that the team generated. Discuss the use of brainstorming as a good way to make sure all possibilities are considered in the team's problem-solving process.

Magic Touch

If using the activity before implementing a team solution and building a plan for holding the gains, compare being on a trip without the needed items to lack of anticipation of resistance to change. Consider what happens if restraining factors are not taken into account before implementation. In addition to this exercise see "Team Tool Carols," p. 257.

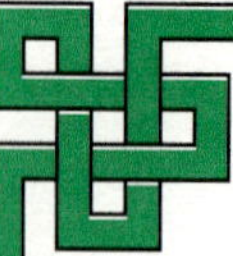
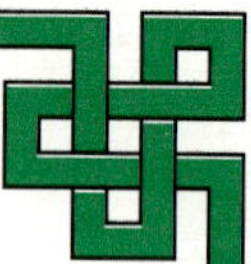

BRAINSTORMING RULES

Brainstorming is used in a group to identify a range of problems or causes and generate ideas for potential solutions or options. The following are ground rules for effective Brainstorming:

1. No idea is evaluated or judged.
2. Say whatever comes to mind. No idea is too crazy. Be creative. All ideas are recorded.
3. Generate as many ideas as possible.
4. Build on others' ideas (piggyback)—one idea sparks another.

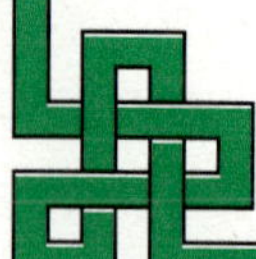
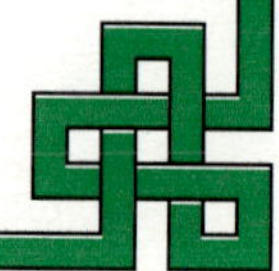

SYNERGY ENERGY

Brainstorming Galore

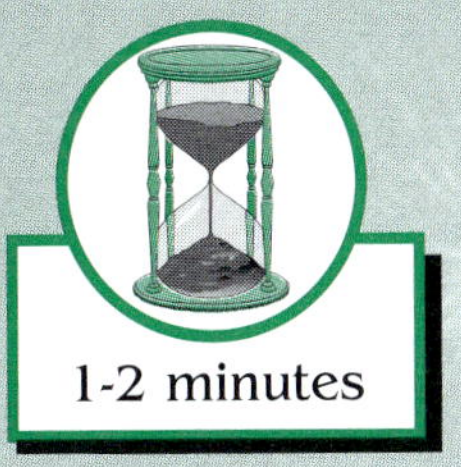

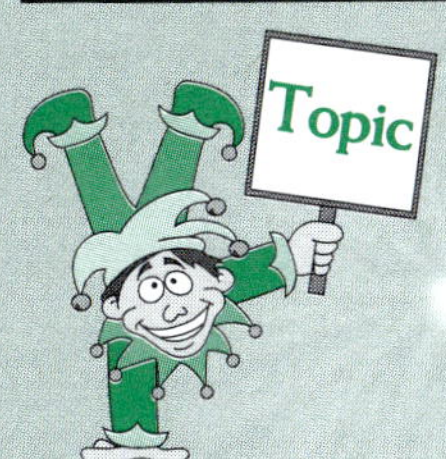

Use to introduce brainstorming or as a quick warmup when brainstorming.

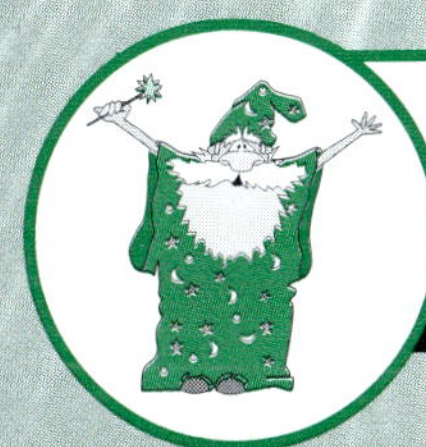

Wizard List

"Synergy Energy," "Brainstorming Rules," flip chart, marker, Koosh ball (optional)

Preparation

1. Select topic to use for brainstorming from "Synergy Energy."
2. Copy "Brainstorming Rules" for each team member (p. 216).

Implementation

1. Distribute "Brainstorming Rules."
2. Review "Brainstorming Rules" with the team.
3. Ask for a volunteer to record ideas. Remember, the recorder does not contribute ideas.
4. Introduce your selected topic.
5. Ask the team to brainstorm on the selected topic.
6. Identify one team member as a starting point. That member calls out his or her idea, and the recorder writes the idea (comment) on the flip chart. The next member responds, and so on. The goal is to call out ideas as quickly as possible. If someone does not have a response, he or she should say "pass," and the next member takes a turn.

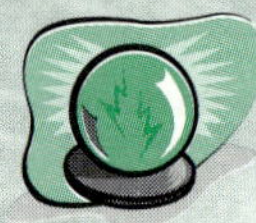

Debriefing

Comment on the benefits of people working together to generate more ideas . . . synergy!

Magic Touch

You may choose to toss a Koosh ball to the next person in line to call out an idea. Use the ball to go around the group with the option to pass.

SYNERGY ENERGY

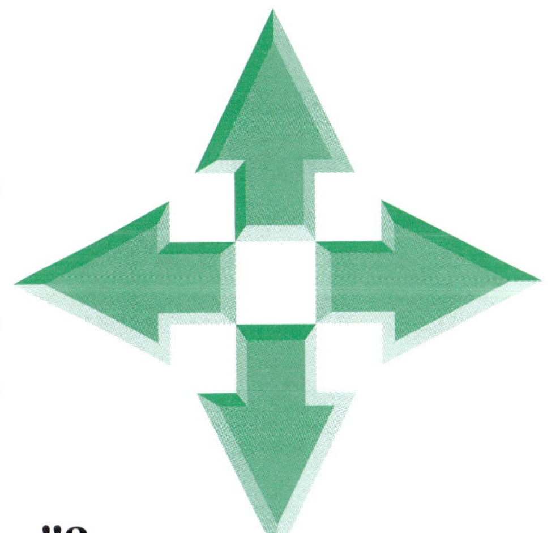

The following are ideas to use to introduce the tool of brainstorming or as a warmup anytime brainstorming is to be used.

1. What are your "pet peeves"?
   Start with one or two of your own, such as people who kick the back of your seat in the theater!
2. List all the uses for a paper cup.
3. List all the uses for a paper clip.
4. List all the uses for a claw-foot bathtub, such as a sofa when the side is cut down.
5. List games you can play with cards.
6. List names of cereals.
7. List models or brands of cars.
8. List game shows on television (current or past).
9. List types of sandwiches.
10. List names of candy bars.
11. List ways to save money at home.
12. List ways to save money at work.

13. If you could provide any kind of special customer service with money no object, what could be done? (For example, one hospital in Washington, D.C., offers valet parking.)
14. What special customer services could be added that would not be expensive?
15. List all the names of the United States of America.
16. List ways to eat peanut butter.
17. List excuses for a poor golf game.
18. List excuses for being late to work.
19. List children's excuses for late or no homework.
20. List all the reasons you should get a raise!

Add your own or collect from colleagues.

21. ____________________
22. ____________________
23. ____________________
24. ____________________
25. ____________________
26. ____________________
27. ____________________
28. ____________________
29. ____________________
30. ____________________

FLOWCHART YOUR WORLD!

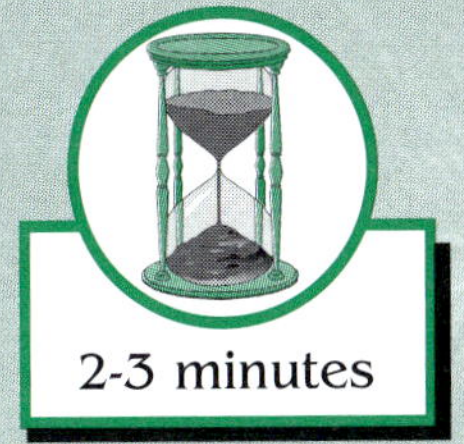

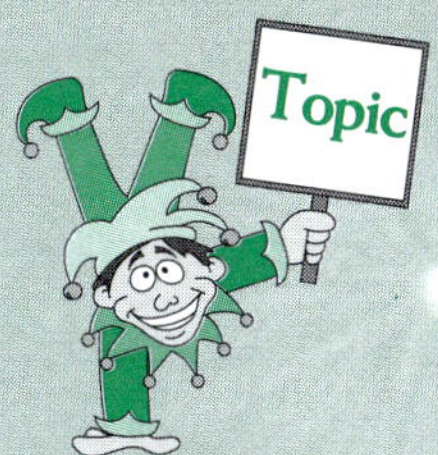

Use to introduce the tool of flowcharting.

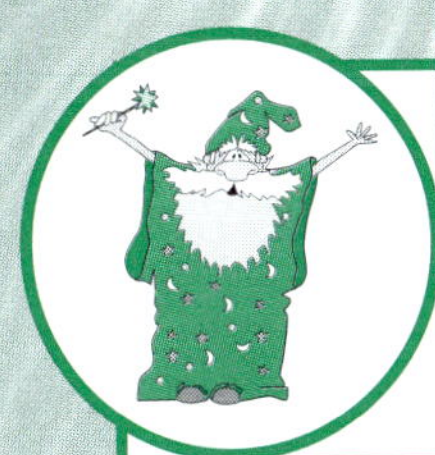

Wizard List "The Flowchart," "Contemporary Oven Cleaning," "The Case of Missing Cat," "To Plan or Not To Plan," "Finding the Surfboard," "A Good Computer Class Is Hard To Get," transparency sheets

Preparation

1. Make flowchart transparencies of the samples provided, pages 224–228.
2. Copy "The Flowchart" for each team member (optional).

Implementation

1. Introduce the flowchart using whatever source you use for teaching quality improvement tools.
2. Distribute "The Flowchart" to each team member (optional).
3. Use one or more of the flowchart examples provided on pages 224–228 for a playful way to demonstrate how easy it is to use this quality-improvement tool. Or have fun constructing your own for a process that can have a humorous twist or for a common process.

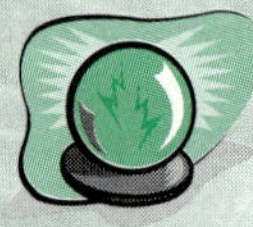

Debriefing

Explain that simple examples demystify the tools that at first can be intimidating.

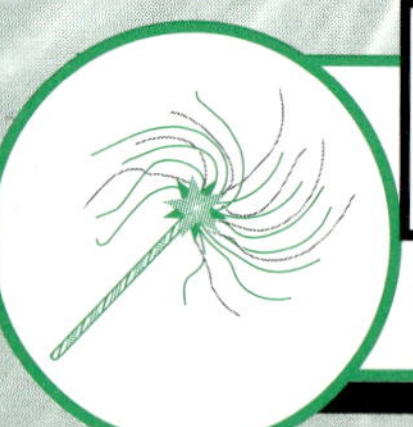

Magic Touch Providing copies of the flowcharts you select can make it easier to follow the process. In addition see "Team Tool Carols," p. 257.

THE FLOWCHART

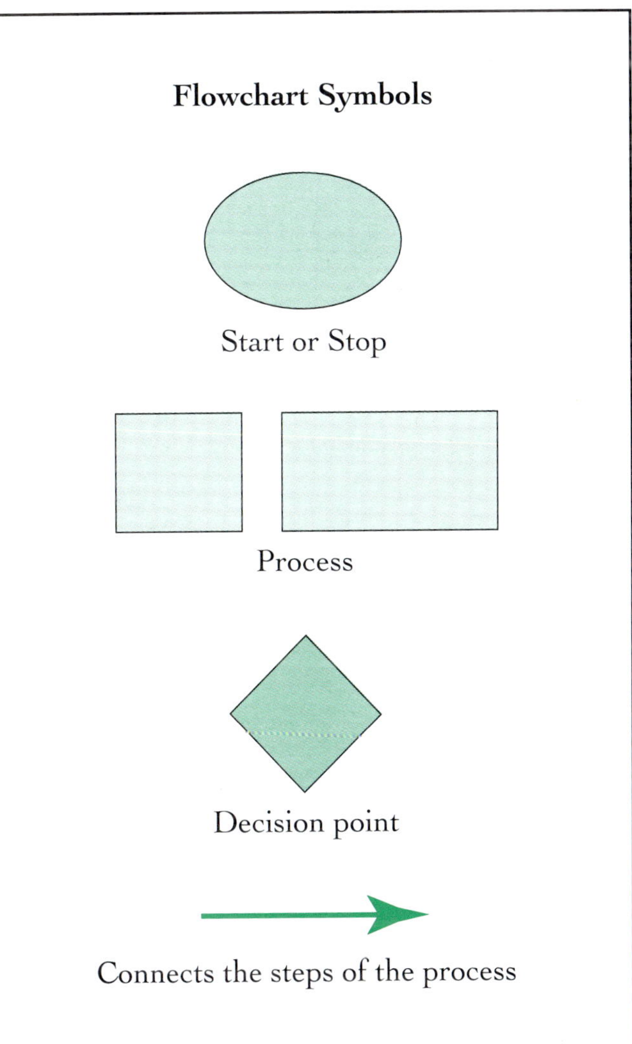

This tool is used to draw a picture of a process of care or service. Creating this picture allows teams to streamline the process, by first creating a picture of the existing process and then creating a picture of an ideal situation. An oval is used for the beginning of the process, a square or rectangle for a step in the process, and a diamond for a decision point with arrows pointing to the options available. (Schroeder, 1994, p. 38)

CONTEMPORARY OVEN CLEANING

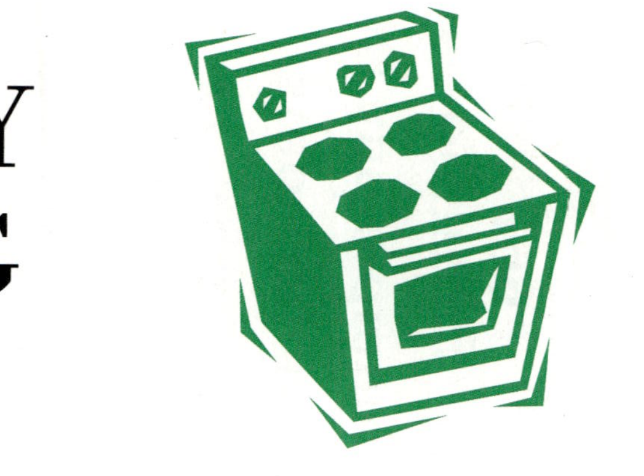

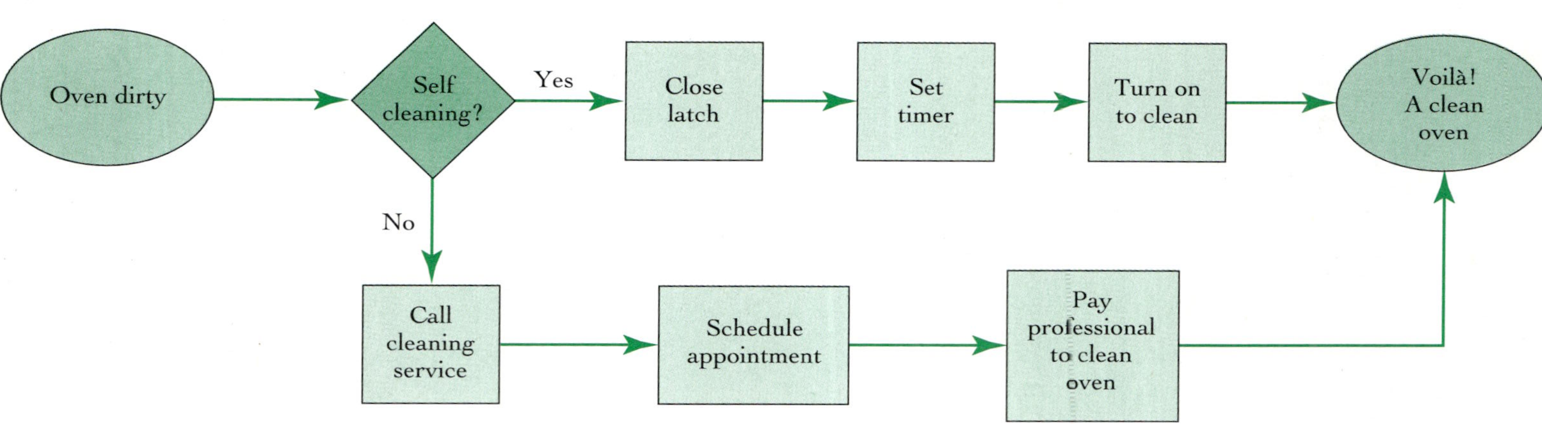

THE CASE OF THE MISSING CAT

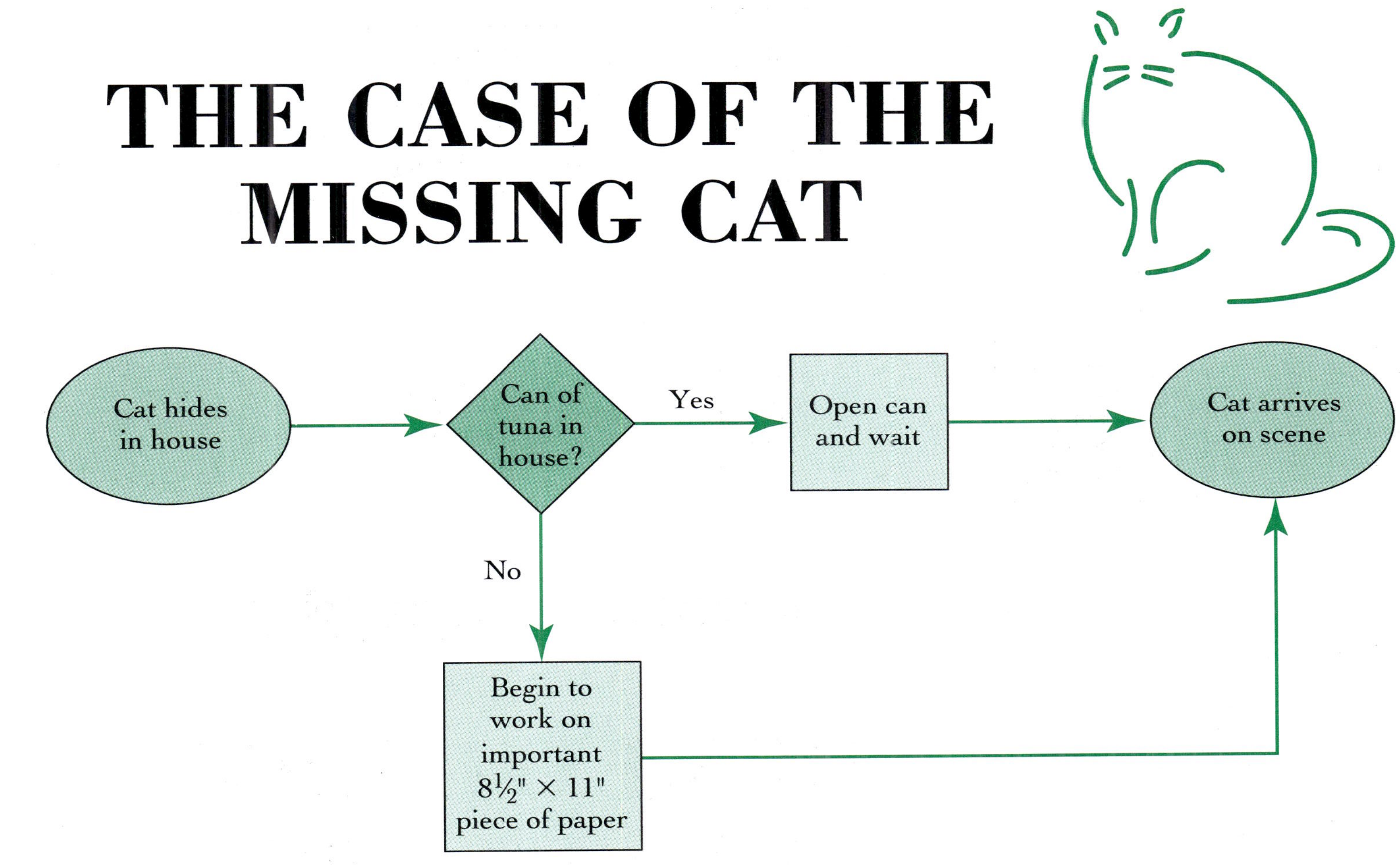

TO PLAN OR NOT TO PLAN

A Potluck Dinner

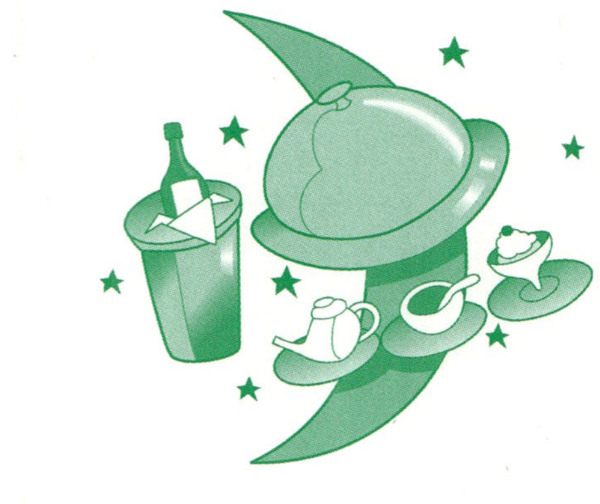

Decide to have a potluck dinner → Organizer-type person available?

Yes → Makes list for menu → Calls and assigns food to be provided or gives choice → Complete menu provided

No → Spontaneous-type person posts "sign-up-for-what-you-want-to-bring list" → Variety of food provided or 25 kinds of brownies

FINDING THE SURFBOARD

Or, Learning How to Access the Internet

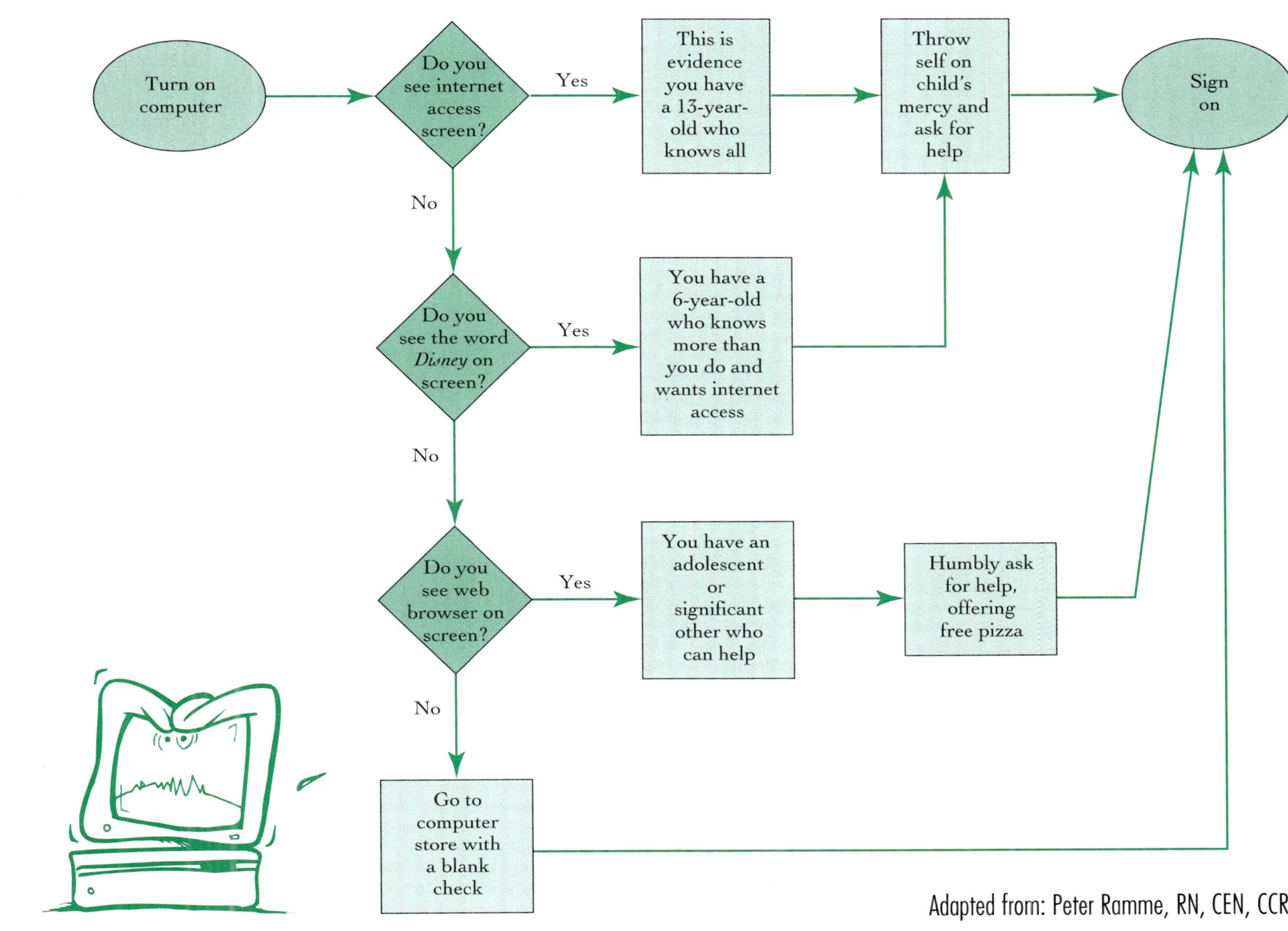

Adapted from: Peter Ramme, RN, CEN, CCRN

A GOOD COMPUTER CLASS IS HARD TO GET

Or, Poor Peggy

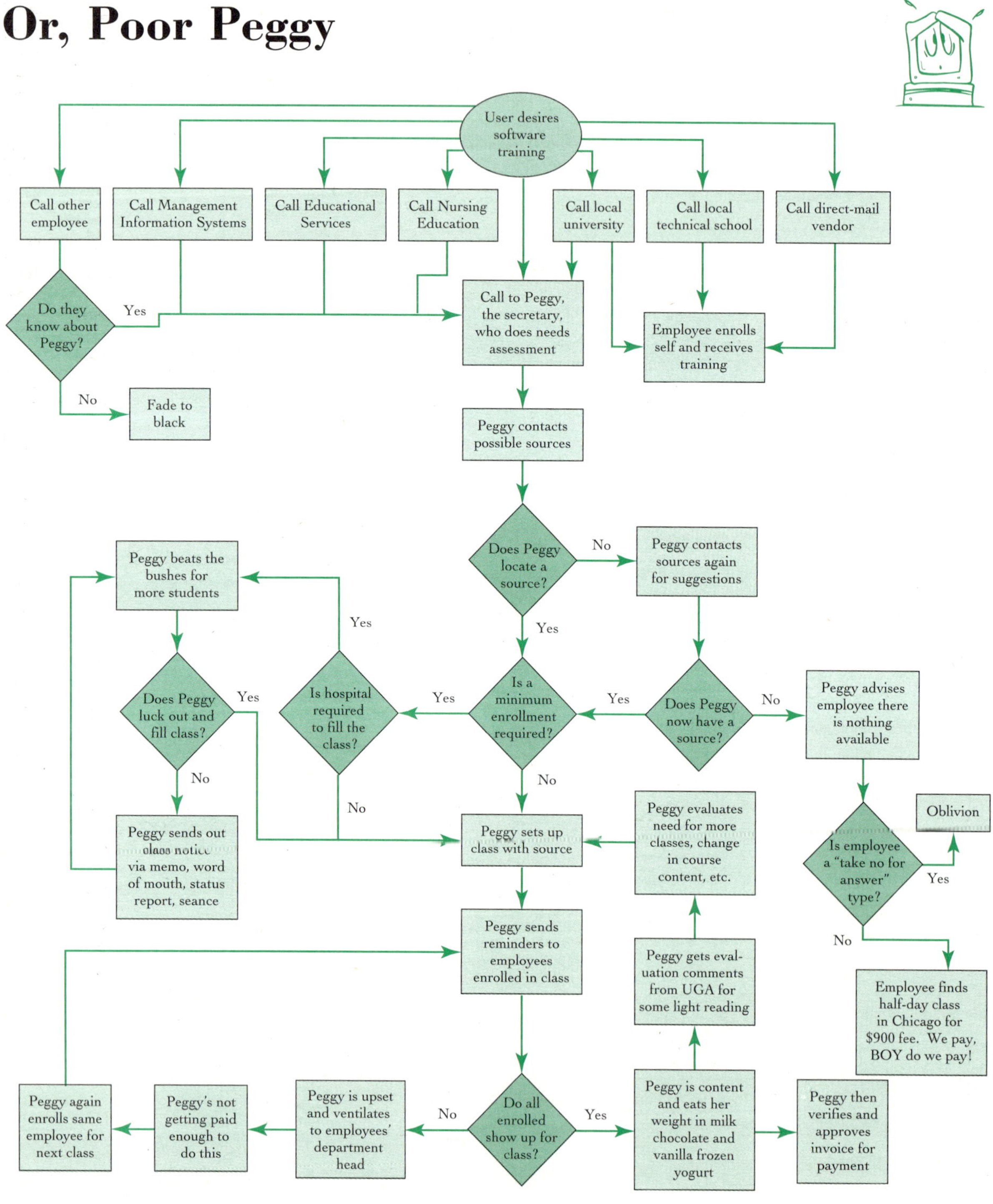

By: Camilla Bracewell, BS, MA, and Beth Warner

THE FLOWCHART BLUES

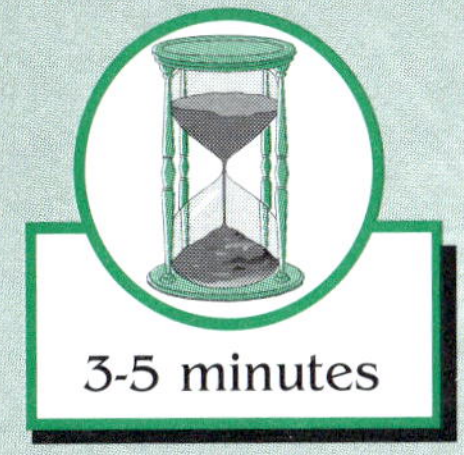

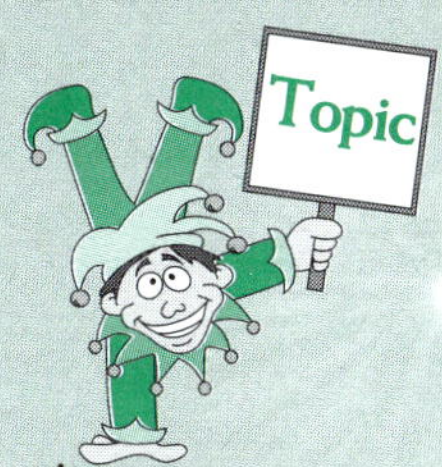

Use when the team is struggling with the process of flowcharting.

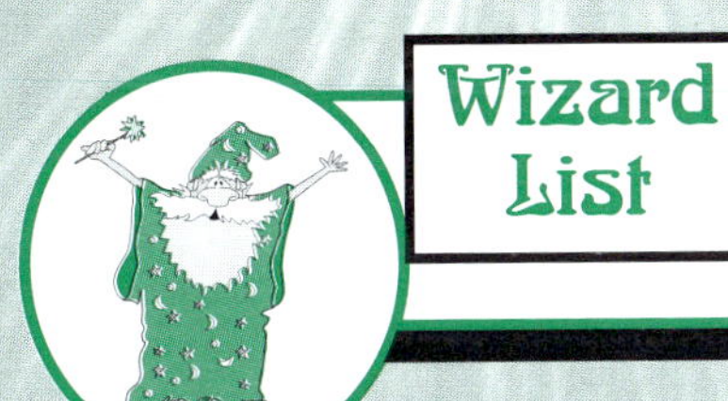

Wizard List "The Flowchart Blues," "The Flowchart" (optional)

Preparation

1. This is a song to be sung to the melody of "I've Been Working on the Railroad." Refresh yourself on the melody, or find a chronologically challenged colleague (this means older than you!) or someone else who can carry a tune and knows the song.
2. Copy "Flowchart Blues" for each team member.

Implementation

1. Acknowledge the team's hard work, and suggest a moment of musical relief!
2. Distribute the "Flowchart Blues," and belt it out with feeling!

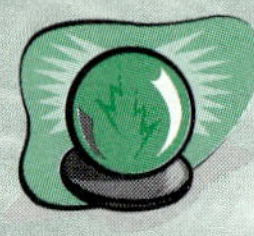

Debriefing

Have a good laugh together, and enough said.

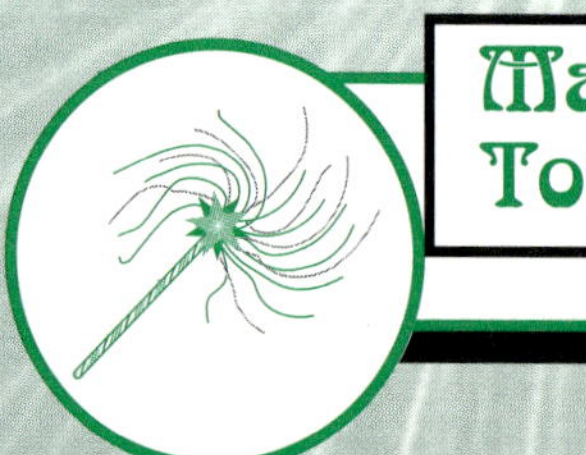

Magic Touch

Use "The Flowchart," p. 223, as a discussion aid. In addition, see "Team Tool Carols," p. 257.

THE FLOWCHART BLUES

I wrote this while facilitating the "Movers & Shakers," a discharge planning team at Baptist Medical Center in Jacksonville, Florida.

(Sung to the melody of "I've Been Working on the Railroad.")

I've been working on a flowchart.
I'm going 'round the bend.
I've been working on a flowchart.
Will it never end?

Can't you tell me when it's over?
How many more meetings will it take?
Can't you tell me when it's over?
I'm afraid my nerves will break!

But wait—It's flowing now more clearly.
I think the next step's in sight.
But wait—It's flowing now more clearly.
We're doing it just right!

The steps we take seem like such small ones.
I want to solve it right now!
The steps we take seem like such small ones.
But we can make it, and how!

As we tidy up this flowchart,
I see the end's in sight.
As we tidy up this flowchart,
I think I see the light.

Can't you see us work together
All along the way?
We can do this all together
And make it seem like play!

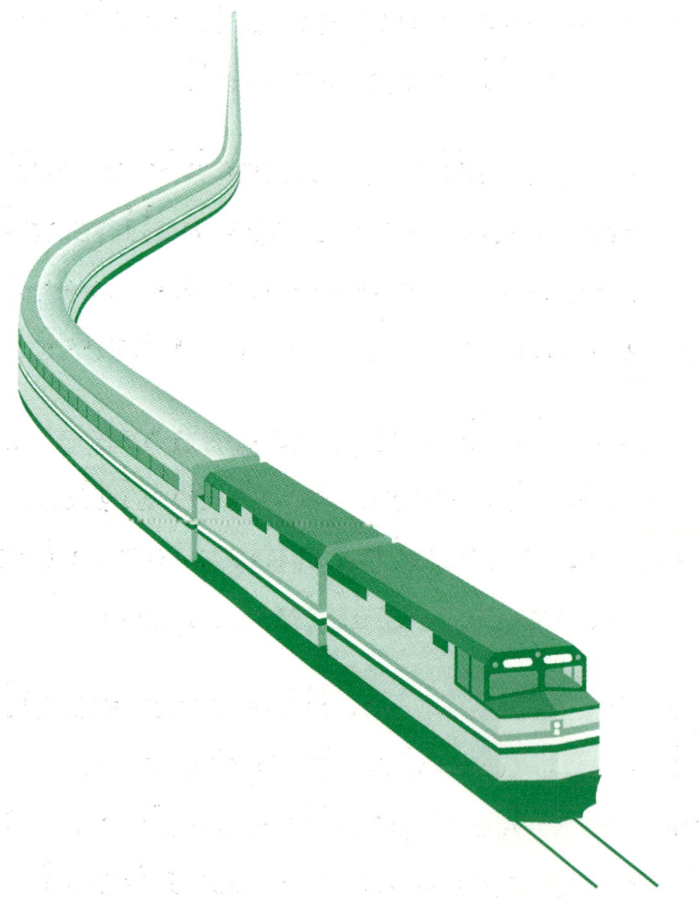

CAUSE-AND-EFFECT DIAGRAMS

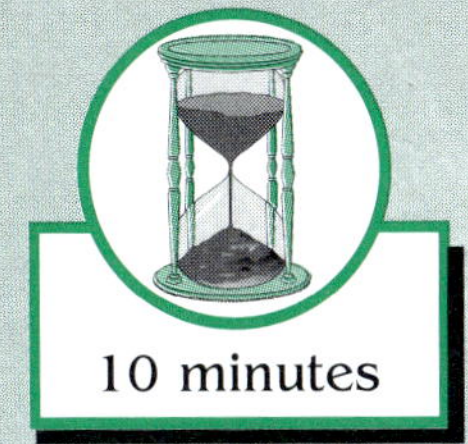

Suffering Is Optional

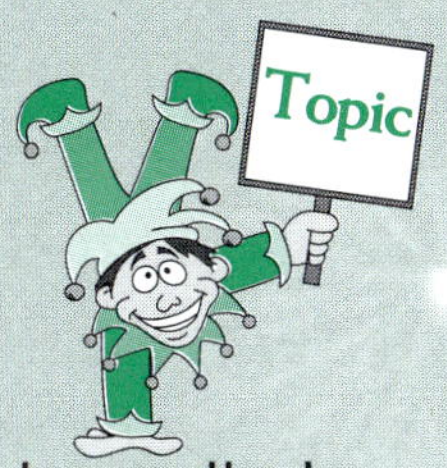

Use to introduce the tool of cause-and-effect diagrams, also called fishbone diagrams.

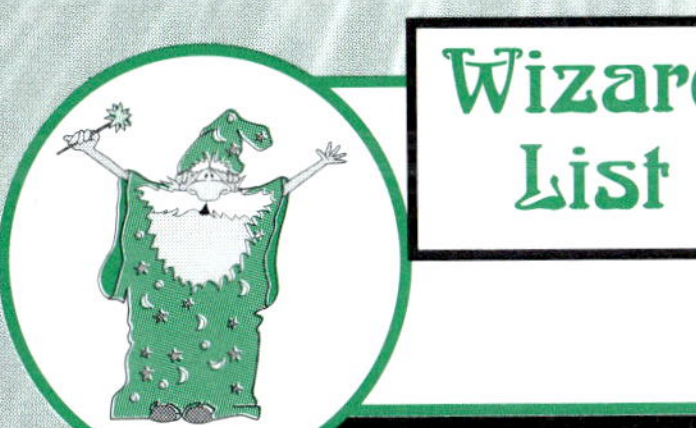

Wizard List

"Cause-and-Effect Diagram Tool," "Cause-and-Effect Diagram," "Fishbone Shell," "Who, Me?," "Likely Stories"

Preparation

1. Make overhead transparencies of "Who, Me?" and "Likely Stories" (use one or both).
2. Copy "Cause-and-Effect Diagram Tool" for each team member. (You may want to provide extra copies for additional practice.

Implementation

1. Distribute "Cause-and-Effect Diagram Tool."
2. Introduce the cause-and-effect diagram to the team using whatever resource you use for teaching quality improvement tools.
3. Use "Who, Me?" and "Likely Stories" for a playful way to show the ease of use of the fishbone diagram.

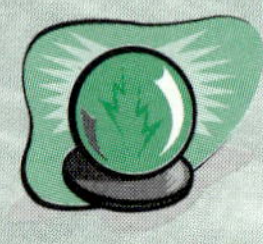

Debriefing

Explain that simple examples demystify the tools that otherwise may be intimidating. Or, as the hospital administrator quipped, "It isn't rocket science." This quote calmed me considerably before my own CQI training!

Magic Touch

Use the "Cause-and-Effect Fishbone Shell" for a transparency, and construct your own fishbone diagram. You may want to use a current life issue or holiday topic. In addition, see "Up on the Cause-and-Effect Diagram," p. 260.

CAUSE-AND-EFFECT DIAGRAM TOOL

The cause-and-effect diagram (also called fishbone or Ishikawa diagram) is a tool used to find the multiple causes, or root causes, for any problem. Identify the problem or result, positive or negative, to be examined. Write this at the end of the central spine. Identify the categories of possible causes and put these in boxes at the end of the bones angled off the spine in the diagram. Along these bones, list the reasons for the causes, which are generated by brainstorming. (Schroeder, 1994, pp. 36–38)

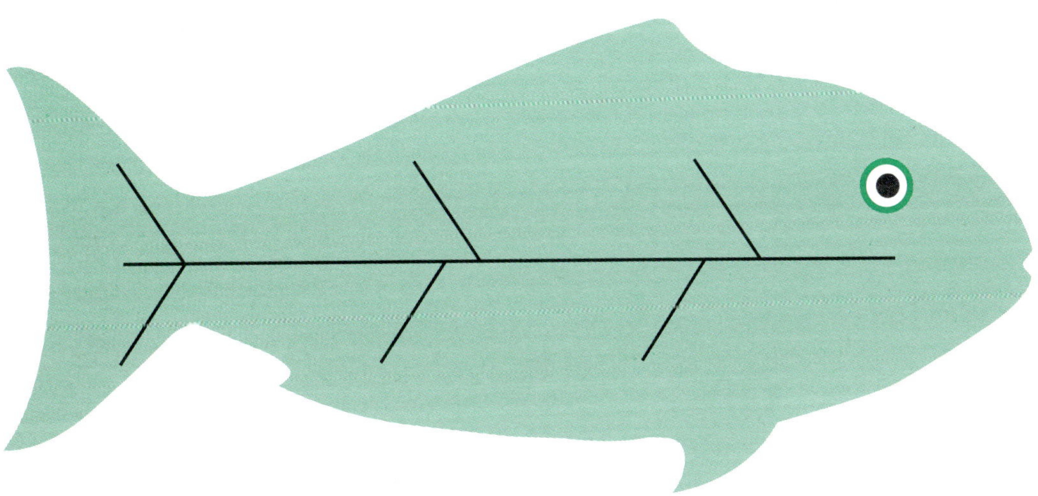

CAUSE-AND-EFFECT DIAGRAM FISHBONE SHELL

WHO, ME?

Cause-and-Effect Diagram

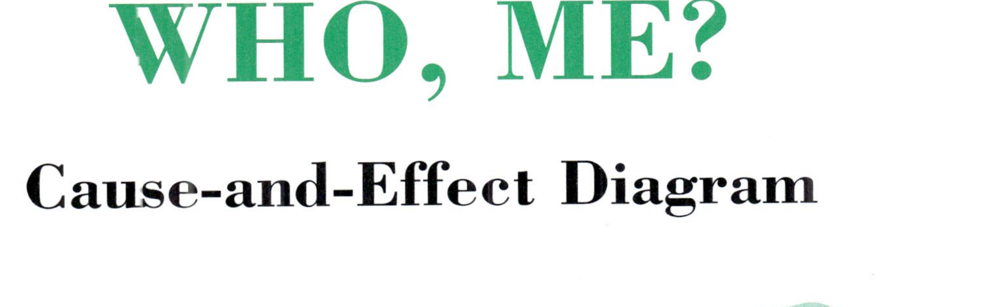

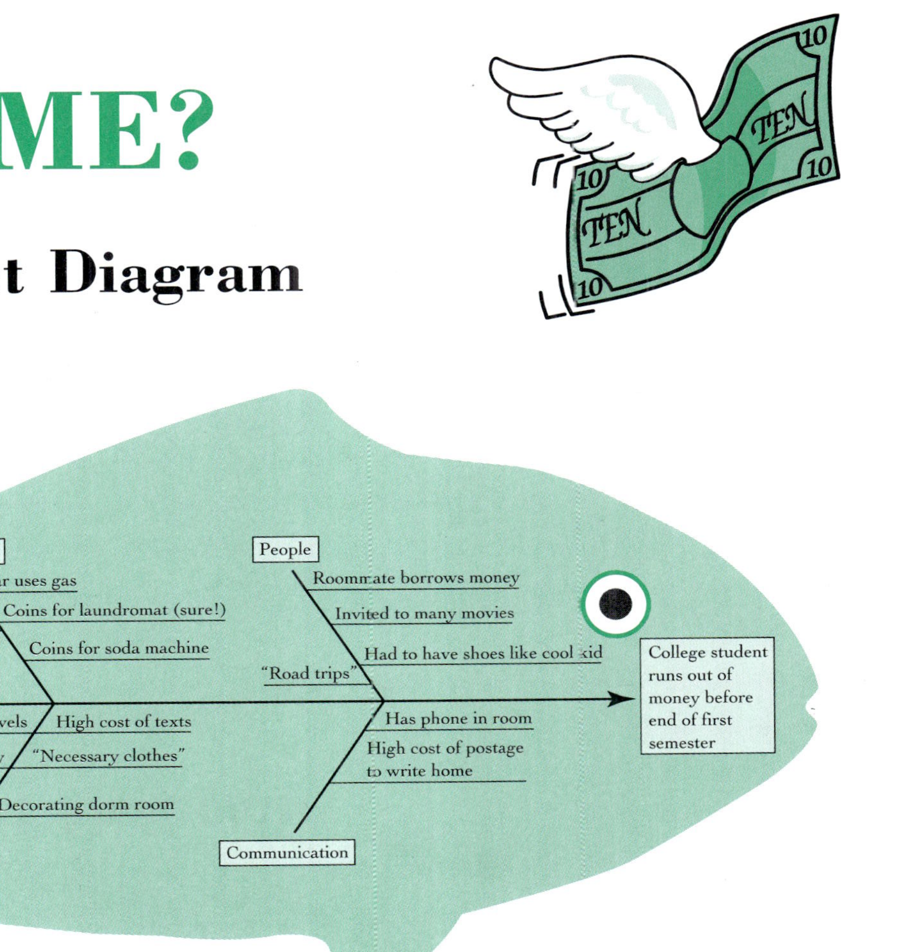

LIKELY STORIES

Cause-And-Effect Diagram

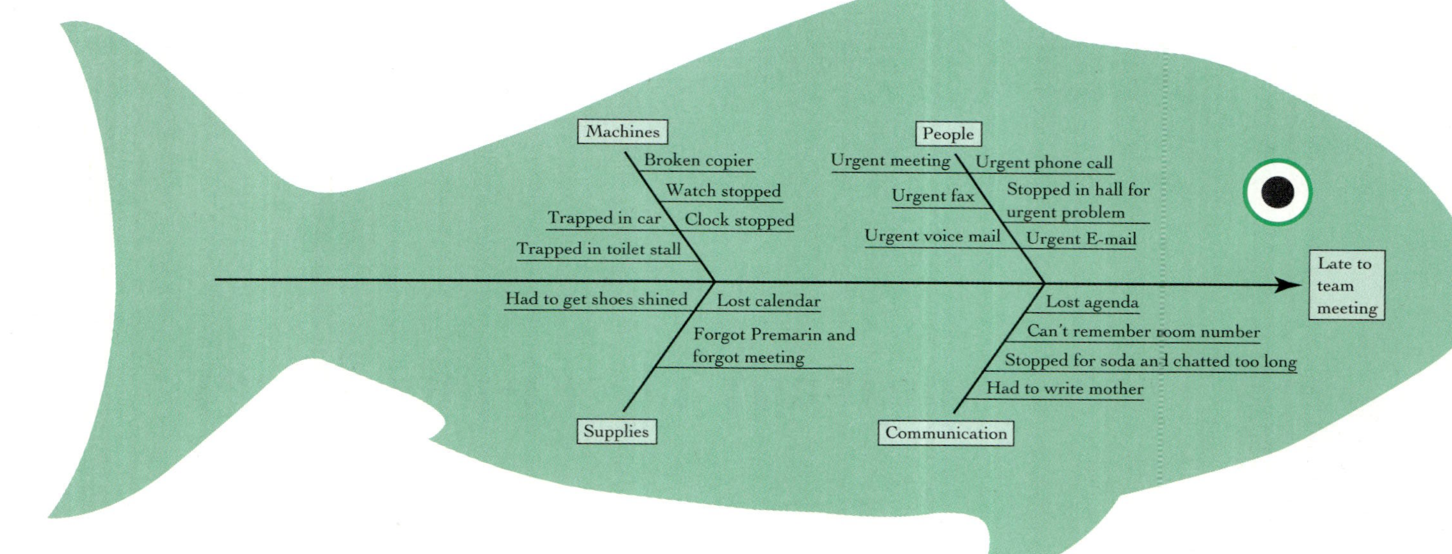

HASTE MAKES WASTE

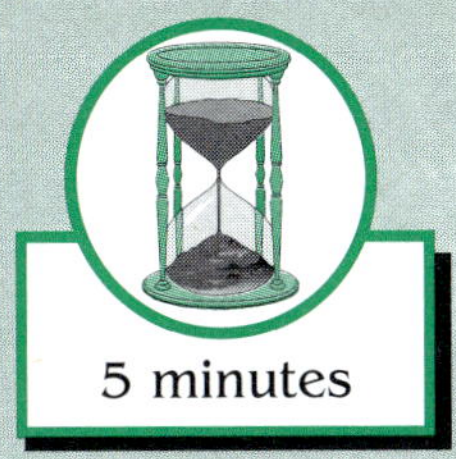

Or, Collect Data In Haste and Repent at Leisure

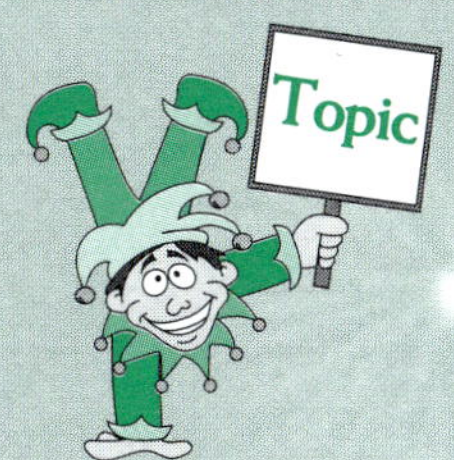

Data collection. Use to teach data collection or when designing data collection tools.

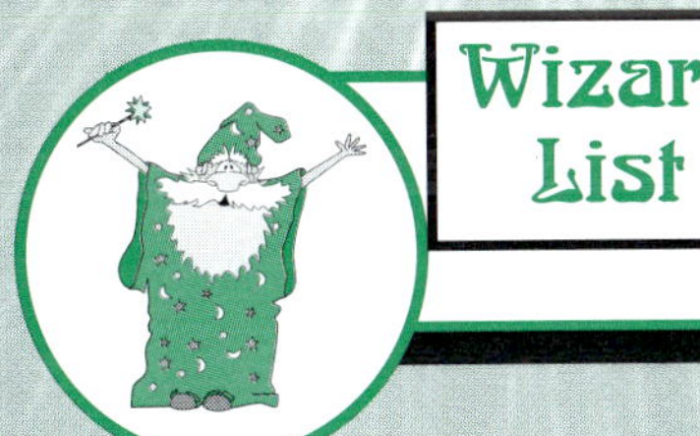

Wizard List "Haste Makes Waste"

Preparation

1. Copy "Haste Makes Waste" for each team member.

Implementation

1. Discuss the process of data collection if using this activity to accompany team training.
2. Distribute "Haste Makes Waste."
3. Ask for a volunteer to read it aloud.
4. Ask for discussion of the poem.
5. Ask if the poem illustrates anyone's prior experience with data collection.

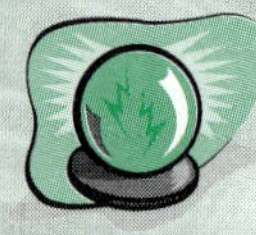

Debriefing

Explain that data collection always seems so easy, but that it is easy to miss important data or not have an adequate plan for analysis.

Magic Touch

Team members may become impatient with the process of designing data collection tools, piloting the tool, and analyzing the data. These steps take time. This activity and "Stuck in the Data Again" are designed to refocus the team on the importance of appropriate data collection and the purpose of the process, that is, improving patient care—the very purpose of all of our work!

HASTE MAKES WASTE

Or, Collect Data in Haste and Repent at Leisure

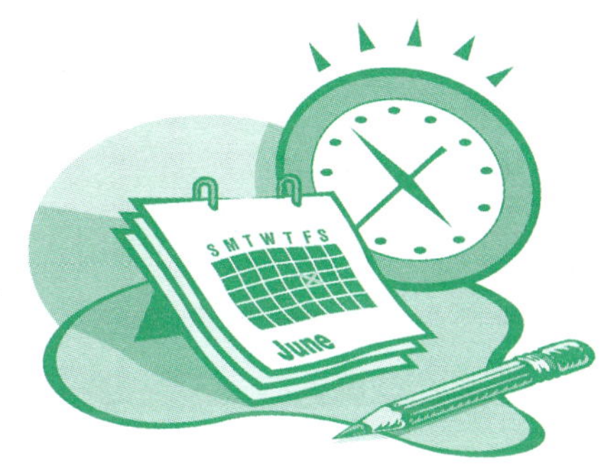

Collecting the data
Is no easy task.
The first time you do it
May not be your last.

Review what you're asking
And pilot collection
So your mission and the data
Can make a connection.

Ask yourself how
The numbers will be used.
Be thoughtful at first
And quite thoroughly peruse.

Be kind to each other
In data analysis
So you don't succumb
To analysis paralysis.

Lighten the load
With humor and play,
Minds refreshed,
Less likely to stray.

STUCK IN THE DATA AGAIN

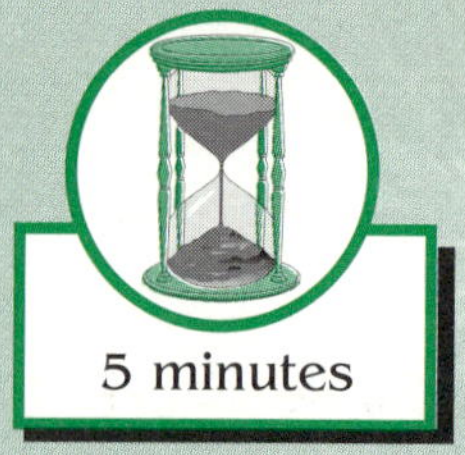

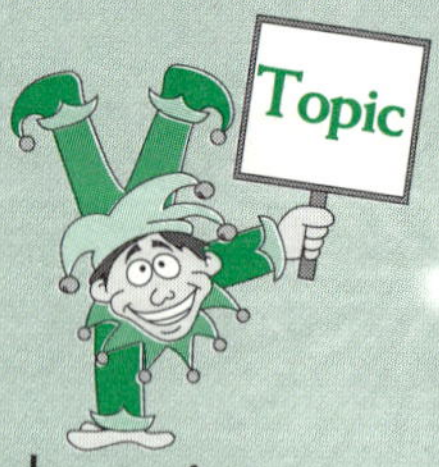

Use when bogged down in designing data collection tools or in analysis of data to refocus to the customer as the reason for the process.

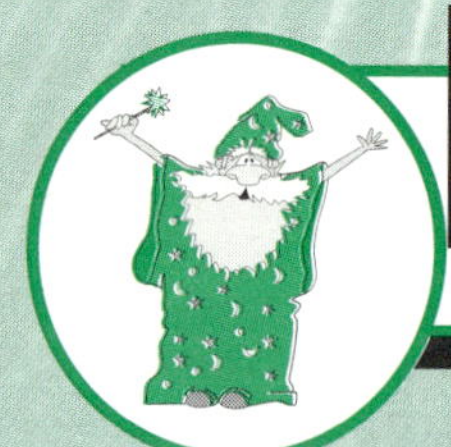

Wizard List "Stuck in the Data Again," flip chart and marker, paper, pens or pencils

Preparation

1. Make one copy of "Stuck in the Data Again."
2. Review "Stuck in the Data Again" and bring it to the meeting.
3. Provide, or make sure you have access to, a flip chart and marker.
4. Provide one sheet of blank paper for each team member and a pen or pencil.

Implementation

1. Explain to the team that you want to take a few minutes to shift in a way that might be helpful to remembering why we are here.
2. Set the stage for this customer expectation exercise. Suggest that each member has just fulfilled a lifelong dream; every one of them has become the owner of an upscale retail store.
3. Distribute blank paper and a pen or pencil to each team member.
4. Ask all team members to think about and write how they would want customers to describe their products and service. Tell them to keep in mind that this store is their sole source of income.

5. Have the team members share their ideas; write them on a flip chart.
6. Review the team's responses. Point out that their desires—for excellent service, high quality products, and professional staff—are very similar to the desires of the hospital's customers as well.

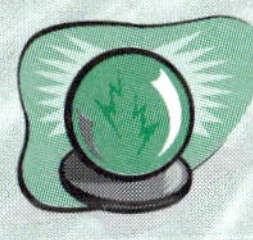

Debriefing

Our customers, whether patients, physicians, or other employees, are looking for the same type of products and services. We all want high quality, great value, and excellent service. Providing this gives us the competitive edge. And although using quality tools and collecting data sometimes is tedious, this venture is aimed at continuous quality improvement.

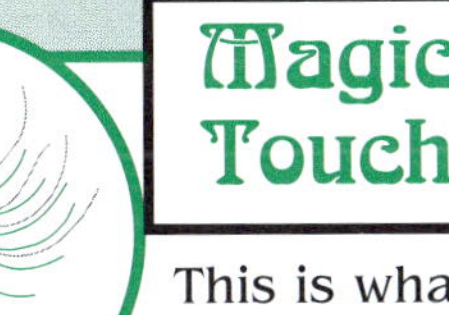

Magic Touch Sometimes we get a break to restore our energy and refocus on what is important—quality patient care. This is what makes these struggles worthwhile.

By: Camilla Bracewell, BS, MA

STUCK IN THE DATA AGAIN

Discussion Guide for Customer Expectations

If you owned an upscale retail store, how would you want your customers to describe your products and services?

Typical team responses:

- High quality
- Knowledgeable staff
- Great value
- Excellent customer service
- Convenient hours, access, and parking
- Exclusive—you can't get merchandise elsewhere

How would you want store employees to treat the customers?

Typical team responses:

- Courteous
- Professional
- Knowledgeable
- Helpful
- Creative
- Takes initiative
- Positive attitude

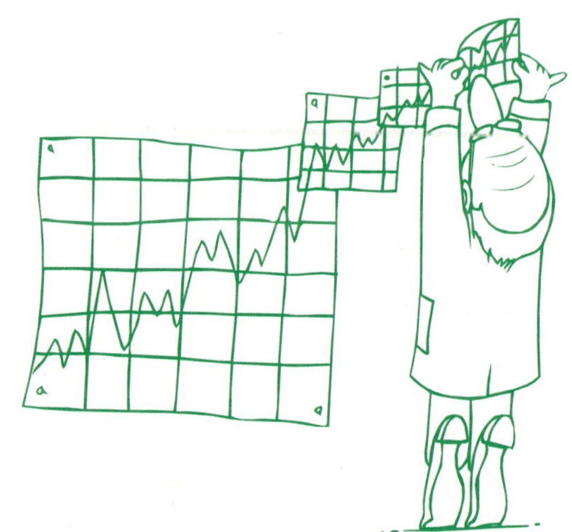

PARETO CHARTS FOR FUN AND PROFIT!

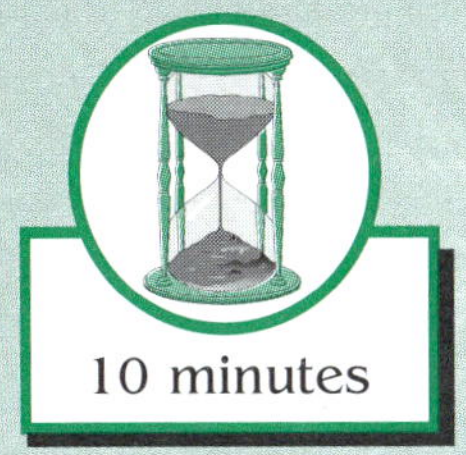

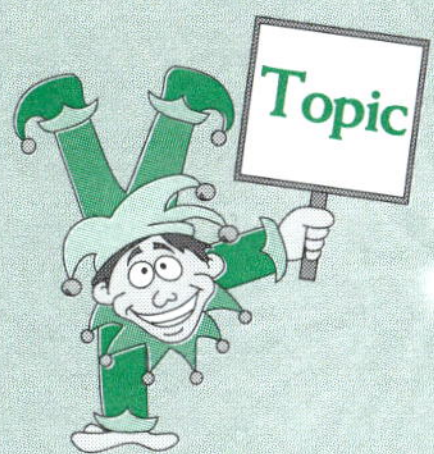

Selection process. Use to introduce Pareto charts to display data and select the vital few issues for focus.

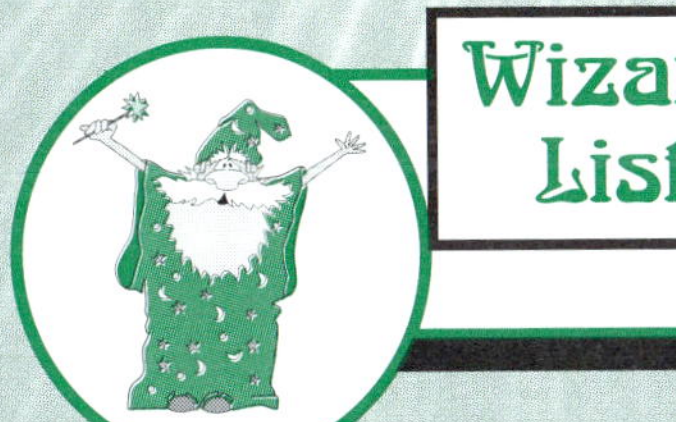

Wizard List

"Pareto Chart Handout," "Pareto—of a Weighty Issue," "Delays in Completing Homework"

Preparation

1. Copy of "Pareto Chart Handout" for each team member.
2. Make overhead transparency of "Pareto—of a Weighty Issue" or "Delays in Completing Homework," or both, as time limitations allow.

Implementation

1. Distribute "Pareto Chart Handout."
2. Introduce the Pareto chart using whatever resource you use for teaching quality improvement tools.
3. Use "Pareto—of a Weighty Issue" or "Delays in Completing Homework," or both, for a playful way to show the ease of use of the Pareto chart.
4. Discuss the Pareto charts as a group, but also allow some time for individual review of this new topic.

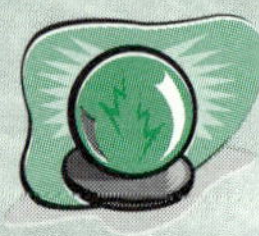

Debriefing

Explain that simple examples demystify the tools that otherwise may be intimidating.

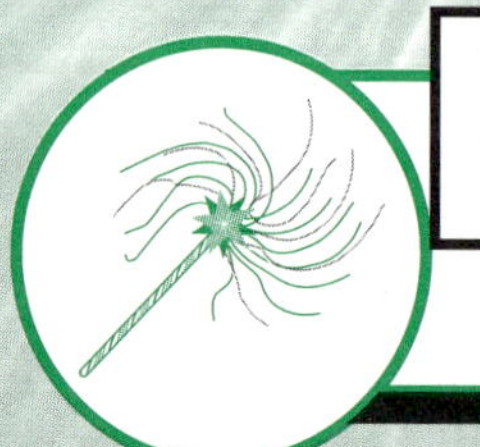

Magic Touch

Have fun! Construct a chart with made-up data that might get a laugh. Also, see "Team Tool Carols: Oh Pareto," p. 261.

PARETO CHART HANDOUT

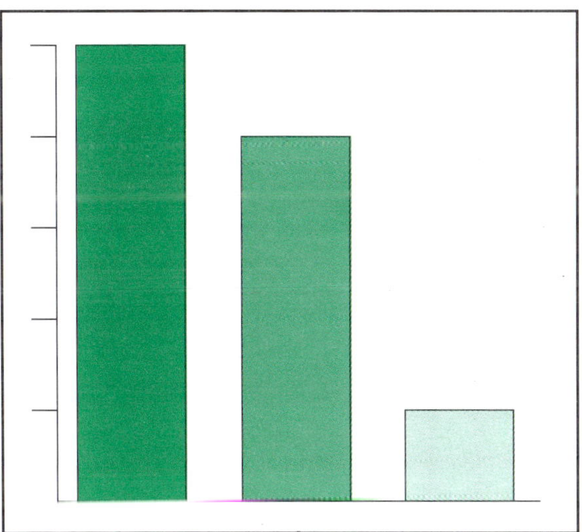

A Pareto chart is a bar graph used to prioritize the causes of a problem. Priority is exhibited in decreasing order, with the highest priority on the left and the least on the right. This illustrates the phenomenon of the "80-20" rule, that is, 80% of the problem is from 20% of events. Consider an elementary school classroom where 80% of the disruption is instigated by 20% of the children in the room; action plans to modify the behavior of these few children can have a major impact on reducing the total disruption in the class. This tool was created by Vilfredo Pareto, an eighteenth-century economist, to identify the vital few causes of a problem. Focusing problem solving on the few causes that create the biggest part of the problem gives more "bang for your buck" in formulating solutions. (Schroeder, 1994, p. 35)

PARETO—OF A WEIGHTY ISSUE

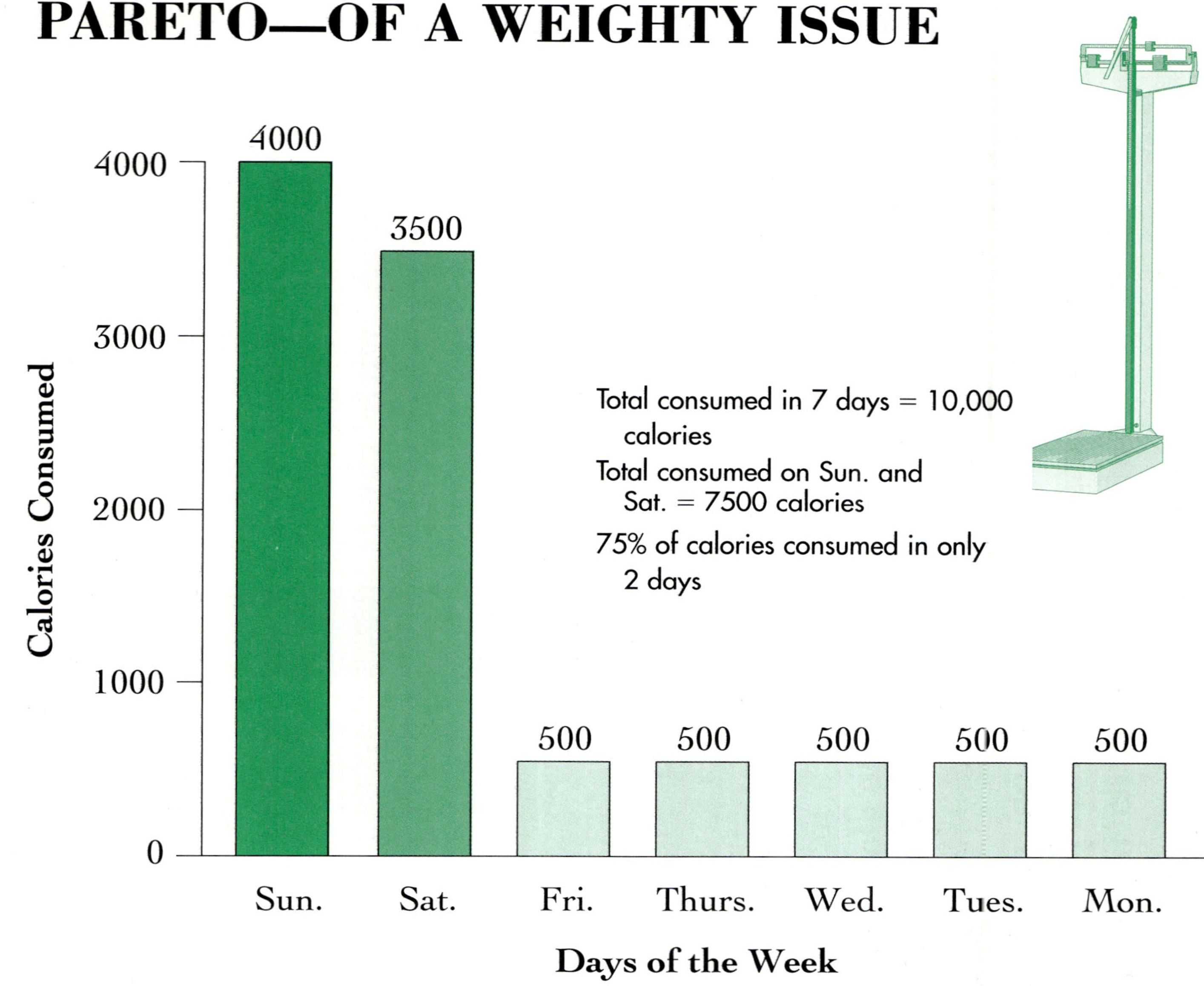

PARETO DIAGRAM

Delays in Completing Homework

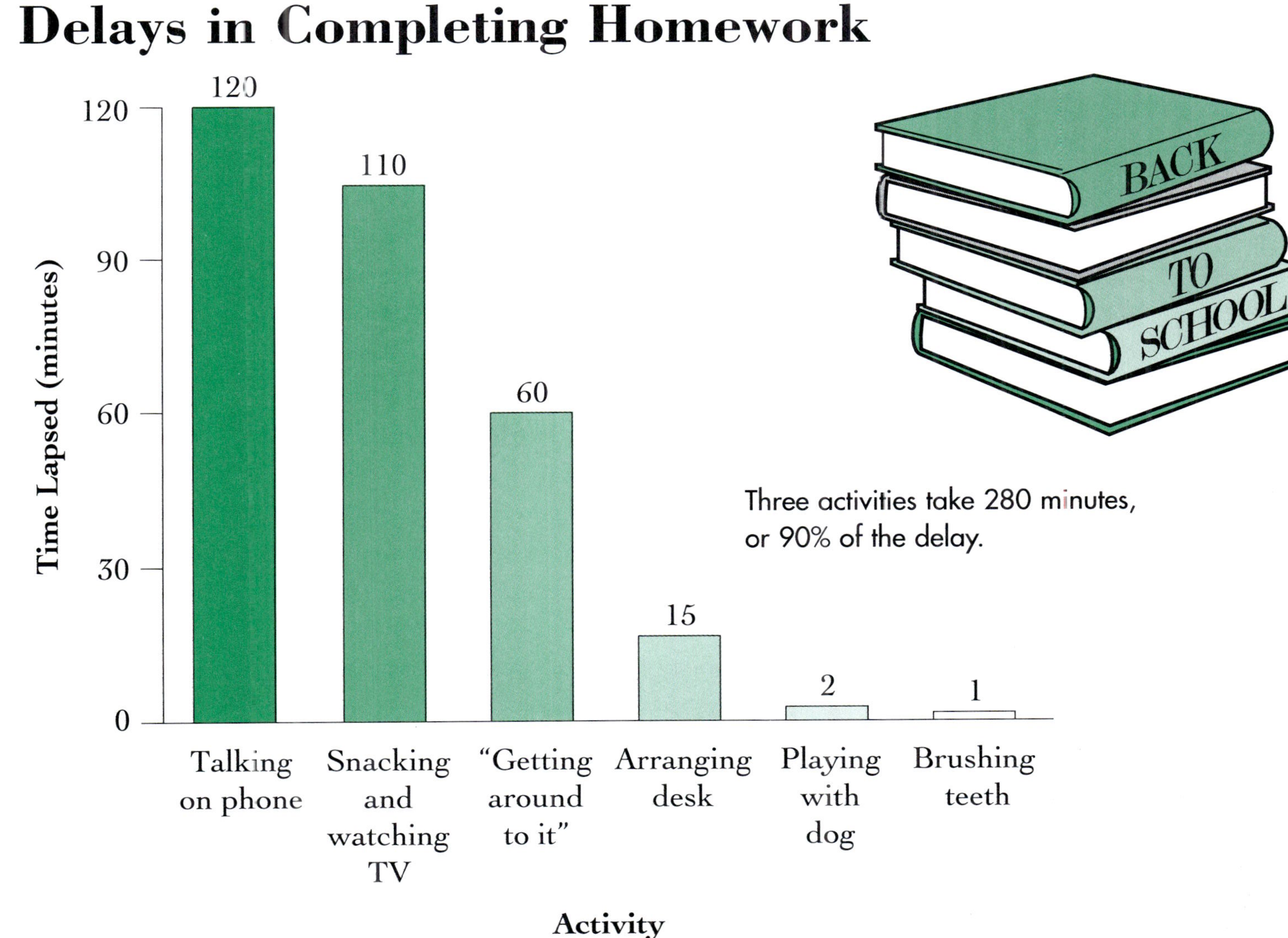

We're All Thumbs!

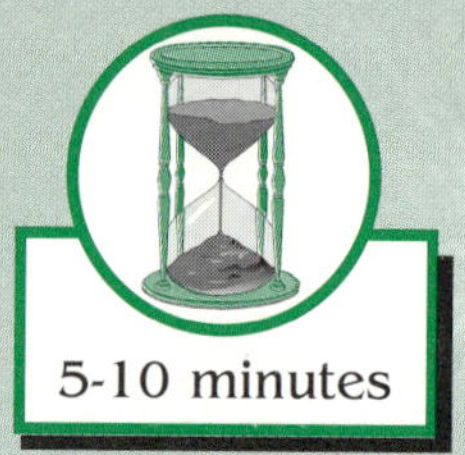

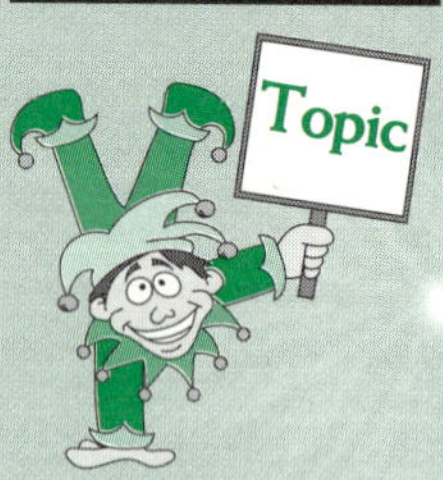

Decision making. Use to introduce this quick method for voting on recommendations early in the life of the team before critical decisions must be made. Coming to a consensus is a critical team skill.

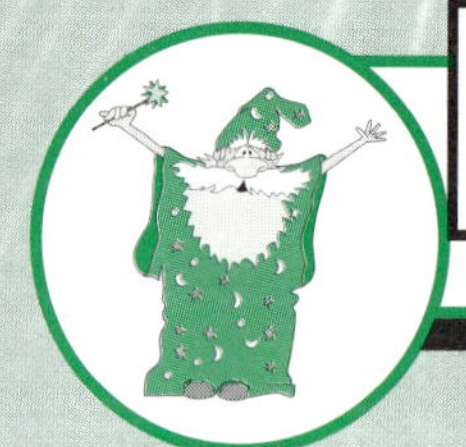

Wizard List

"Thumbs: Voting and Team Consensus"

Preparation

1. Copy "Thumbs" for each team member.

Implementation

1. Distribute copies of "Thumb."
2. Explain that when decisions or recommendations are made, team members will be asked to vote with their thumbs.
3. Review "Thumbs: Voting and Team Consensus" with the team.

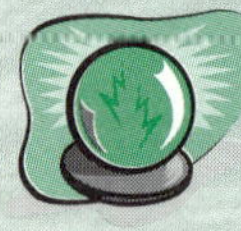

Debriefing

Why use the thumbs approach?

1. It quickly clarifies the team's position on an issue. A "Thumbs Down" or a few "Thumbs Across" indicate that further dicussion or data is needed.
2. It requires people to take a stand on an issue, rather than falling back on a "no comment" approach.

3. It solidifies support for decisions, minimizing later backtracking or waffling.
4. Most important, it establishes a norm for reaching consensus. Instead of using a majority rule or autocratic approach to decision making, when a team uses thumbs voting they *must* achieve a level of consensus to move forward.

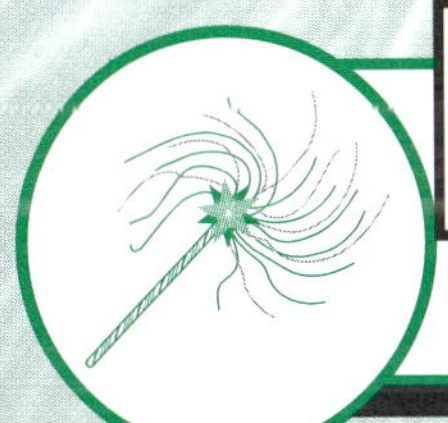

Magic Touch Coming to an agreement is essential throughout the life of a team. See "Team Tool Carols: Consensus Wonderland," p. 262.

"THUMBS"

Voting and Team Consensus

When decisions or recommendations are made, team members are asked to vote with their thumbs.

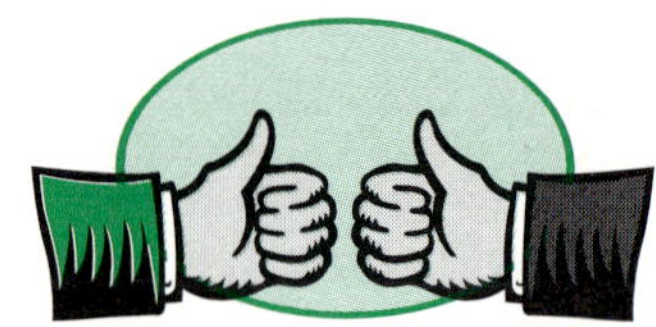

"Thumbs Up" signifies agreement and support.

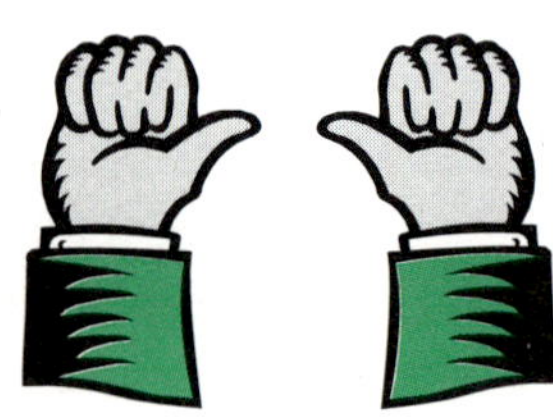

"Thumbs Across" indicates that while the member may not be crazy over the idea, he or she agrees that the idea is acceptable and will support it.

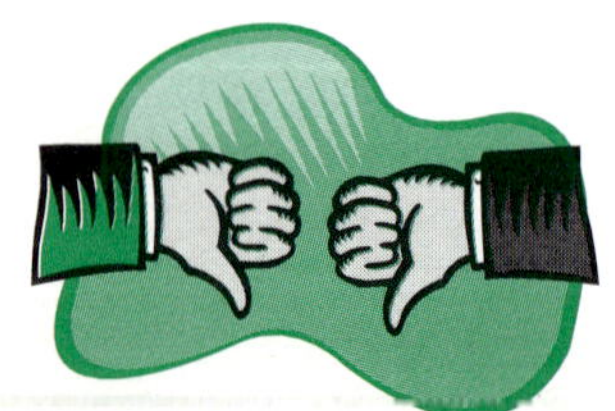

"Thumbs Down" signifies that the team member absolutely disagrees with the decision and would leave the team because he or she cannot support the idea. Anytime this vote is cast, the dissenting member(s) must discuss the reasons for this position. In addition, those supporting the idea must also help the dissenter(s) understand why they support the idea. The team will be expected to work through the issues until all thumbs are "Thumbs Up," "Thumbs Across," or until the decision is changed.

HOUSE HUNTING

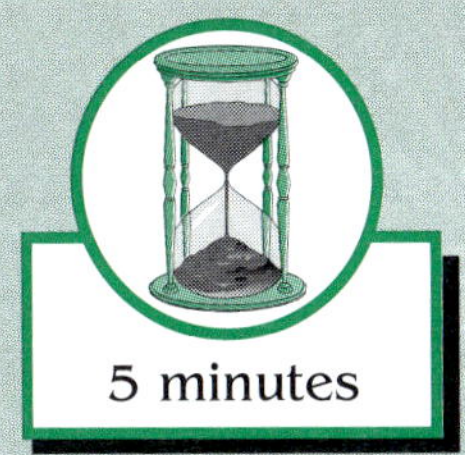

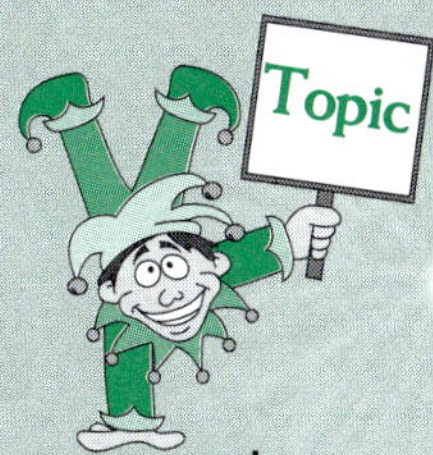

Decision making. Use as a practical example of a selection grid.

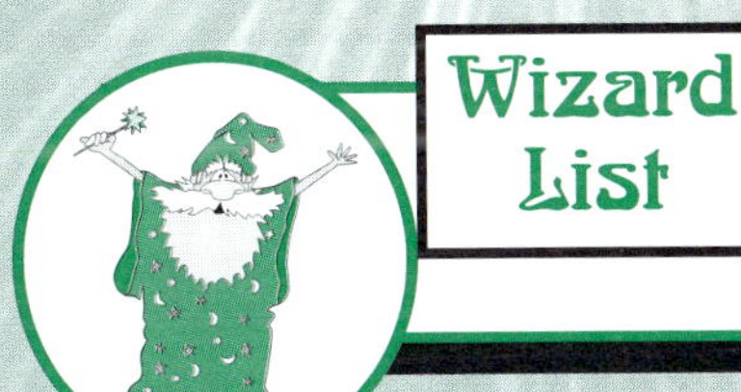

Wizard List

"House Hunting Selection Grid," "The Family Decision"

Preparation

1. Copy "House Hunting Selection Grid" and "The Family Decision" for each team member.
2. Carefully review "House Hunting Selection Grid" and "The Family Decision."

Implementation

1. Distribute "House Hunting Selection Grid" and review with the team.
2. Distribute "The Family Solution," noting that the house selected was number 4, with a high score of 120.

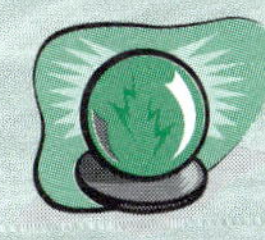

Debriefing

Reviewing this example illustrates how time consuming it can be to identify and weigh important characteristics or criteria to make a decision, but how clearly a decision can be made and substantiated with quantitative data, that is, real numbers!

Magic Touch

"House Hunting" provides a real-world example of using a selection or decision grid. A decision-making grid allows the team visually to examine alternatives and compare them based on the same criteria. To use a selection grid, decide on the necessary criteria for the decision (in this example, house characteristics) and weigh the importance of each. In *Leadership Roles and Management Functions in Nursing,* by B. L. Marquis and C. J. Huston (Philadelphia, 1996, Lippincott, p. 48), a learning exercise illustrates the use of a decision grid for selecting staff. The reader is asked to construct a grid in order to choose one of six applicants for a position in an open heart unit by selecting and weighing essential selection criteria. This makes the decision one based on quantitative data. As you use these and other decision-making strategies, design examples that are easily understood and illustrate common concerns.

By: Kathy Beck, RN, MSN

HOUSE HUNTING SELECTION GRID

A family of seven decides to buy a new house. The parents, proponents of the democratic process, decide to involve the children in this purchase and promptly call a family meeting. The following items are presented as needs in a new house:

- The children each want to have a bedroom for themselves with an adjoining bathroom.
- The father insists he must have a garage for his new Porsche.
- All agree that it must be large enough to allow everyone to have personal space.
- The mother wants a one-story house.
- Because of the parents' hectic work schedule, both would like to be near work and schools.

(Of course, the parents met with a mortgage company and were preapproved.) All of these characteristics were presented to a real estate agent, who shows them the following five houses:

House Characteristics	*House 1*	*House 2*	*House 3*	*House 4*	*House 5*
Size (sq. ft.)	2300	3000	2800	3200	2600
Number of bedrooms	4	5	4	6	3
Number of bathrooms	3	3	4	4	3
Garage	No	Yes	No	No	Yes
One story	Yes	No	No	Yes	Yes
Distance from school (miles)	12	5	15	20	10
Distance from work (miles)	15	20	15	15	5

After the family viewed each house, they have another family meeting. During the meeting, they determine the weights of the charcteristics.

House Characteristics	*Weights*
Size (sq. ft.)	20%
Number of bedrooms	20%
Number of bathrooms	20%
Garage	5%
One story	5%
Distance from school (miles)	15%
Distance from work (miles)	15%

THE FAMILY DECISION

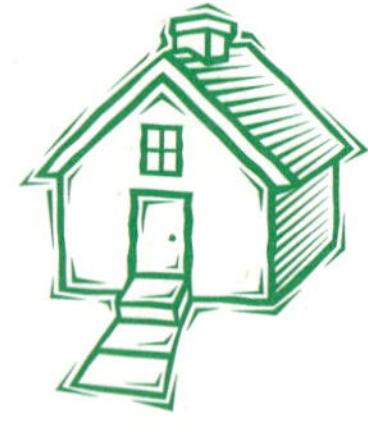

House Characteristics	*House 1*	*House 2*	*House 3*	*House 4*	*House 5*
Size (sq. ft.) High ≤ 3000 Score 2 Med 2600–2900 Score 1 Low ≥ 2500 Score 0 Weight: 20%	0	2	1	2	1
Number of bedrooms High ≤ 6 Score 2 Med 4–5 Score 1 Low ≤ 3 Score 0 Weight: 20%	1	1	1	2	0
Number of bathrooms High ≤ 6 Score 2 Med 4–5 Score 1 Low ≤ 3 Score 0 Weight: 20%	0	0	1	1	0
Garage Yes Score 1 No Score 0 Weight: 5%	0	1	0	0	1
One story Yes Score 1 No Score 0 Weight: 5%	1	0	0	1	1
Distance from school (miles) High ≤ 5 Score 2 Med 6–15 Score 1 Low ≤ 16 Score 0 Weight: 15%	1	2	1	0	1
Distance from work (miles) High ≤ 5 Score 2 Med 6–15 Score 1 Low ≤ 16 Score 0 Weight: 15%	1	0	1	1	2
Score	55	95	90	120	75

TEAM TOOL CAROLS

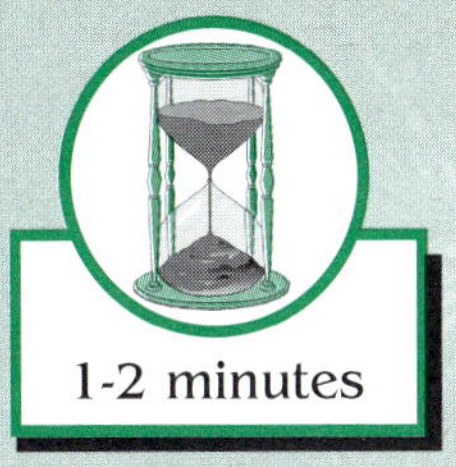

New Lyrics to Amazingly Familiar Songs!

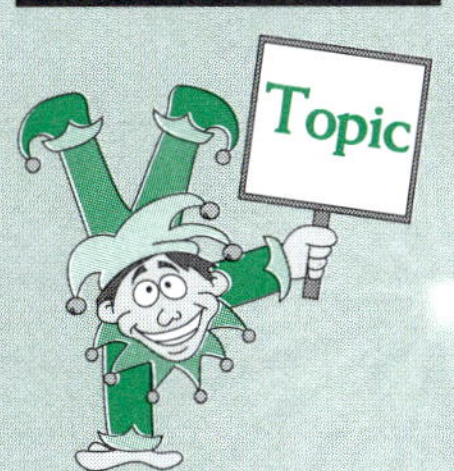

Use for an energizer or a bit of comic relief when working with one of the statistical tools.

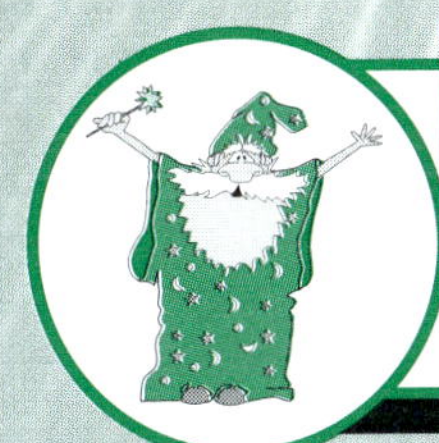

Wizard List

"Deck the Walls with Brainstorming," "Up on the Cause-and-Effect Diagram," "Oh Pareto," "Consensus Wonderland"

Preparation

1. Copy the selected carols for each team member.
2. Make a transparency for a visual demonstration.

Implementation

1. Ask the team if they would like to lighten up for a minute. Invite the team to sing a customized team carol and to sing it with gusto.
2. Distribute the appropriate carol(s) to team members.
3. Sing!

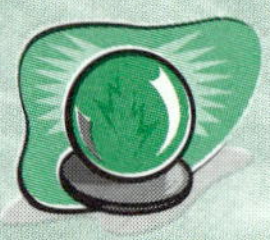

Debriefing

Admit that although some of these ideas seem wild, a bit of amusement can often revitalize and stimulate creativity. Whose idea could be questioned after one of these carols?!

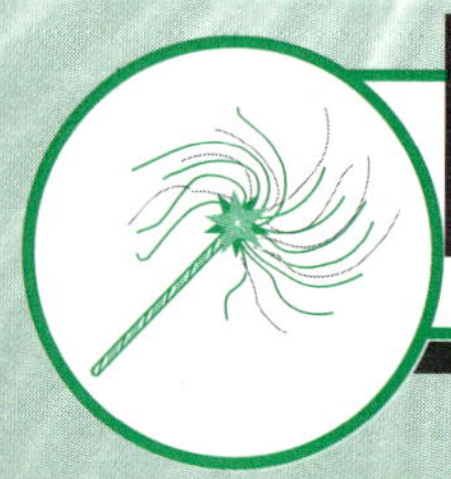

Magic Touch

Enthusiasm is contagious! Spread it to the team members!

DECK THE WALLS WITH BRAINSTORMING

(Sung to the Tune of "Deck the Halls")

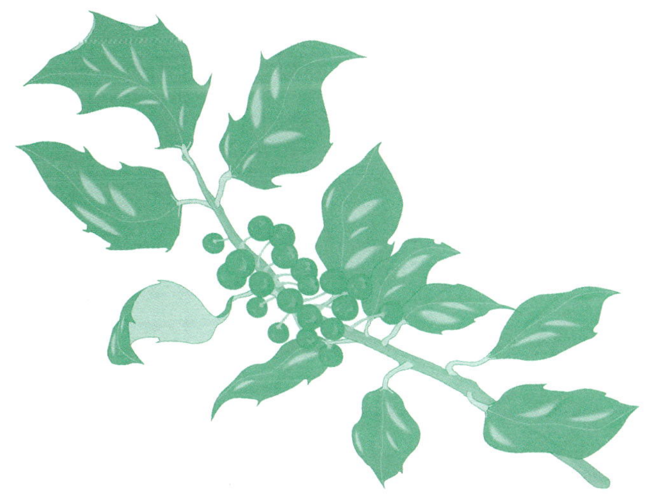

Brainstorm til your minds are weary!
Fa la la la la, la la la la!
All around the team we query!
Fa la la la la, la la la la!
Never judging contributions.
Fa la la, la la la, la la la!
This is where we find solutions!
Fa la la la la, la la la laaaaaaaaaah!

UP ON THE CAUSE-AND-EFFECT DIAGRAM

(Sung to the tune of "Up on the Rooftop")

Up on the cause-and-effect diagram,
All our ideas we try to cram.
Will something useful come from this?
To solve our mission, oh what bliss.

Whine, whine, whine!
Who wouldn't whine?
Whine, whine, whine!
Who wouldn't whine?

Quality tools we try to apply,
And work to keep our spirits high!

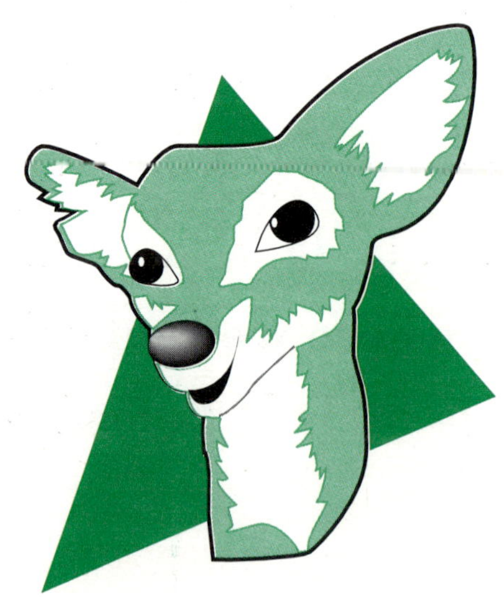

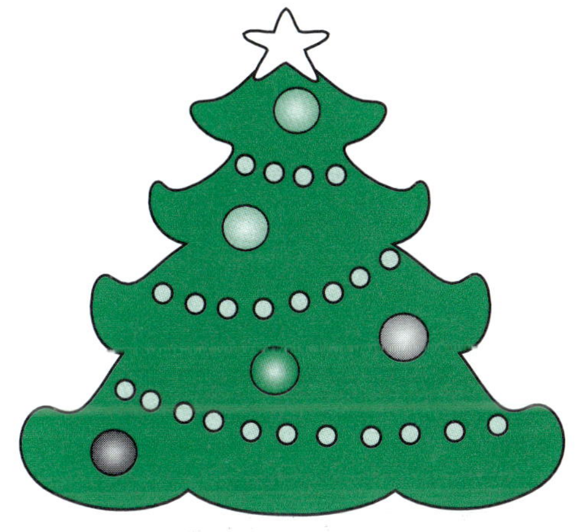

OH, PARETO

(Sung to the tune of
"Oh, Christmas Tree")

Oh, Pareto,
Oh, Pareto,
The things you try to teach us!

Oh, vital few,
Oh, vital few!
The data come to greet us!

We'll try to focus on the few,
Not led astray by each thing new!

Oh, Pareto,
Oh, Pareto,
The things you try to teach us!

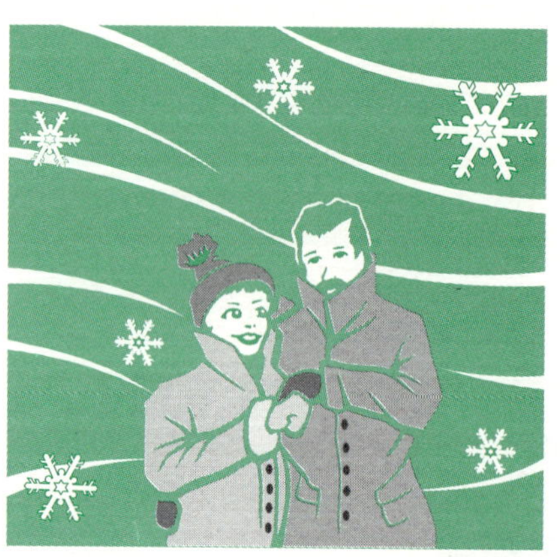

CONSENSUS WONDERLAND

(Sung to the tune of "Winter Wonderland")

Consensus time, are you listening?
Things unsaid, are you listening?
Openness we seek, from strong and from meek.
Let's find a way to make our voices heard.

Sometimes it is easy just to sit there,
Waiting for the vocal ones to share.
They assume in silence, we agree.
But what if you must implement solutions?
Then you'll find yourself up in a tree!

Consensus time, are you listening?
Things unsaid, are you listening?
Openness we seek, from strong and from meek.
Let's find a way to make our voices heard.

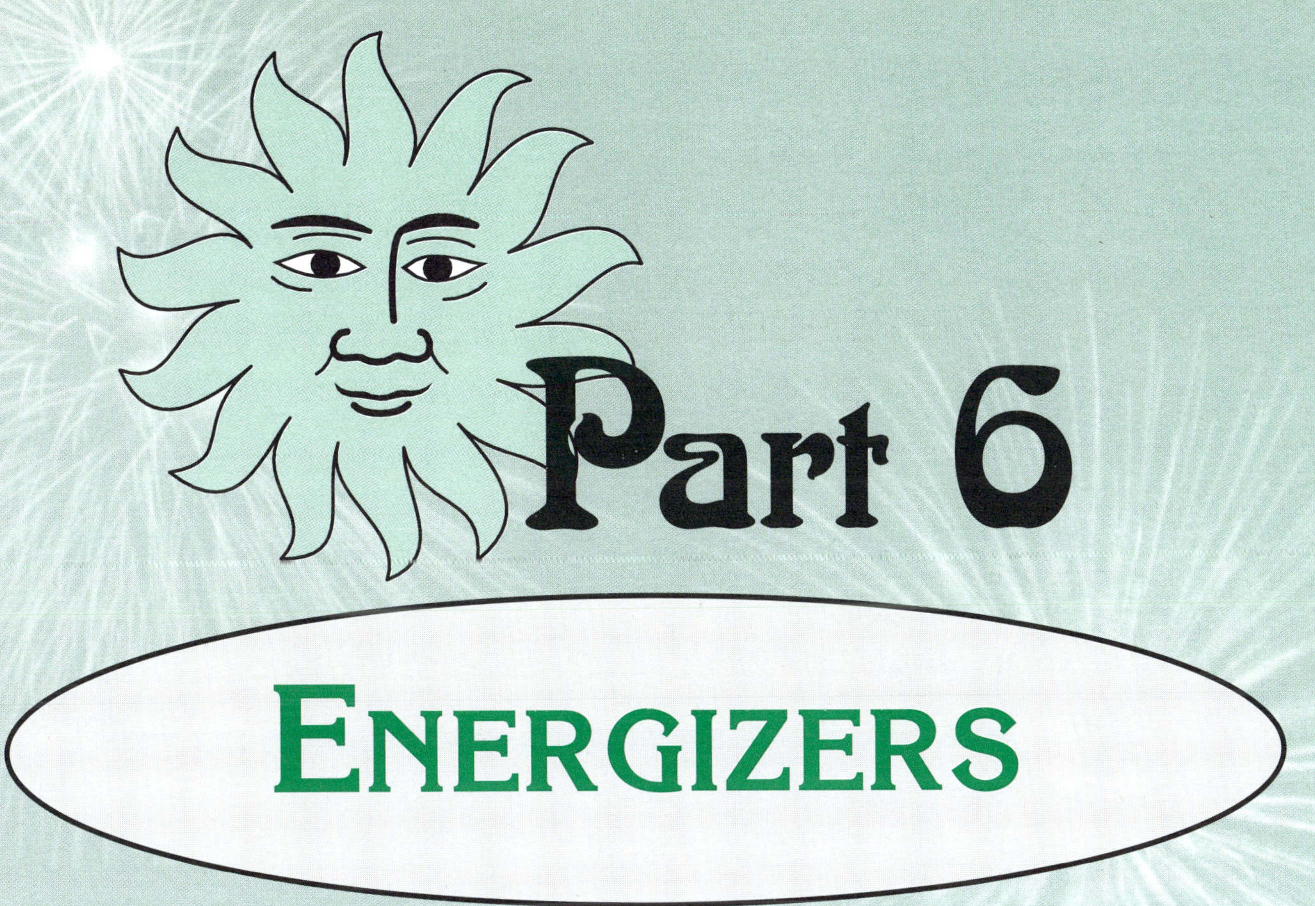

Part 6

ENERGIZERS

Teamwork is a challenge. Participants come to yet another meeting, facing busy schedules and work that waits patiently or impatiently for them during the time spent working with the team. Brief activities designed to energize members can contribute to team efficiency. As always, debriefing is important to keep the focus on work. There are many exercises in this section from which to choose. They are divided into the following categories:

- provides fun
- distracts from stress before the meeting
- refocuses attention to teamwork
- moves beyond a team impasse
- provides food for fun
- helps to learn even more about team members
- chooses a leader for an activity
- gets team feedback

Take your magic wand in hand and get ready to energize!

LOOSEN' UP

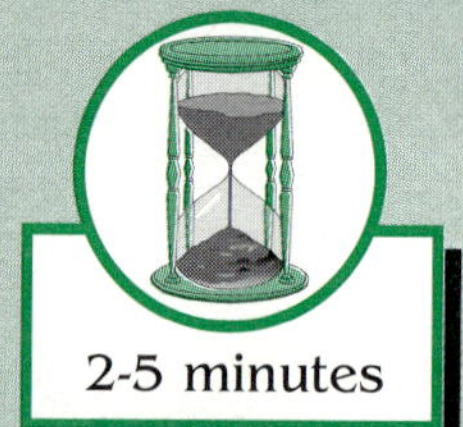

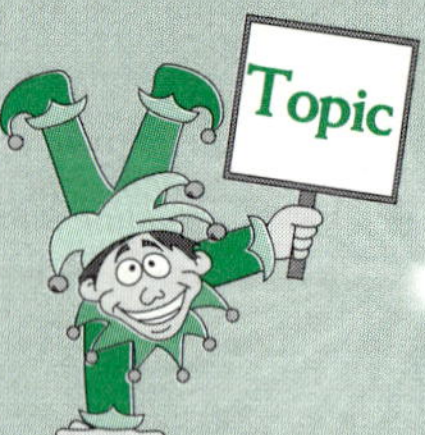

Involvement. Use this exercise for fun and stress relief.

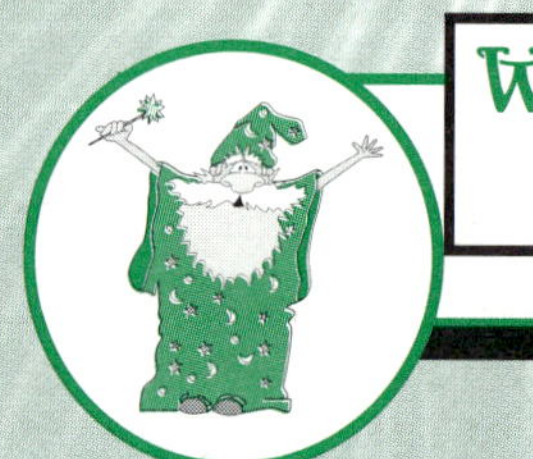

Wizard List

a Koosh ball or soft, squeezable ball

Preparation

1. Supply a Koosh ball or soft, squeezable ball.

Implementation

1. Instruct the group that it is time to loosen' up a bit.
2. Toss the ball to a team member and ask the team to toss the ball among themselves to relax for a moment before the team meeting.
3. You can start this activity for early arrivals.
4. Ask the team for feedback about tossing the ball.

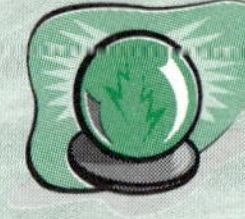

Debriefing

Ask if they note any difference between the behavior of the group before the activity and after. Usually there is more noise, involvement, laughter, and a sense of anticipation about who will get the ball next. If someone has raised a hand to signal the desire to receive the ball and was thrown the ball, then use this as an illustration of getting what you want in life if you ask for it, expect it, or go after it. If the team expects to be successful, it is more likely that it will be. Someone who sat back and wanted the ball, but did not take the risk to show he or she wanted to come out and play, might not have received the ball. This also illustrates that we may have a fear of looking foolish in front of our peers if we show enthusiasm, although this is a feeling we should try to overcome because it's okay to show enthusiasm.

Magic Touch

Variation: Incorporate "Loosen' Up" into a lesson. For example, tell the team that each team member has to come up with a good quality that each team member should possess. They have to say the quality when the ball is tossed to them. The ball should be tossed around among all team members or until all qualities have been mentioned.

MAN YOUR PADDLES!

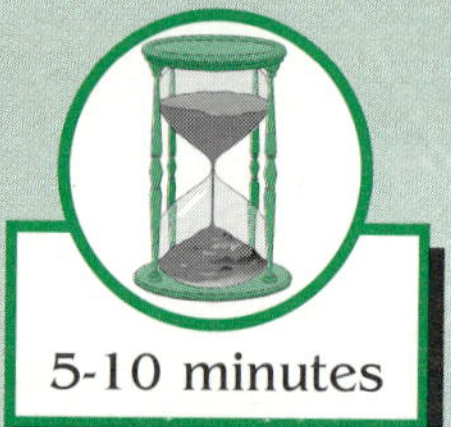

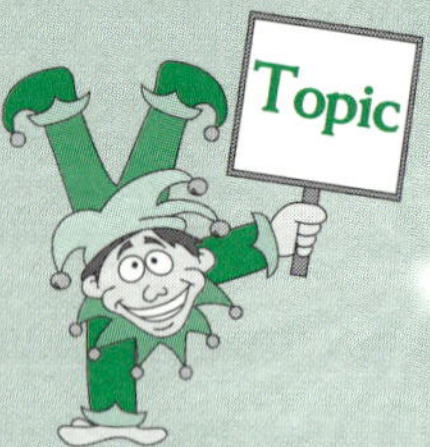

Use for fun and stress relief.

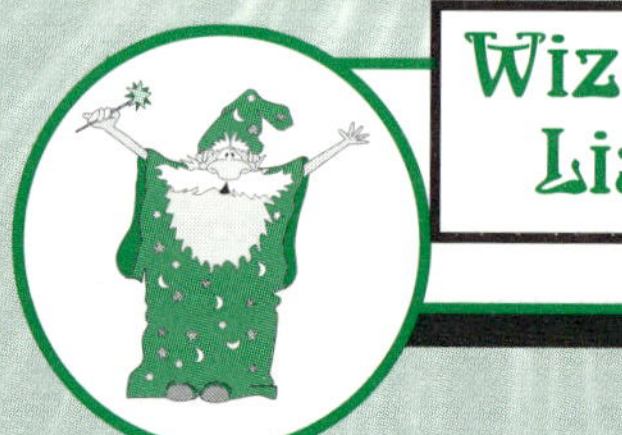

Wizard List

Paddle ball, watch with a second hand, whistle, prizes

Preparation

1. Purchase paddle balls for each team member. (These are wooden paddles with a small ball attached by a rubber band.)
2. Bring a watch with a second hand and a whistle.
3. Purchase a prize for the winner and small prizes for each member.

Implementation

1. Explain that the group is in for a treat, a brief contest in which prizes *might* be involved!
2. Demonstrate how to use the paddle ball. Try to keep the ball in motion for as long as possible. If you can't get the hang of it, ask for a volunteer to demonstrate.
3. Invite the group to participate in a contest to see who can keep it going for the longest time without missing. Distribute the paddles and give everyone one minute to practice and warm up . . . it may have been a while! (Clear tables of any breakables!) If anyone is not willing to participate, ask that person to be a judge (counter), or the group can count each paddle hit. If the group is large, divide into small groups and have each small group cheer for their representative.

4. Explain to the group that each member is allowed 30 seconds for the contest and that you will blow the whistle to start and stop. You can increase the time if you choose.
5. Award a prize to the member with highest number of continuous hits.
6. Award a small prize to each member for participation.

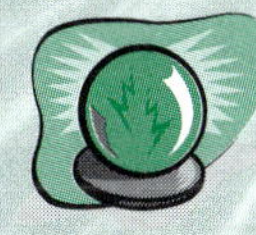

Debriefing

Ask for comparisons between the behavior of the group and the atmosphere in the room before and after the exercise. Comment on the laughter and increased energy in the room. Ask if anyone felt awkward or a little foolish. Point out that sometimes we are a bit uncomfortable with something new or something we have not done in a while. It is okay not to be perfect, or skilled at the same things, and to lighten up a little!

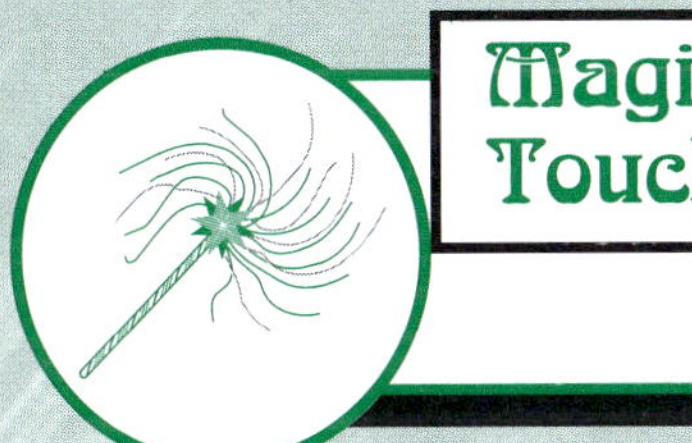

Magic Touch

Reintroduce the toys for brief stress relief in later meetings after the group has participated in this activity.

MY VERY OWN TENT

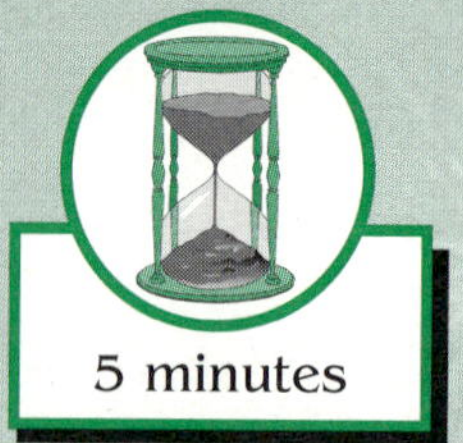

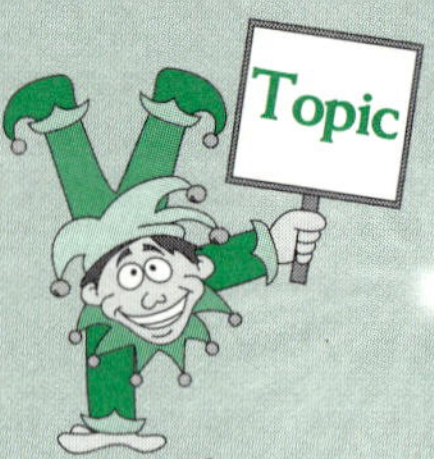

Use for fun and stress relief. It should be used when team members are seated at tables.

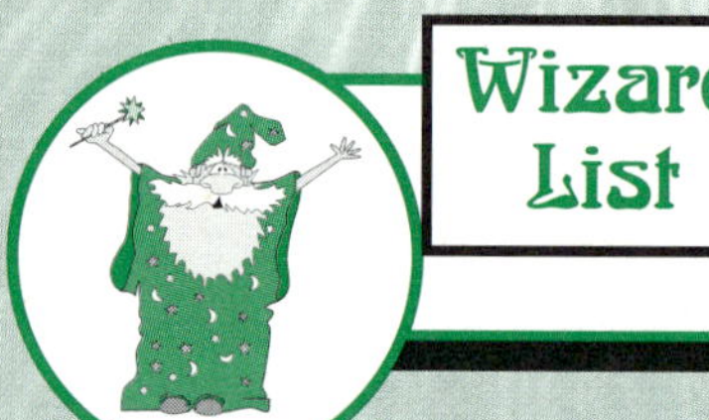

Wizard List A heavier stock paper, poster board, or copy paper; colored markers

Preparation

1. Choose a heavier stock paper, poster board, or copy paper folded twice to double the thickness to create a table tent nameplate.
2. Cut paper or poster board to the desired size. (A good size is $8\frac{1}{2}'' \times 11''$.) Provide one for each team member.
3. Provide multicolored markers.

Implementation

1. Place the table tent nameplates and multicolored markers at each table.
2. As team members arrive, ask them to create their own table tent name and art!

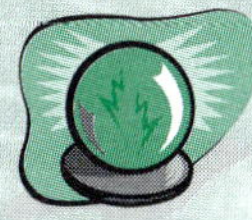

Debriefing

Point out that this exercise was just to energize and have some fun.

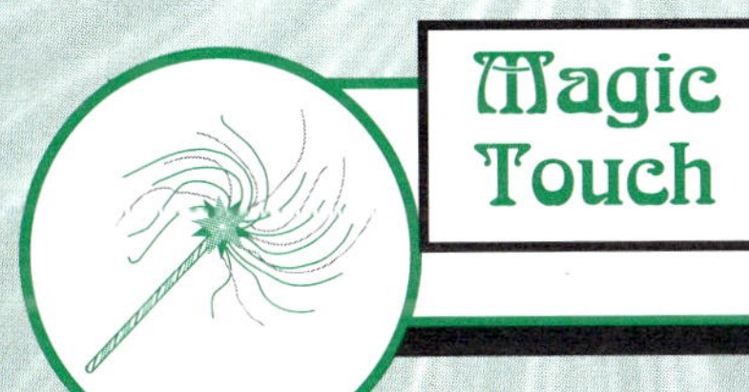

Develop a personalized atmosphere. Call each member by his or her name.

ONE-LINERS TO LIVE BY

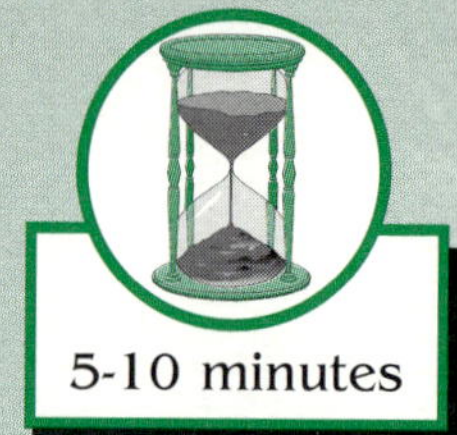

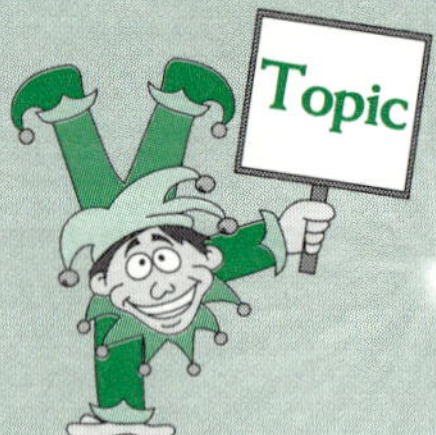

Use for fun and stress relief.

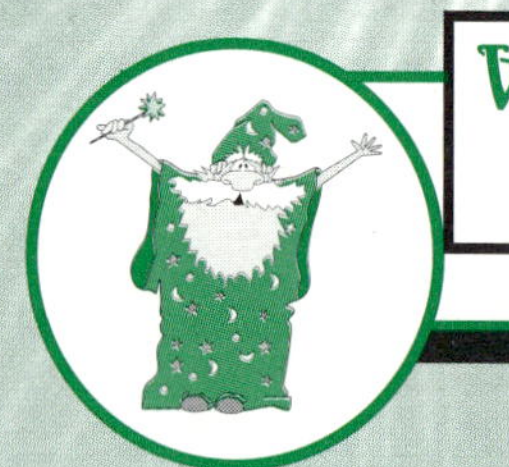

Wizard List

"One-liners To Live By" quotes, index cards

Preparation

1. Review the "One-liners To Live By" quotes, and add some of your own.
2. Provide index cards, one for each team member.

Implementation

1. Ask the team to take a minute to think of their favorite one-liners that they can share. Suggest they try to recall favorite bumper stickers, buttons, or T-shirts they have seen.
2. Give a few examples from the list or from your own research.
3. Ask team members to share theirs just for fun, but not to embarrass anyone!
4. Pass out index cards and ask participants to record their one-liners.
5. Collect the index cards and read the one-liners to the team.

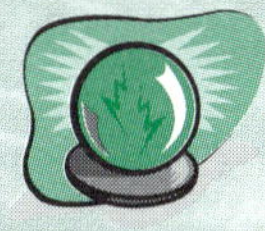

Debriefing

Explain that sometimes a little perspective helps us get through the day.

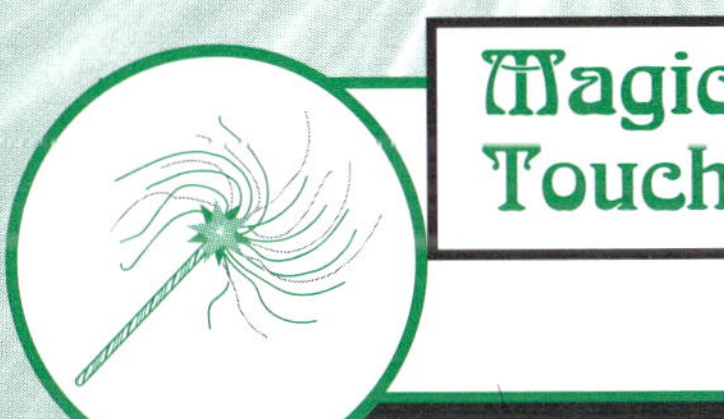

Magic Touch

Ask colleagues, friends, and family to add their favorites. Put out a request on E-mail, "Wanted: One-liners to live by."

ONE-LINERS TO LIVE BY

1. "Toto, I don't think we're in Kansas anymore." (*The Wizard of Oz*)
2. "I won't think about it today. I'll think about it tomorrow at Tara." (*Gone with the Wind*)
3. "He who laughs last."
4. "They said, 'Cheer up. It could get worse.' So I cheered up and sure enough, it got worse."
5. "Within every problem there is a lesson. Release the problem and embrace the lesson."

Add others:

6. ______________________________
7. ______________________________
8. ______________________________
9. ______________________________
10. ____________________
11. ____________________
12. ____________________
13. ____________________
14. ____________________
15. ____________________

CARTOON CAPERS

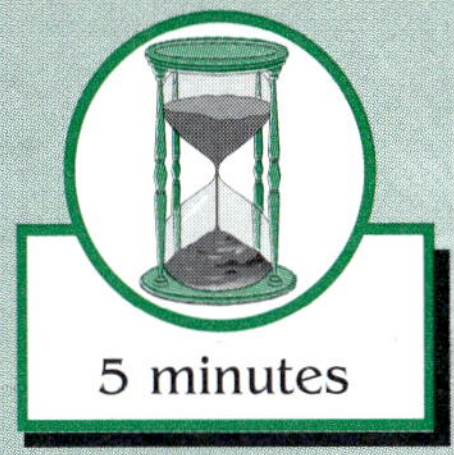

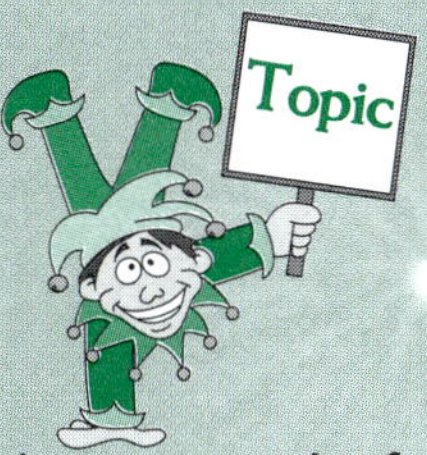

Laughter. Use for fun and stress relief.

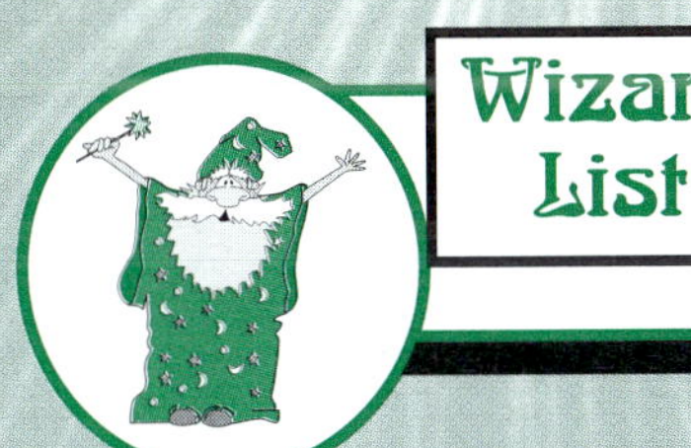

Wizard List

Cartoon collection

Preparation

1. Save comic sections from Sunday and daily newspapers or begin to collect a variety of cartoons that you think apply to work. Collect cartoon books.
2. Place the individual cartoons in a photo album. This allows you to pass around the cartoons without violating copyright laws.

Implementation

1. Explain that sometimes a cartoon can help us acquire a fresh perspective or help us know we are not alone.
2. Pass around a variety of cartoons. To move things along, you can provide more than one cartoon album.
3. Ask each team member to choose one cartoon to share with the group and explain why it tickles his or her fancy.

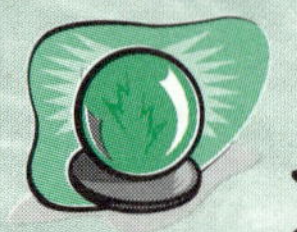

Debriefing

Discuss how some of the cartoons apply to team dynamics.

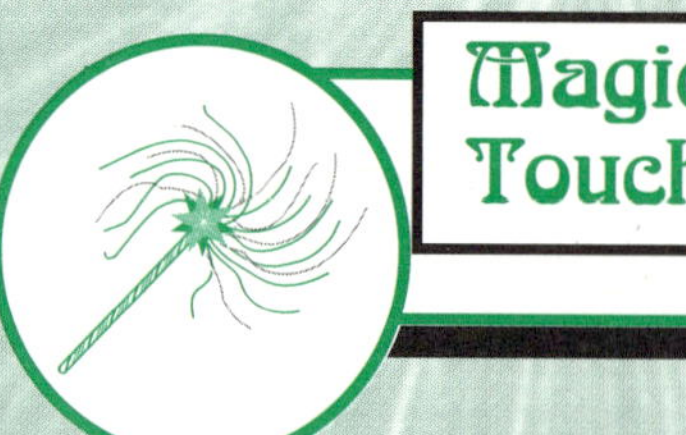

Magic Touch

Laughter lightens the load! It relaxes and diminishes the effects of stress.

It's Written in the Stars

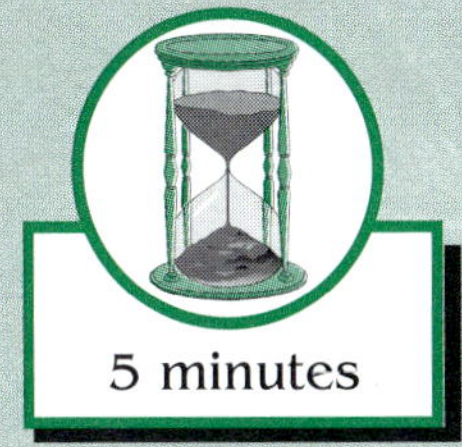

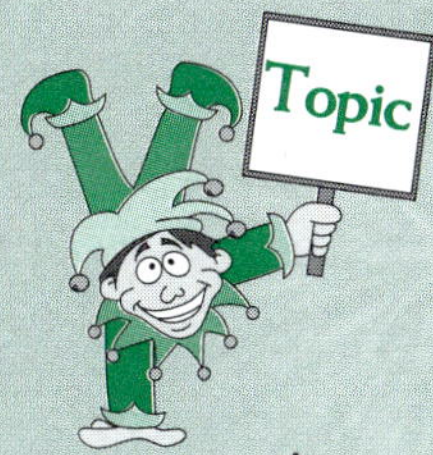

Use for fun and to learn more about team members.

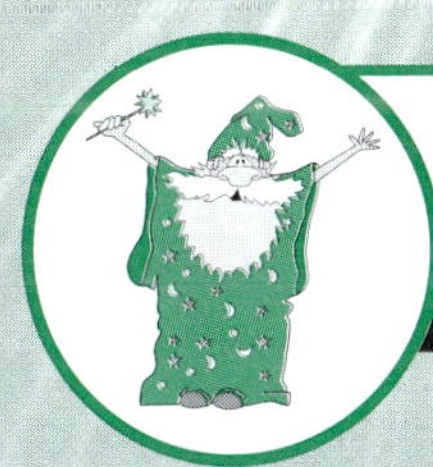

Wizard List Horoscopes from current newspaper, magic wand

Preparation

1. Bring the horoscopes to the meeting.

Implementation

1. Ask the group if they will give you several minutes to have a little fun.
2. Pass the newspaper around and have each team member read aloud his or her horoscope for the day. To save time, you can ask someone to volunteer his or her sign and read the appropriate horoscope.

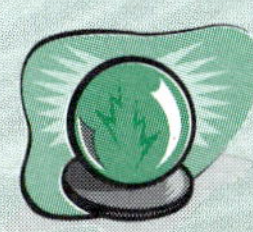

Debriefing

This activity is just for fun and to get people talking and in the mood for sharing.

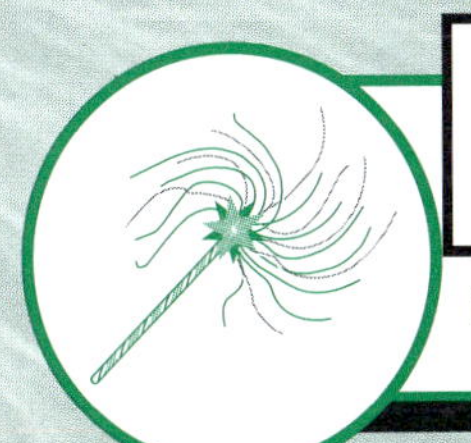

Magic Touch Start the first reading while holding the magic wand, then pass it to the next member for his or her reading. For each horoscope reading, pass the magic wand.

CAN YOU TOP THAT?

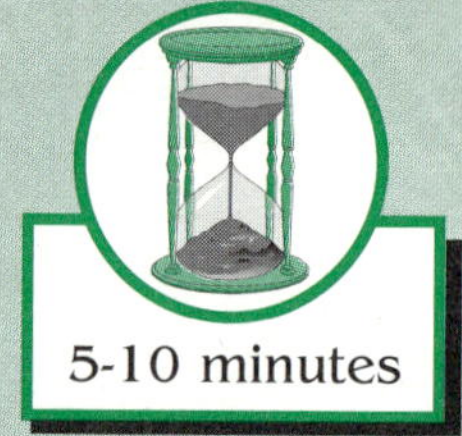

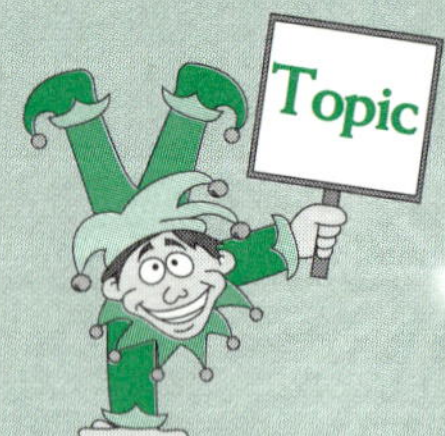

Hats we wear. Use this exercise for fun and to get to know one another better.

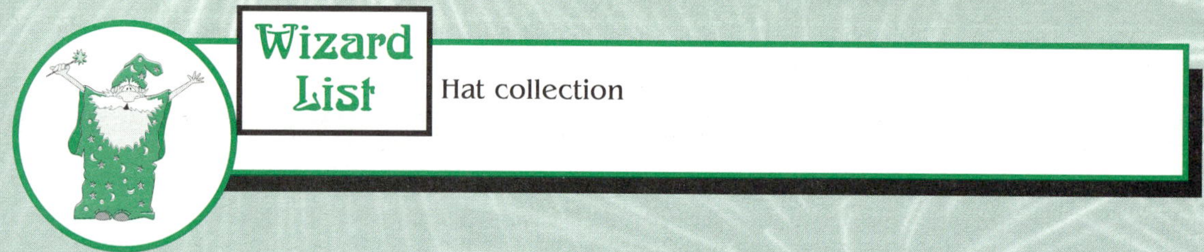

Preparation

1. Conclude a meeting with instructions for this activity to be used at the next team meeting.
2. Explain that we all wear different hats in our lives. Ask team members to wear a hat to the next meeting that says something about their job or personal interests.
3. Announce that if anyone shows up without a hat, one will be provided and fellow team members will make the selection.
4. Gather a hat collection. Look for castoffs or go to a party, costume, or toy store.
5. Select a hat for you to wear.

Implementation

1. At the next meeting, ask the group to choose a hat from the hat collection for anyone who didn't wear one.
2. Explain what the hat you are wearing represents.
3. Invite each team member to explain his or her hat and what it represents.

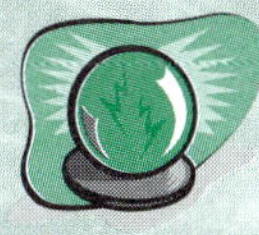

Debriefing

Ask for feedback about the activity and then explain that a bit of fun and creativity energizes the team.

Magic Touch

Look for hats for group roles, such as firefighter (facilitator/team leader), police officer (gatekeeper), and coach (team teacher), and create an activity developed around the team roles.

STARTING OFF ON A POSITIVE NOTE

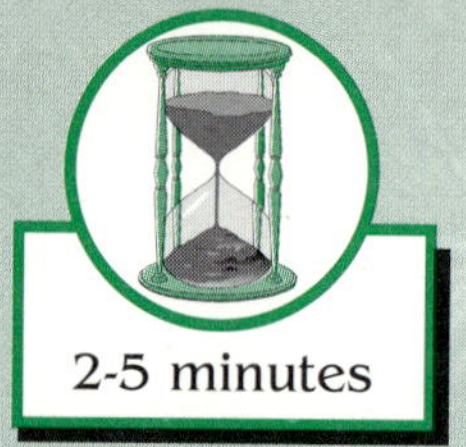

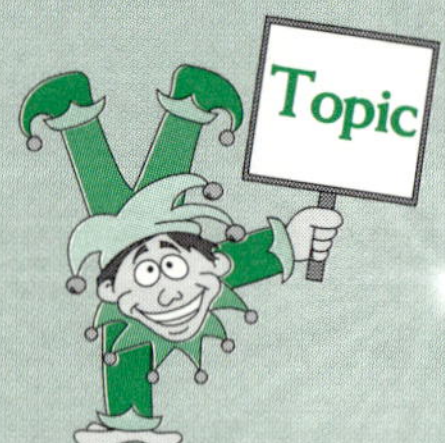

Use to generate a positive atmosphere with a little fun.

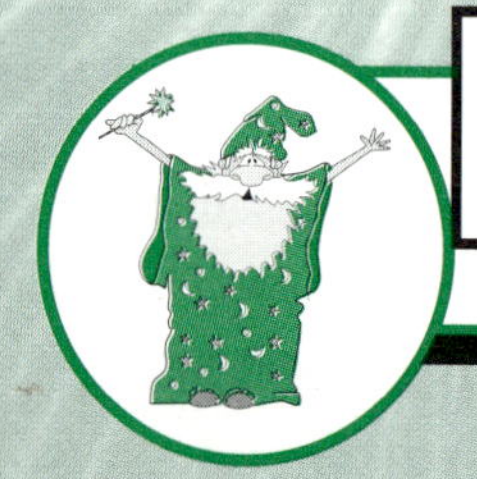

Wizard List

"Starting Off on a Positive Note" topics sheet, magic wand (optional)

Preparation

1. Review "Starting Off on a Positive Note."
2. Think about the comfort and security children and adults gain from a bedtime ritual or a morning ritual that launches the day. Consider what you know about team members and choose from the ideas on the "Starting Off on a Positive Note" topics sheet or generate your own questions.

Implementation

1. Explain to the group that you want to create a ritual to give the group a way to start each meeting, something for them to think about to answer at each meeting.
2. Choose one question or read all questions from "Starting Off on a Positive Note" to the group and have the group come to a consensus about which one they desire.
3. Ask each team member to answer the question and set the expectation that each meeting will start with the same question.

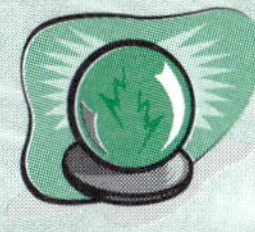

Debriefing

Remind the group of the comfort that children receive from a bedtime ritual and that adults have in a morning or evening ritual that starts or ends the day on a positive note. Explain that in stressful times sometimes a brief moment to focus on something positive can add joy to the day. Suggest that even thinking in advance about an answer can set the expectation of doing or watching for something positive in the workplace.

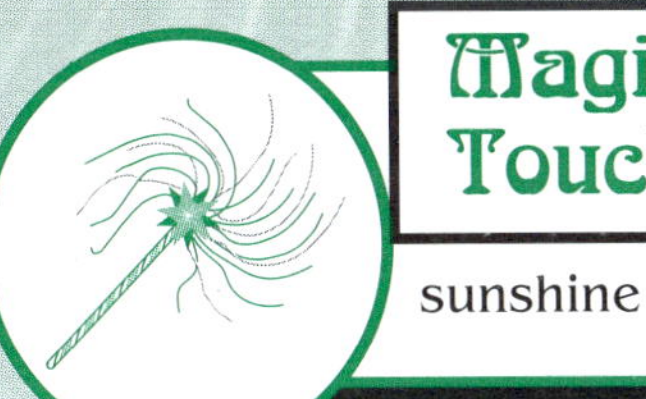

Magic Touch Close this activity by waving your magic wand and saying something positive, such as "May you all have sunshine in your life today."

STARTING OFF ON A POSITIVE NOTE

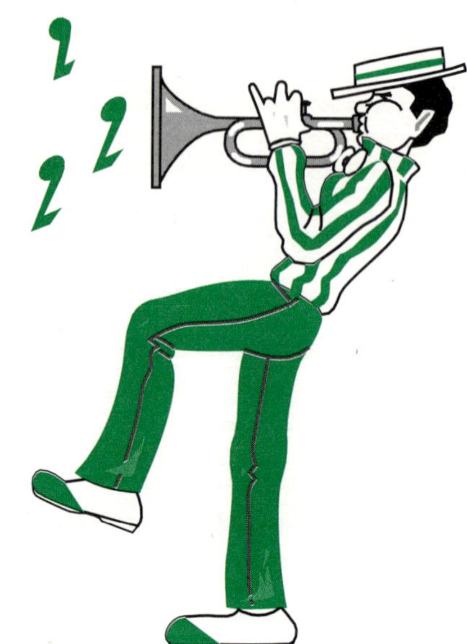

Topics

1. Name one thing you learned today.
2. Identify one positive thing that happened today.
3. Identify one goal for your week.
4. Tell one positive thing you did today.
5. Share one compliment you gave today.
6. Identify one example of positive internal customer service today, either something you or someone else did. (Remember, internal customers are your co-workers.)

Others

7. ______________________________
8. ______________________________
9. ______________________________
10. ______________________________

ROLLIN' IN THE DOUGH

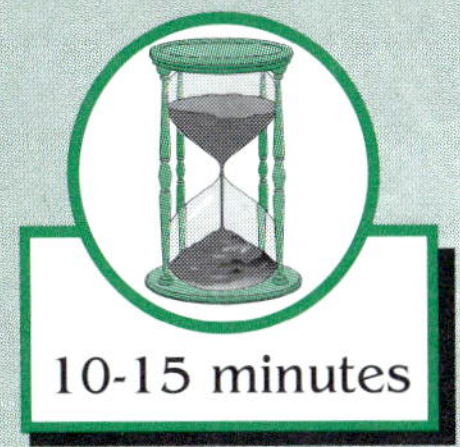

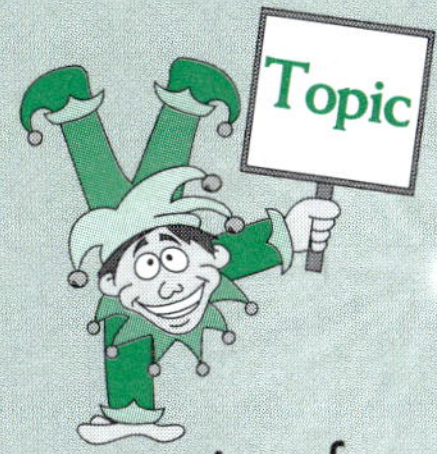

Use for hands-on, creative fun.

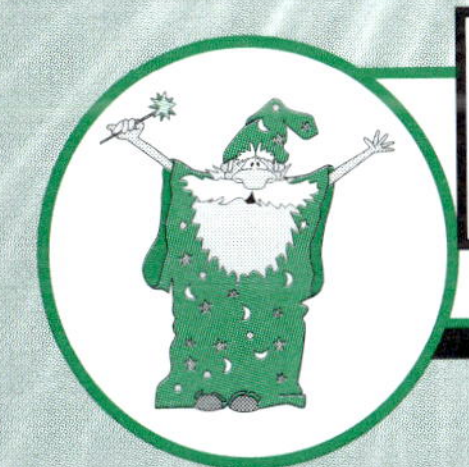

Wizard List Modeling clay or dough, containers (optional)

Preparation

1. Purchase clay or dough.
2. Place in large covered container or provide a small covered container for each team member.

Implementation

1. Tell the group that they are in for some fun . . . honest!
2. Distribute the clay and instruct team members to make something that represents who they are or something important about them that they will share.
3. Let the fun begin!
4. Have each person explain his or her creation to the group.

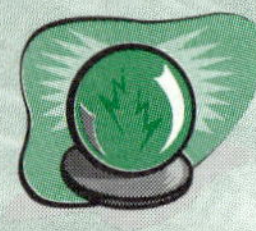

Debriefing

Ask for feedback and shape your debriefing from this. Comments might include not wanting to do it but having fun anyway . . . not unlike teams!

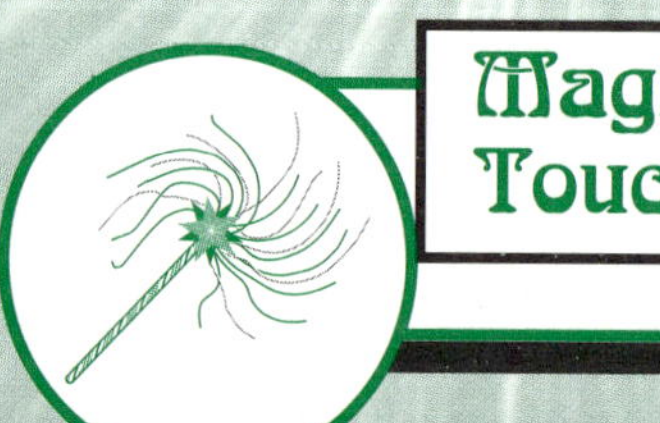

Magic Touch

Join the fun! Create one for yourself.

HELLO . . . MY NAME IS JOE

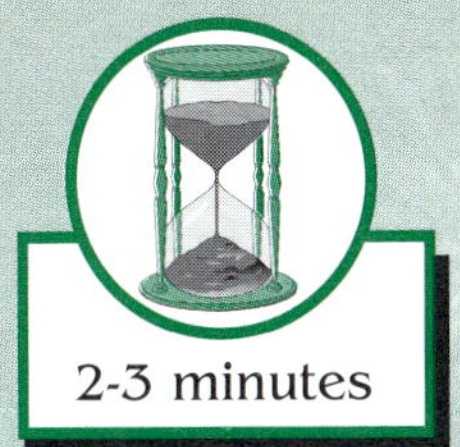

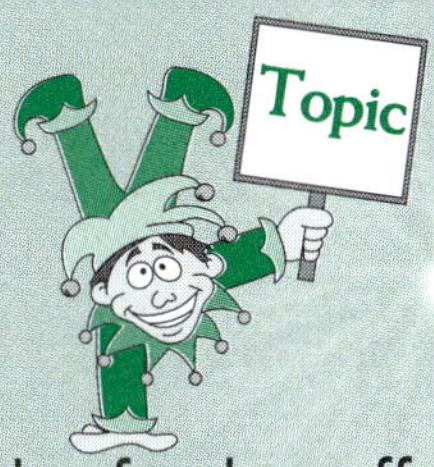

Energizer. Use this to change the mood and refresh staff.

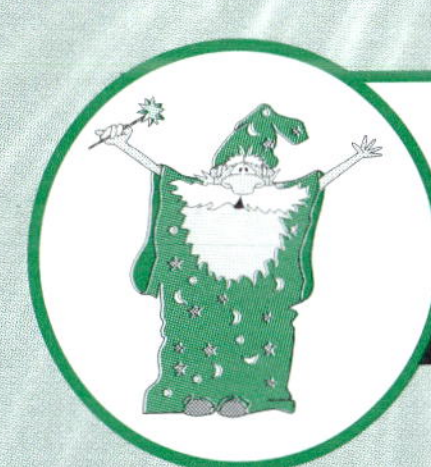

Wizard List

"Hello . . . My Name Is Joe"

Preparation

1. Copy "Hello . . . My Name Is Joe" rap sheet for each team member.
2. Review and practice "Hello . . . My name Is Joe" using a moderate beat.

Implementation

1. Distribute "Hello . . . My Name Is Joe" to each team member.
2. Review the instructions included on the "Hello . . . My Name Is Joe" rap sheet with the group, and demonstrate the movements that accompany the song.
3. Ask for volunteers to assist you with leading the group.
4. Ask everyone to stand and join in.

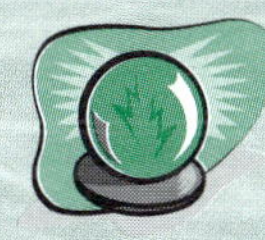

Debriefing

Be sure to practice. Staff, especially those who participate in the singing and dancing, return to work with a smile and a positive attitude. You do risk several things by doing this exercise:

- being called "Joe" by staff from time to time
- having staff from other units request a performance
- having others catch the mood and share some of their favorite tension breakers
- disbelieving look of nonparticipants

Magic Touch

Everyone can relate to the frantic feeling of having more to do than one can handle. This exercise is a rich example of risk-taking that works magic.

By: Enoch Albert, RN

HELLO . . . MY NAME IS JOE

(A Rap Song)

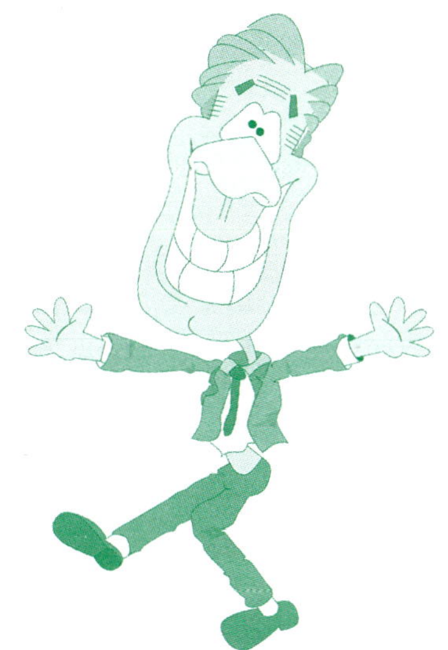

Perform to a moderate beat, and pause when you see ellipses.

Hello . . . my name is Joe . . .
And I work . . . in a button fac-tor-y.
I have a wife . . . and a dog . . . and a fam-i-ly.
One day . . . my boss came up to me . . .
She (or he) said Joe . . . are you busy?
I said no . . .
Then push . . . the button with your right hand.

[Using your right hand, push your open palm out away from your body, and keep this motion going throughout the song. Other body motions will be added.]

2nd verse—Repeat the first verse and change the last line.

Then push . . . the button with your left hand.

[Using your left hand, push your open palm out away from your body, and keep this motion going throughout the song.]

3rd verse—Repeat the first verse and change the last line.

Then push . . . the button with your right foot. [Using your right foot, tap the floor, and keep this motion going throughout the song.]

4th verse—Repeat the first verse and change the last line.

Then push . . . the button with your left foot. [Using your left foot, tap the floor, and keep this motion going throughout the song.]

5th verse—Repeat the first verse and change the last line.

Then push . . . the button with your head. [Move your head in a forward-backward motion. By this time you will probably be discombobulated and laughing uncontrollably, but keep going—you're almost finished.]

6th verse—Repeat the first verse and change the sixth line.

I said YES!

Do you know your ABCs

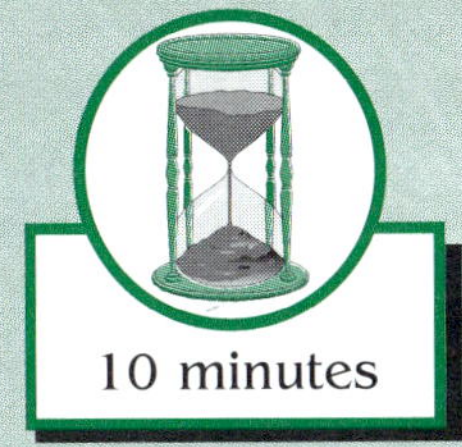

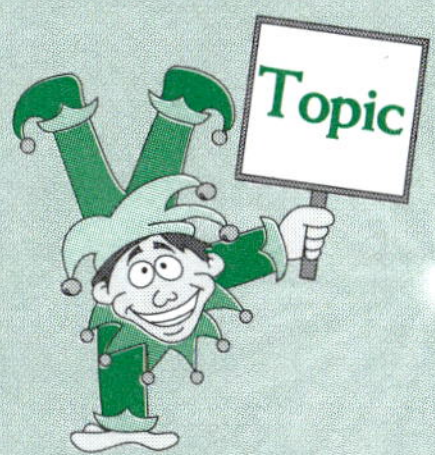

Attributes. Use to distract from stressors before a meeting.

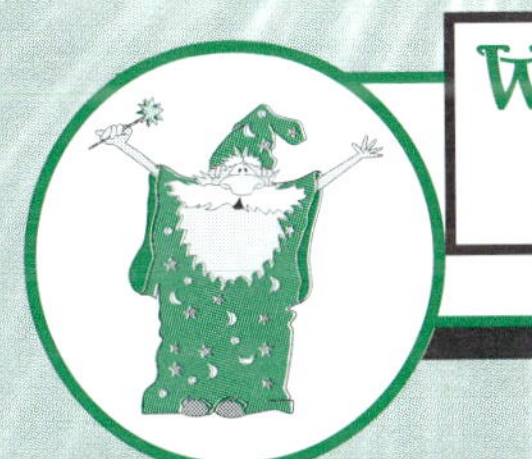

Wizard List Flip chart, markers, whistle

Preparation

1. Write the ABCs on the flip chart in bold letters in a single column.
2. Supply a marker and a whistle.

Implementation

1. Ask the team to give you five minutes to add a little energy and be creative.
2. Ask the team to think of one attribute of each team member that starts with each letter of the alphabet. Give examples, such as: Jane is *A*rtsy! John make *B*old contributions! Carla leads us to *C*onsensus!
3. Ask for a volunteer to write the attributes on the flip chart.
4. Announce that the time allowed is five minutes and that the sound of the whistle is the signal to start and stop.

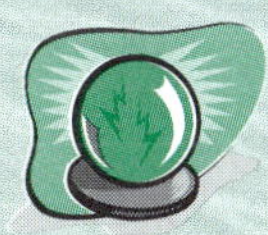

Debriefing

Ask the group to comment on the process of completing the task and ask for feedback about the activity. Recognizing attributes of

other team members helps us to realize that everyone has something to contribute.

Magic Touch

Variation: If the group is large, divide it into small groups and have each group identify attributes of the members within that group.

A novel task can energize and distract team members from stressors that preceded the meeting.

QUESTIONING MINDS

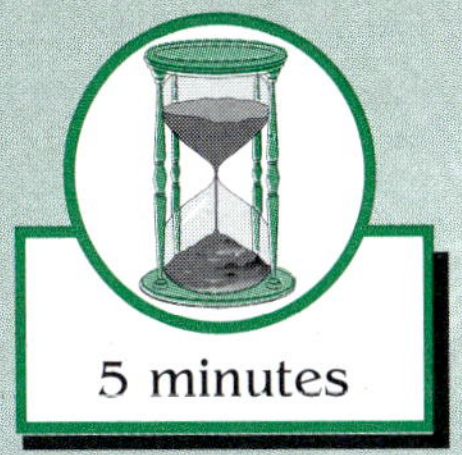

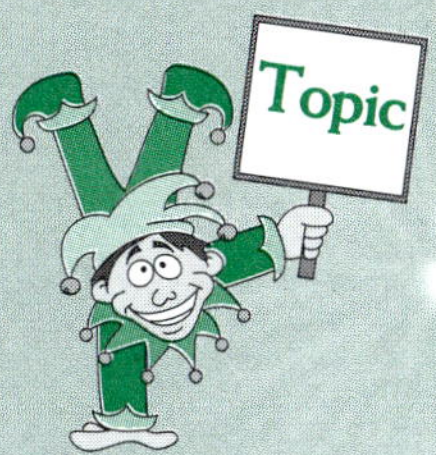

Stress distractor. Use this at the beginning of a meeting.

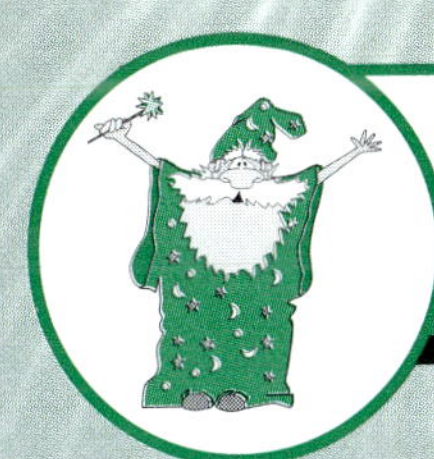

Wizard List

"Questioning Minds," flip chart, marker, transparency and felt-tip pen (optional)

Preparation

1. Select one question from "Questioning Minds."
2. Write the question you have selected on a flip chart or transparency.

Implementation

1. Invite the team to have some fun.
2. Announce the question displayed on the flip chart or transparency.
3. Ask the group to think about the answer. (Allow about one minute.)
4. Explain that they will be asked to share their answer with the group.
5. Ask for feedback about how the team liked the activity.

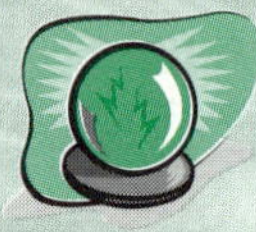

Debriefing

Explain that this exercise serves to distract from other commitments and stressors, and helps to refocus the group to get to the teamwork.

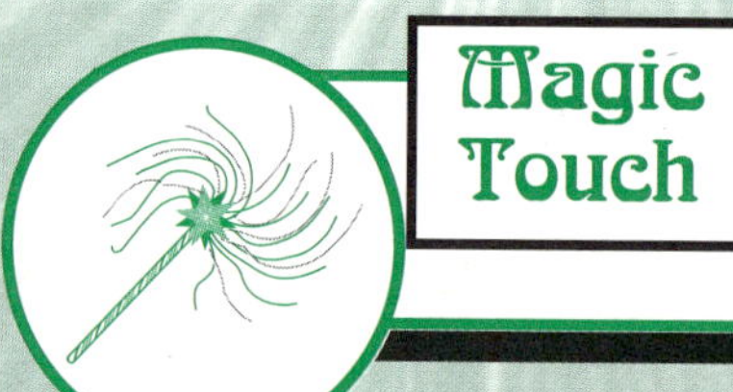

Ask each team member to submit one question for future meetings.

QUESTIONING MINDS

1. What is an ideal pet for you? Why?
2. What is your favorite car? Why?
3. What is your favorite color? Why?
4. Do you change clothes when you go home from work? If so, what do you wear?
5. What was your favorite vacation? Why?
6. If you won the lottery, what is the first thing you would do?
7. Who is the one person, living or deceased, whom you admire most? Why?
8. Name a favorite possession. Why is it a favorite?
9. If you could speak a language in addition to your native tongue, what would it be? Why?
10. What is your favorite dessert?
11. Name one comfort food.
12. If you could have free tickets to any event, what would you choose?
13. Name a favorite book or movie. Why is it a favorite?
14. Did you ever go on a blind date? What was it like?
15. If you could live anyplace in the world, where would it be? Why?
16. Name one personal characteristic you would like to have.
17. Have you ever had a mentor? If so, share one thing you learned from this person. If not, what would you look for in a mentor?
18. If you found a $20 bill and could not find its owner, what would you do with it?
19. How many different states have you lived in? Name them.
20. If you could have any career, assuming you already had the education and preparation, what would it be?
21. Are you a detail person or a big picture person? How has this affected your work?
22. Do you think to talk or talk to think? How does this affect the way you work with other staff in your department?
23. What is your favorite kind of weather? Why?
24. What do you see yourself doing if you retire?
25. What is one question you would like to ask the top administrator of this organization? Why?

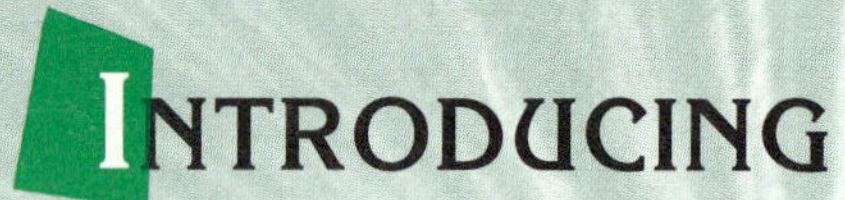

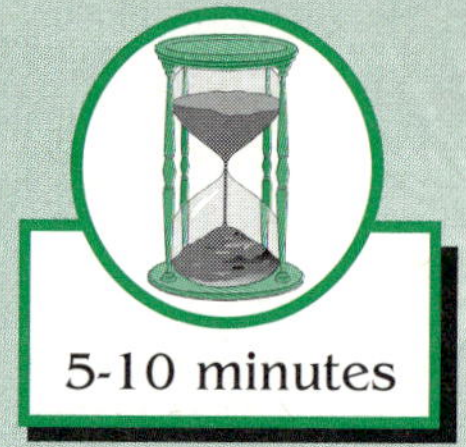

The Real Me

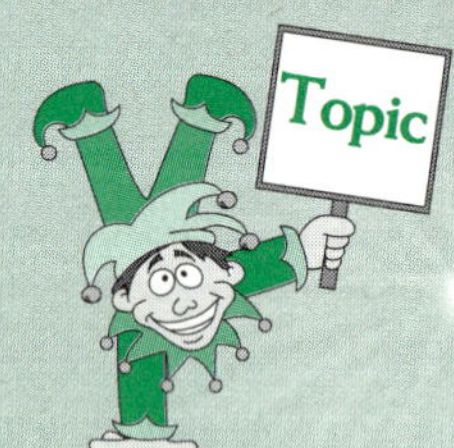

Use this after people have worked together to learn something new.

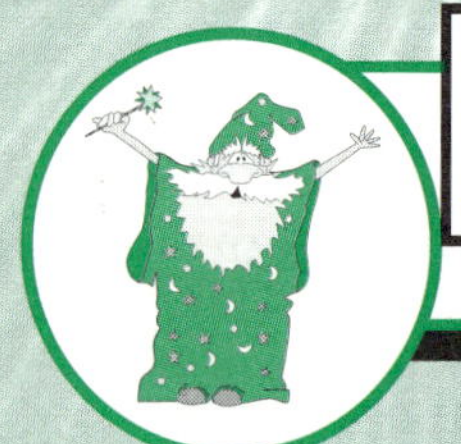

Wizard List

A collection of toys and objects, such as hats, sports equipment, and plastic flowers—the wilder the better.

Preparation

1. Collect garage-sale type items. Involve staff by asking them several days before the meeting to bring in various items to use.
2. Arrange the collected items on a table at the entrance to the meeting room.

Implementation

1. As team members enter the meeting room, ask each to choose an item that represents something about them that they will share and take into the meeting room with them.
2. Ask team members to introduce themselves and explain why they chose the object. (For example, one person chose a roller skate and said she felt like she needed skates to get all her work done.)

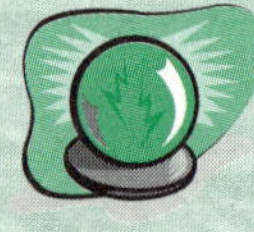

Debriefing

Explain that this activity is a way to get to know one another, have a bit of fun, and energize the group.

Magic Touch

Challenge the team members. Assign any object to each team member or have them draw out of a hat one of many objects listed on small pieces of paper. Instruct the team members to explain how their object represents something about them.

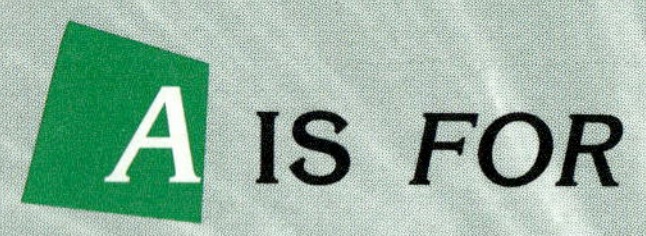

A IS FOR

. . . Wait a Minute . . . I GOT IT—*A* is for Armadillo

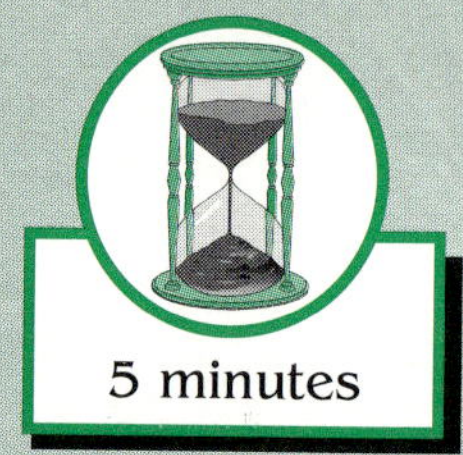

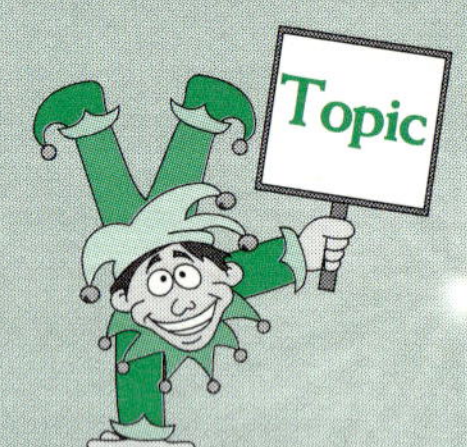

A challenge. Use to distract from stress before a meeting.

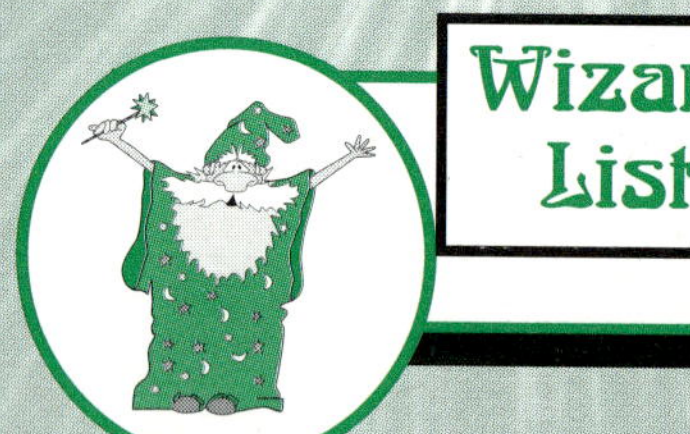

Wizard List

"*A* Is For" category examples, flip chart, markers

Preparation

1. Choose a category (animals, plants, music, history) and begin to make an alphabetical list of items that fall in the selected category.
2. Review "*A* Is For" category examples.

Implementation

1. Ask team members to clear their minds and get ready to work, because you are going to issue a team challenge.
2. Introduce the specific category and ask that they work as a team to come up with at least one item related to the identified category beginning with each letter of the alphabet as quickly as possible.
3. Ask for a volunteer to be scribe at the flip chart and get started!
4. Post the flip chart sheet, leaving any letters blank that the team could not fill, and request that additions be made during breaks or at the end of the meeting.

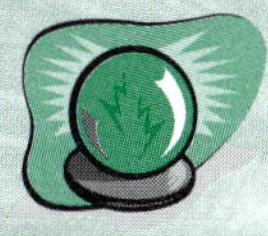

Debriefing

Ask if they enjoyed the activity. Ask if it took their minds off the stressors of the day, the intent of the exercise! Ask for a volunteer to come up with a category with which to begin the next meeting, but not to share it until the start of the next meeting.

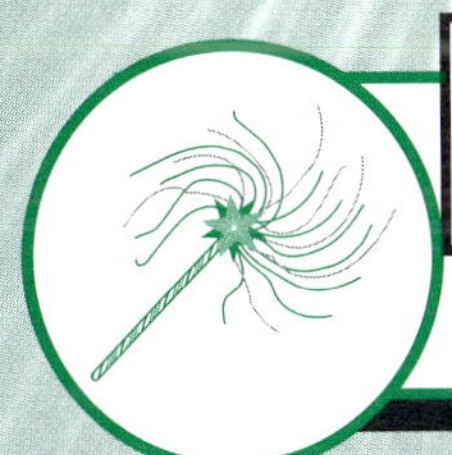

Magic Touch

Mind challenges keep things interesting and allow members to switch from stress-related activity to light-hearted fun.

A IS FOR

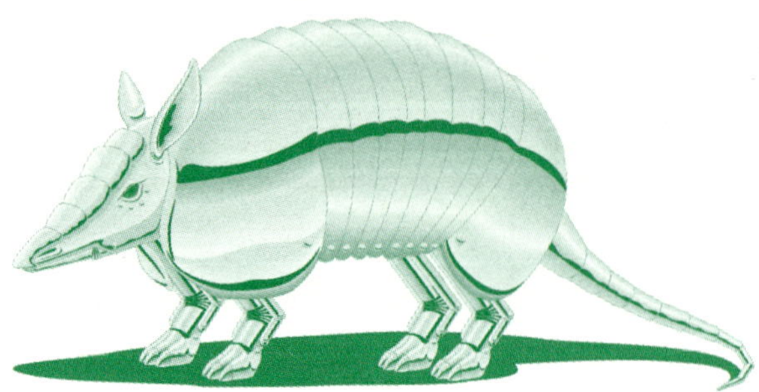

. . . Wait A Minute . . . I Got It . . . A Is For Armadillo

Category Examples

PLANTS

azalea, bamboo, chrysanthemum, daffodil, Easter lily, fern, geranium, hyacinth, iris, jasmine, kalanchoe, lavender, magnolia, narcissus, orchid, palm, quince, rose, scarlet sage, tulip, umbrella plant, violet, wisteria, xerophyte, yucca, zebra plant

ANIMALS

armadillo, baboon, cat, deer, elephant, fox, giraffe, hamster, iguana, jackrabbit, kangaroo, lamb, mouse, newt, otter, parakeet, quail, raccoon, skunk, turtle, unicorn, Vietnamese potbellied pig, walrus, ox (okay, so *x* isn't the first letter), yak, zebra

Just the Facts, Ma'am

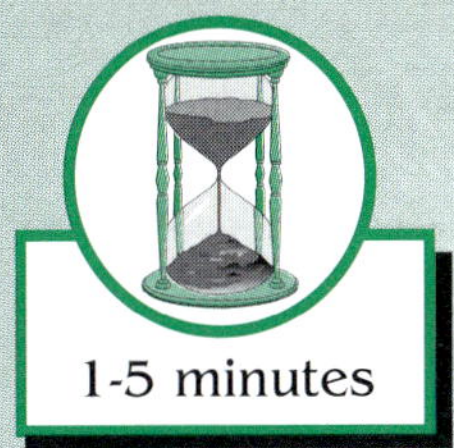

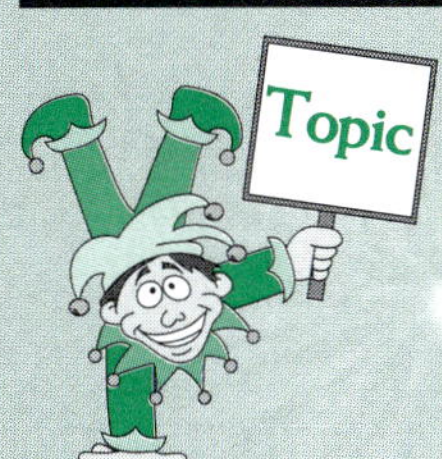

Fun facts. Use just for fun.

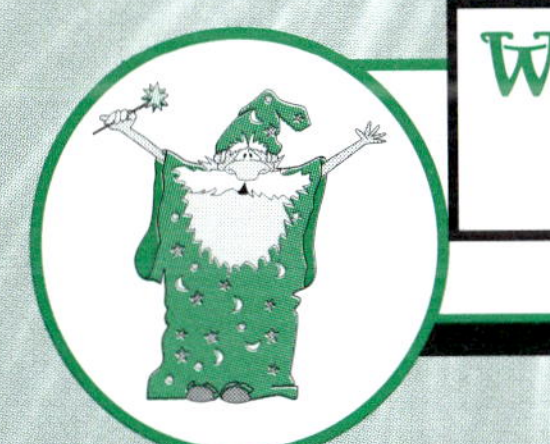

Wizard List "Just the Facts, Ma'am," small prizes

Preparation

1. Review "Just the Facts, Ma'am."
2. Select a question from "Just the Facts, Ma'am" or collect interesting statistics, especially about common events.

Implementation

1. Pose the question at the beginning of the meeting.
2. Give a prize for the correct answer or closest to the correct answer. Give additional prizes if you choose.

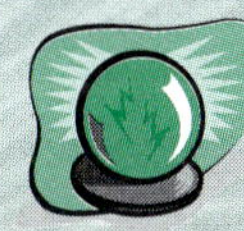

Debriefing

Ask the group for feedback about the exercise. This helps you to see what kind of exercises this team is likely to find energizing. Explain the use of the activity as an energizer.

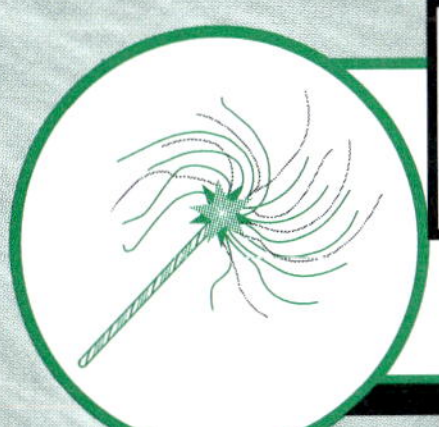

Magic Touch Ask team members to contribute interesting examples that can be added to your collection. Also ask for suggestions of books or sources.

JUST THE FACTS, MA'AM

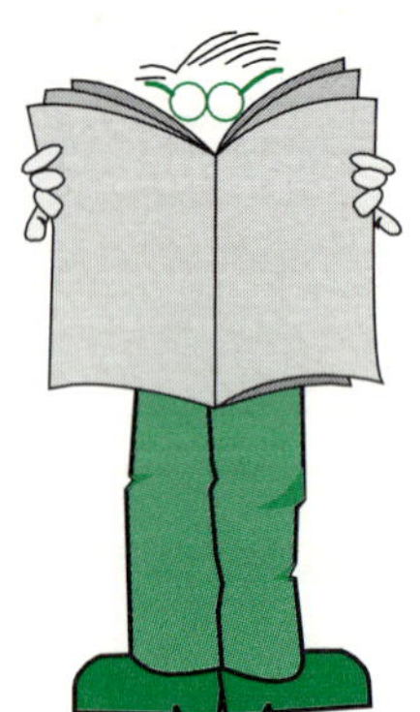

1. How many streets in Atlanta contain the word "Peachtree"? (This statistic came from an American Express ad in the Atlanta, Georgia, airport at the time of the 1996 Olympics.)

    42

2. What percentage of Americans can work a microwave oven?

    58%*

3. What percentage of Americans use ATMs?

    53%*

4. What percentage of Americans report they can use ALL the features of a VCR?

    37%; about the same number say they have no idea how to fix the flashing red light.*

5. What do you really know about fat grams? The good, the not so bad, and the unbelievable†:

    How many fat grams are in one soft pretzel ($2\frac{1}{2}$ oz)?

    0 grams

    How many fat grams are in $\frac{1}{16}$ of a 10″ tube (2 oz) of angel food cake?

    0 grams

    How many fat grams are in one fortune cookie?

    0 grams

    How many fat grams are in 3 oz of cooked flounder?

    1 gram

How many fat grams are in three crisp slices of bacon ($^{3}/_{4}$ oz)?

9 grams

How many fat grams are in 14 potato chips (1 oz)?

10 grams

How many fat grams are in $^{1}/_{8}$ of a 9″ one-crust pie?

15 grams

How many fat grams are in one slice of a pepperoni pizza, thin or thick crust ($^{1}/_{12}$ of 14″ to 16″ pie)?

11 grams

How many fat grams are in one reuben sandwich?

51 grams

How many fat grams are in one grilled cheese sandwich?

38 grams

6. What do you know about measurements in cooking?

How many ounces in a cup?

8

How many cups in a pint?

2

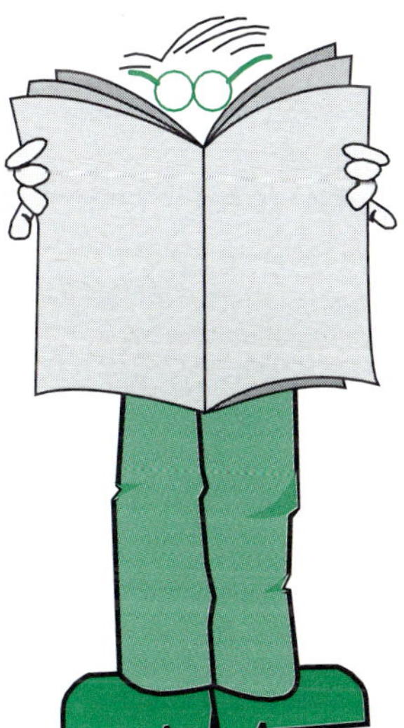

How many pints in a quart?

2

How many quarts in a gallon?

4

How many ounces in a pound?

16

How many teaspoons in a tablespoon?

3

7. In which state did the American Revolution begin?

   Massachusetts[‡]

8. What is the average distance between the earth and the sun?

   93 million miles[‡]

9. Who was the oldest president of the United States?

   Ronald Reagan, at 78 years of age.[‡]

10. Who was the youngest president of the United States?

    Theodore Roosevelt at 42 years of age.[‡]

11. In one day in America[§]:

    How many babies are born?

    10,901

    How much money is spent on health expenditures?

    $2.6 billion ($1.1 billion by the government)

    How many doctor's office visits are made?

    1.87 million

    How many emergency room visits are made?

    256,000

    How many transplants are performed?

    2 lung, 6 heart, 10 liver, and 29 kidney transplants

    How many fishing licenses are purchased?

    104,000

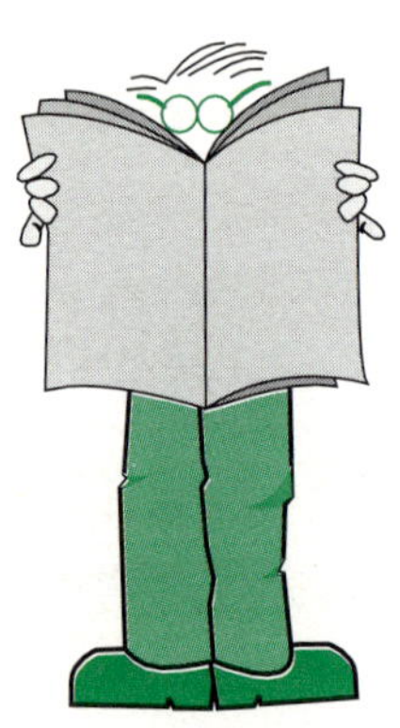

* Kanner, B. *Are You Normal?* New York, 1995, St. Martin.
† Weight Watchers, Fat and Fiber, 1996, Weight Watchers International.
‡ World Almanac Books. *The World Almanac for Kids.* Mahwah, NJ, 1996, World Almanac.
§ *The Washington Post,* I Jan 1996, A17; from Statistical Abstract of the United States, 1996.

A TISKET, A TASKET

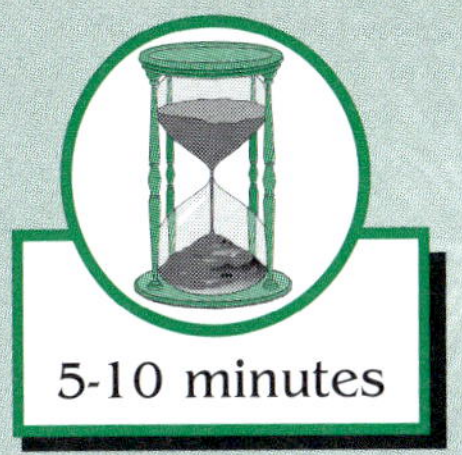

Who Makes the Basket?

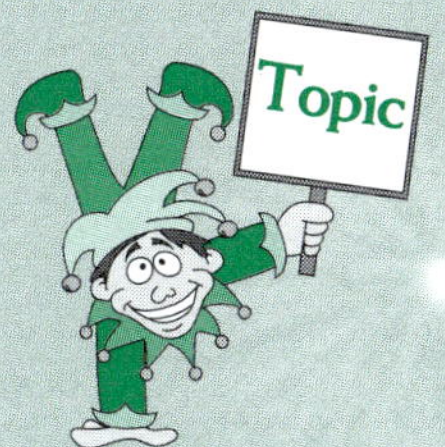

Use for physical stress relief.

Wizard List Toy basketball and hoop or an 8″ ball and a small trash can, a whistle, watch with a second hand, "The Best Rebounder," "The Best Timekeeper," "The Best Scorekeeper," "For Participation with Merit," small prizes

Preparation

1. Set up the basketball hoop before the meeting, and try it out to make sure it will stay attached. These usually have a suction cup. Be cautious about using a painted wall, because the suction cup may leave a mark—not politically correct! (A small 8″ ball and a small trash can big enough for the ball to be thrown into can be used as a substitute.)
2. Bring a whistle and watch with a second hand.
3. Purchase small prizes, such as Cracker Jack, Tootsie Roll Pops, gum, or small packages of peanuts. You can use prizes or the certificates provided with this exercise, or both.
4. Make one copy each of "The Best Rebounder," "The Best Timekeeper," "The Best Scorekeeper," and as many copies as necessary of "For Participation with Merit."

Implementation

1. Ask if there are any ringers in the group; who are the pros? Invite the group to come out and play.
2. Explain that we are going to shoot a few hoops just for fun and that you know they are secretly dying to try it!

3. Ask who is willing to try, and explain that there *might* be prizes involved!
4. Ask nonparticipants to keep track of scores, to keep track of time, to retrieve balls, and so forth. Try to get everyone involved.
5. Ask the group to choose 30 seconds or 1 minute for the time each team member is allowed to shoot.
6. Use the whistle to start and stop the exercise. The whistle can also be used as a reminder that a team member's turn has ended.
7. Tally the scores.
8. Announce the winners. Each person places. Award prizes. Award suggestions: 1st, 2nd, 3rd place and the rest honorable mentions so that all are winners. Announce awards for "Participation with Merit" for helpers so that all get awards.

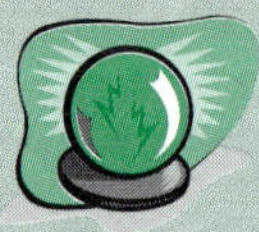

Debriefing

So many activities are cerebral, or at least sedentary. Use a physical activity for a change or in the middle of a meeting when an energizing break seems needed.

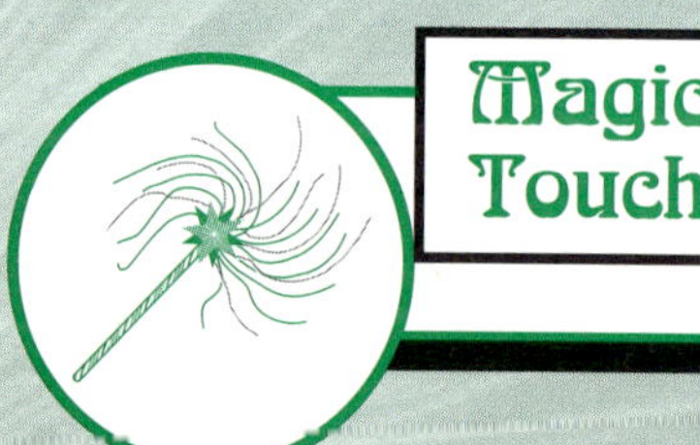

Magic Touch

For added fun, choose teams. For a personal touch, design your own certificates.

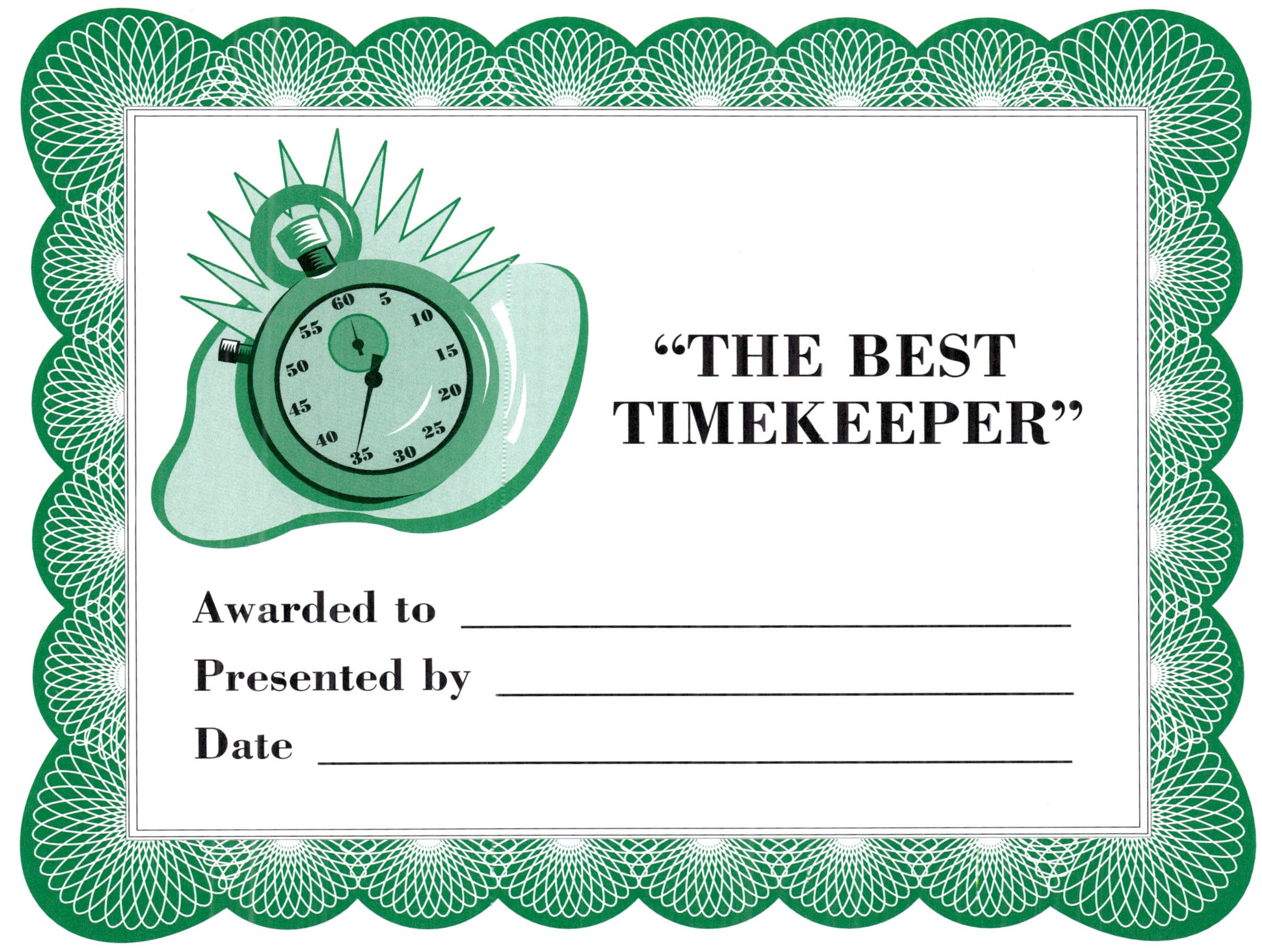
"THE BEST
TIMEKEEPER"
Awarded to
Presented by
Date

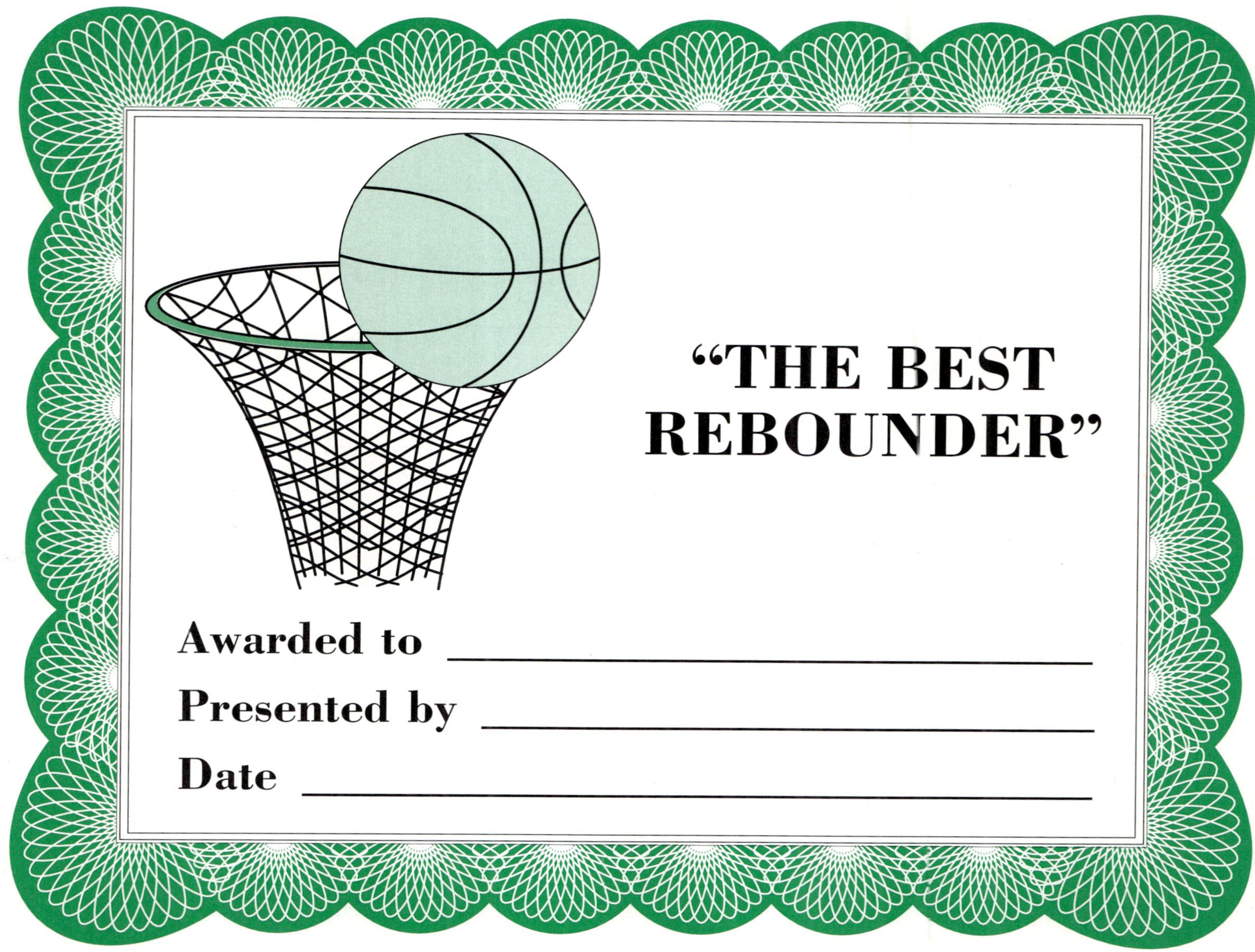

"THE BEST
REBOUNDER"
Awarded to
Presented by
Date

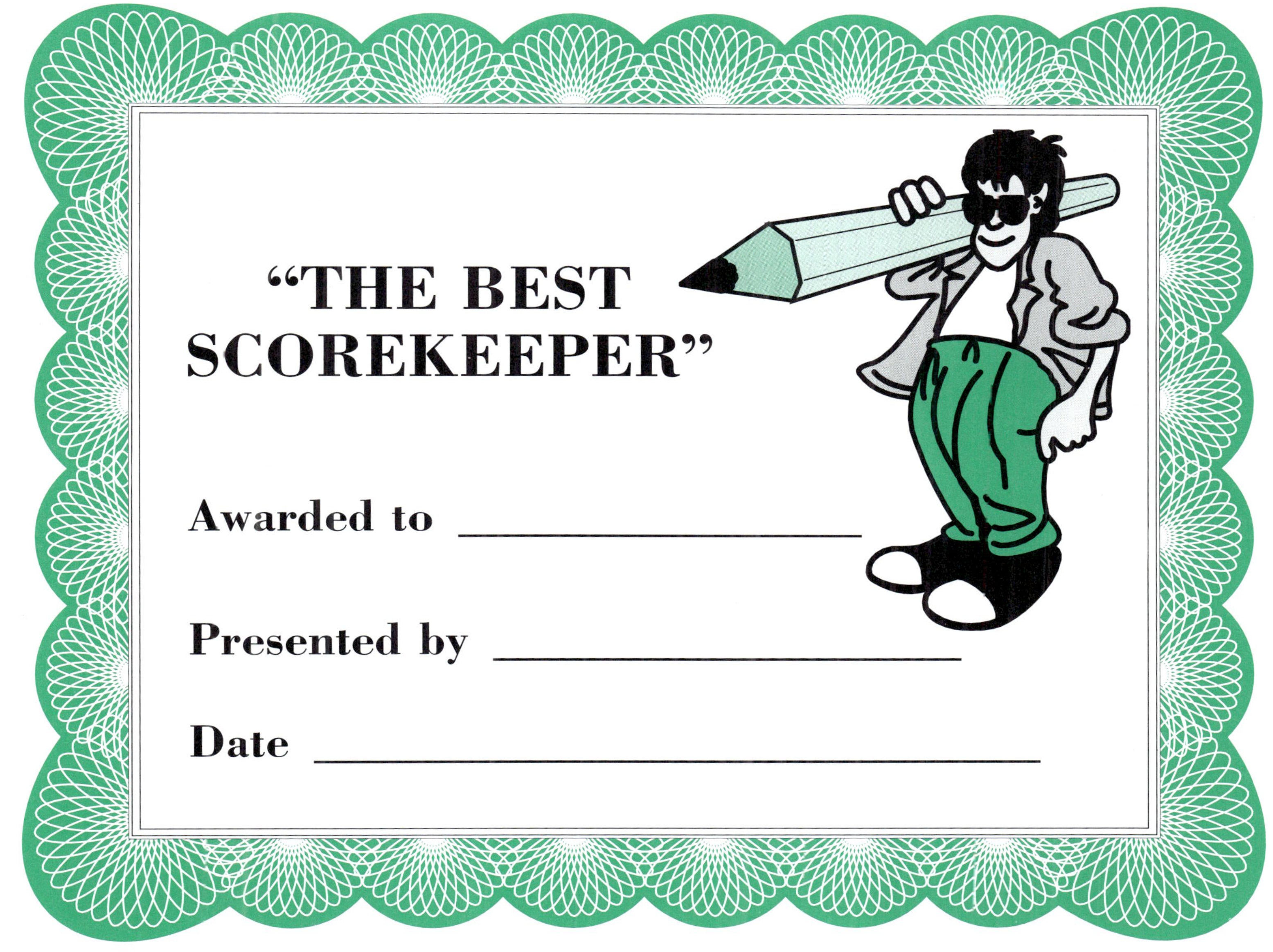
"THE BEST
SCOREKEEPER"
Awarded to
Presented by
Date

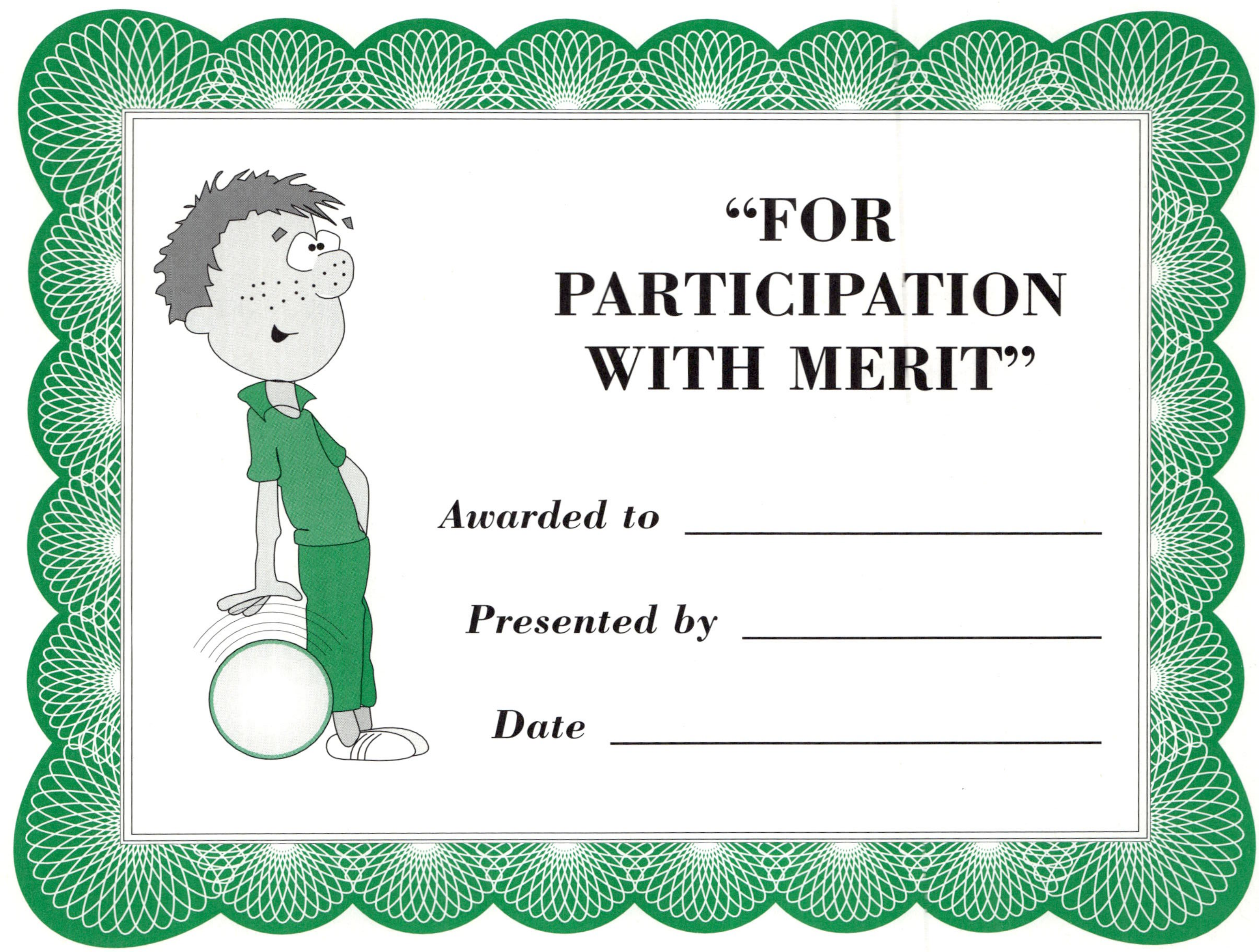
"FOR
PARTICIPATION
WITH MERIT"
Awarded to
Presented by
Date

IN THE NEWS TODAY

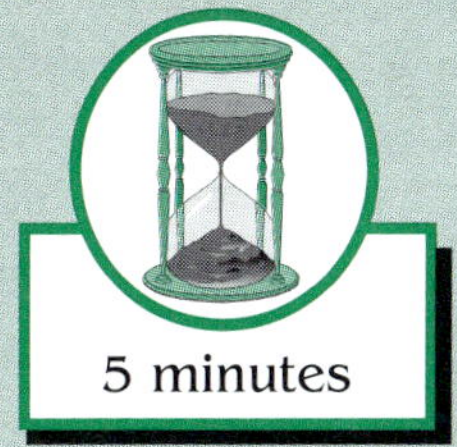

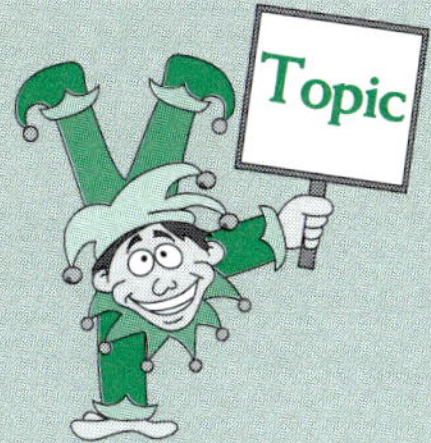

No work-related events. Use this to distract from stress before meeting and add perspective.

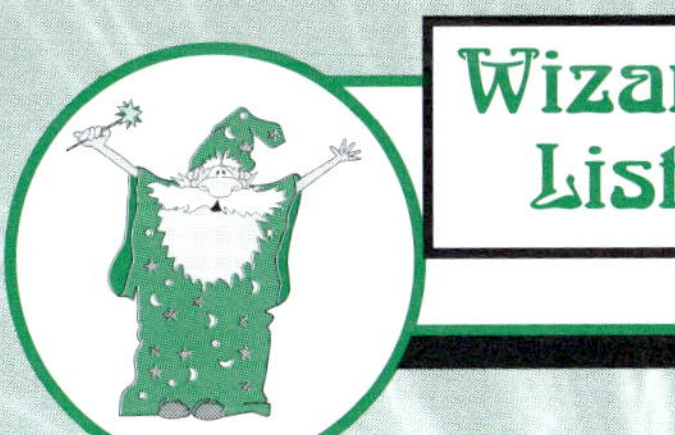

Wizard List

Today's newspaper

Preparation

1. Provide today's newspaper.
2. Make sure you have enough sections for each member in your group.

Implementation

1. Explain that to start the meeting each person is to choose a section of the newspaper and select one headline, the slogan of an advertisement, or a cartoon to read to the group; they should be prepared to share their comments on their selections with the group.
2. Ask for comments on the events reported.

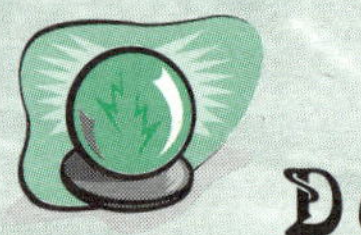

Debriefing

Explain that sometimes we get so caught up in our own world that we forget the big picture, that there is a world outside our work.

Magic Touch

It is interesting to see what team members select and how they react. Do they select something of interest to them? Something they do not usually read? Something positive?

SOMETHING TO THINK ABOUT

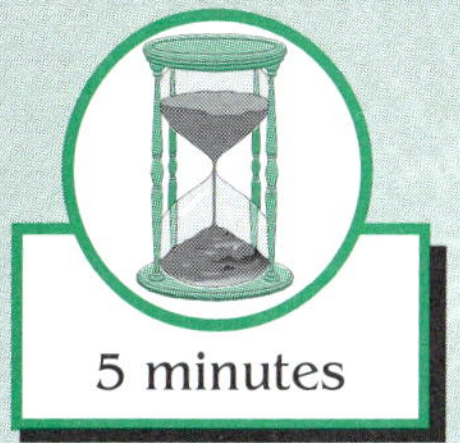

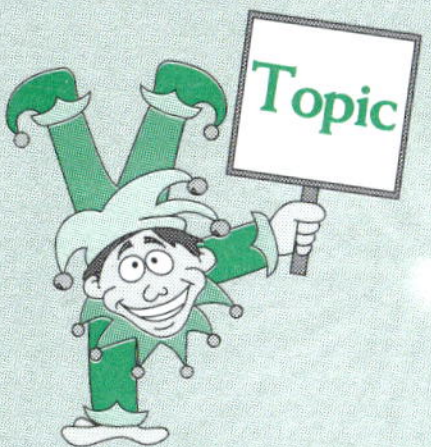

Motivational thoughts. Use this for stress relief and to add perspective.

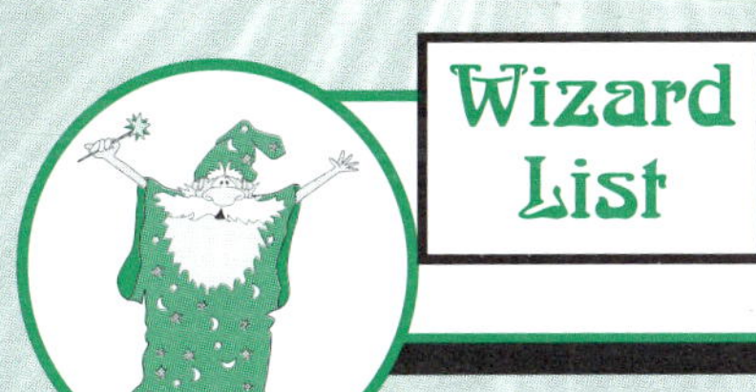

Wizard List

Motivational quotations, magic wand (optional)

Preparation

1. The week before this exercise is to be used, ask each member to bring in a favorite quotation that is personally motivating to share.
2. Bring at least one quick-to-read book of motivational quotes as backup!
3. Remind members of the assignment to bring a favorite quotation by including it on the agenda if the agenda is sent out before the meeting, or remind team members on voice mail or E-mail. (If you have access to voice mail or E-mail, make a mailing list so that it is easy to send a message to all team members at the same time. The wonder of technology!)

Implementation

1. Ask who has brought a quotation to share.
2. Pass around one or several books for people who did not bring one.
3. Ask team members to choose one they will share and note the page number so other team members can use the book, if needed.

4. Ask each person to share one quotation.
5. Generate discussion about the philosophy shared.

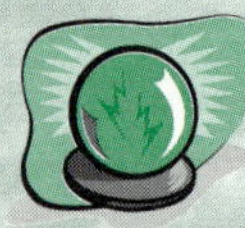

Debriefing

Explain that sometimes seemingly simple truths are, in fact, not so simple, that other people's words of wisdom may be helpful to focus our perspective on the events around us.

Magic Touch

Hand the magic wand to the first team member to share a quotation, and ask that each time a new quotation is shared the magic wand be passed to that team member. Here are some book suggestions: *Live and Learn and Pass It On,* by H. Jackson Brown, Jr., Nashville, Tenn, 1992, Rutledge Hill Press; *Great Quotes from Great Women,* Lombard, Ill, 1984, Great Quotations; *The Soul Would Have No Rainbow if the Eyes Had No Tears and Other Native American Proverbs,* by Guy Zona, New York, 1994, Simon & Schuster; *The House of the Heart Is Never Full and Other Proverbs of Africa,* by Guy Zona, New York, 1993, Simon & Schuster.

PLANT A SEED

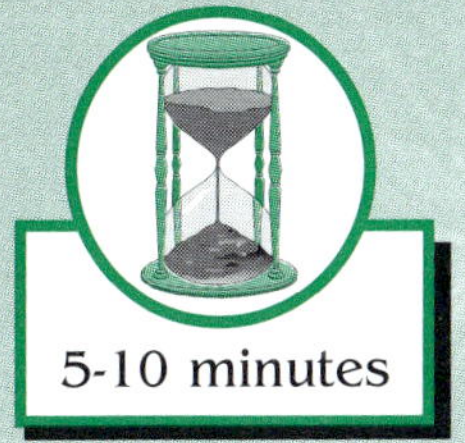

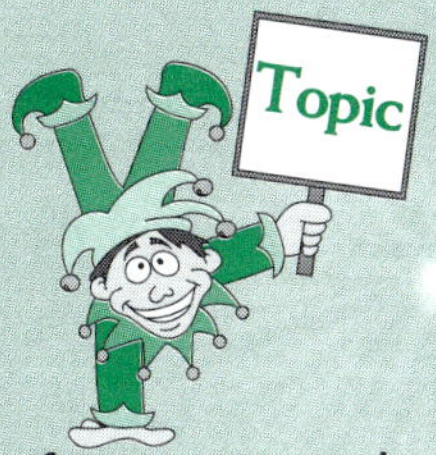

Growth. Use to refocus on ingredients of team work.

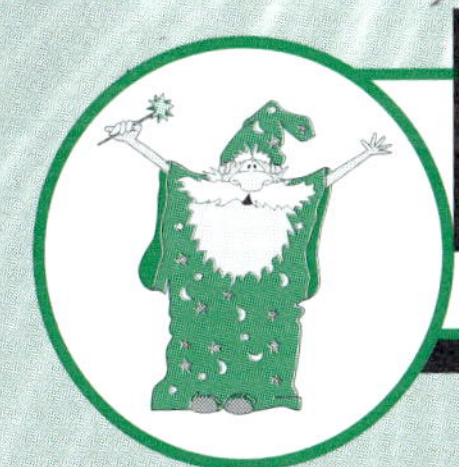

Wizard List

Blooming plant, flowerpot, index cards, pens or pencils

Preparation

1. Provide a blooming plant.
2. Provide an index card for each team member.
3. Provide an empty flowerpot.
4. Provide pens or pencils for each team member.

Implementation

1. Ask the team what it takes to make a plant grow and bloom (light, water, good soil, plant food).
2. Distribute index cards and pen or pencil to each team member.
3. Ask team members to write on the cards what the ingredients are to make the team grow and produce good outcomes. Ask them to sign the card.
4. Collect the cards in an empty flowerpot.
5. Ask for a volunteer to read aloud the ingredients listed on each card, but not the name.
6. Place the cards in the empty flowerpot, and draw a name. Voilà! The winner of the plant!

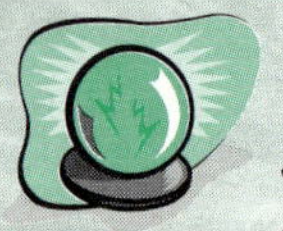

Debriefing

Contributing to the team can pay off!

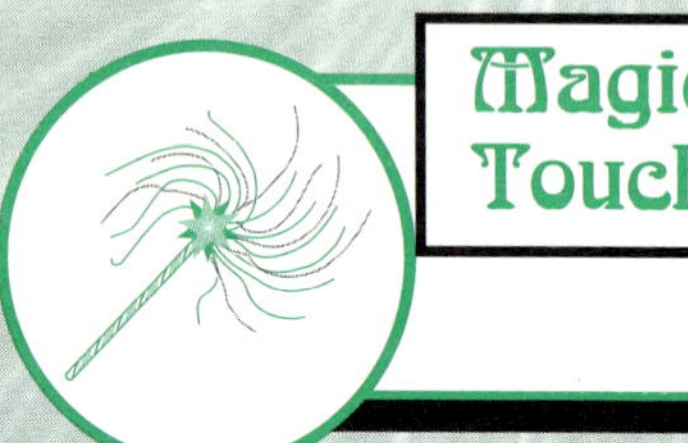

Magic Touch

Variation: For large groups, provide two plants and draw a second name. Be creative—hand paint the flowerpot(s).

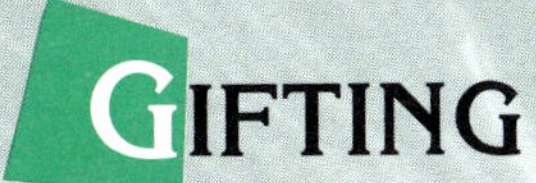

GIFTING

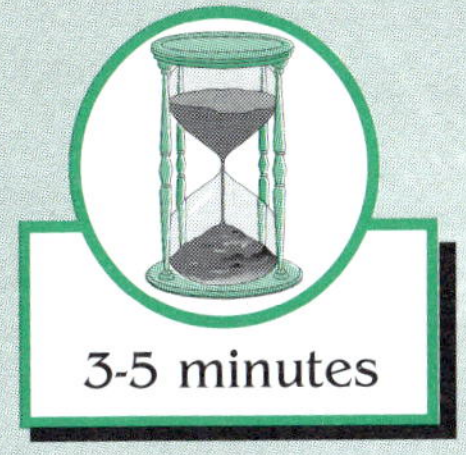

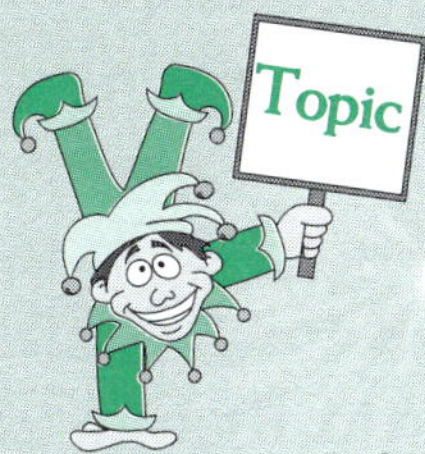

A creative refresher. Use this to refocus on team work.

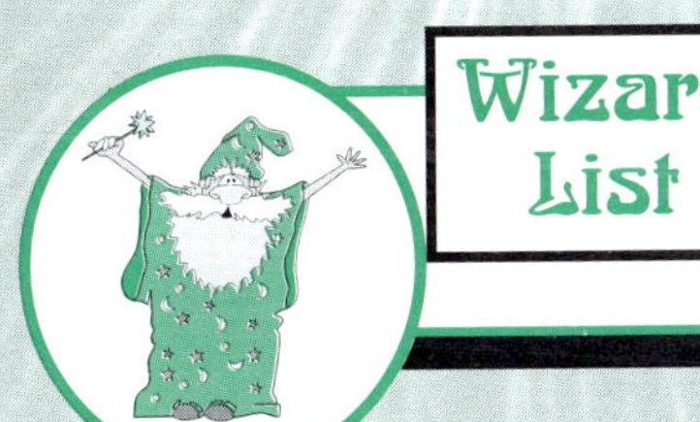

Wizard List "The Custom of Gifting," extra gifts

Preparation

1. Review "The Custom of Gifting."
2. Distribute "The Custom of Gifting" via agenda, E-mail, voice mail.
3. Establish a voting plan to select the "gifting day." This should take place at a meeting before the gifting meeting.

Implementation

1. Have each member place his or her gift on a table at the front of the meeting room.
2. Ask each member to select a gift in order of first to last birthday in the year.
3. Have members unwrap their presents one at a time, and ask the donor to identify himself or herself and ask why this gift was chosen and to share any special meaning it might have.

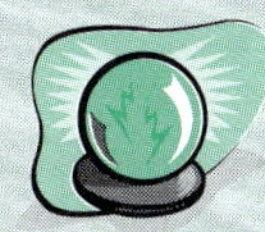

Debriefing

Initiate a discussion of how this activity went, what it was like to choose a gift, what it was like to give it, what it was like to receive it, and what applications they might see for their own department. Mention that giving is easier for some people than receiving. Add that giving gifts can be a bit of fun to energize the group, giving them something to figure out and something that they can look forward to in the meeting. Conclude that the work of the team can be seen as a gift to the organization and that this view may be a way to reframe staff's views of being asked to participate on a team.

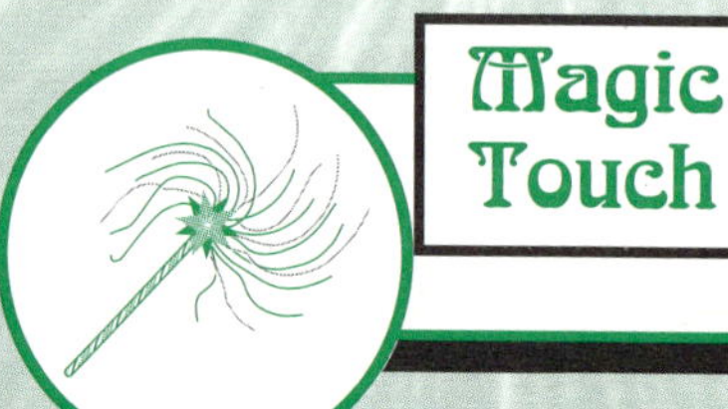

Magic Touch

Bring several extra gifts to make sure each member gets one.

Adapted from: Innovation Thinking Network Conference, attended by Deanna Berg.

THE CUSTOM OF GIFTING

Presenting visitors and friends with small tokens of esteem and friendship is an old Russian custom. Borrowing on the flavor of this tradition, one group at a conference on creativity adopted the custom. They selected gifts that were representative of the participants themselves, or of the companies where they worked. Participants chose a variety of objects, such as key chains, small toys, pins, pens, or novelty items. In addition, participants could write a poem or share a favorite cartoon, quotation, or compliment. The group reported feeling awkward at first, but soon got the hang of it. They gave a gift whenever it seemed appropriate.

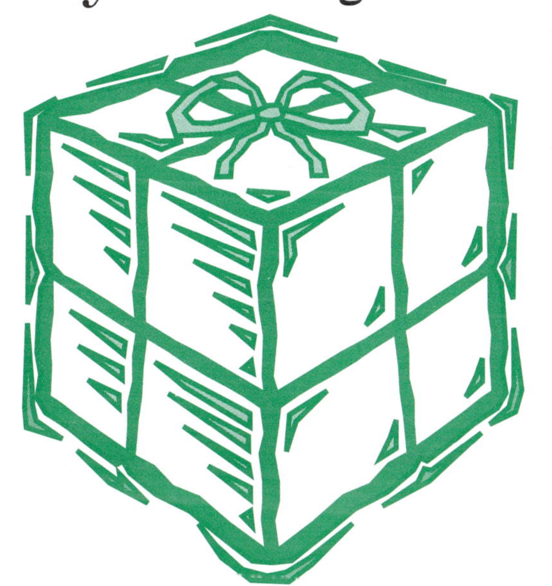

We are requesting that our team try this activity as a way to honor our work together. Although it is not necessary for each member to participate, we are encouraging your participation. Think about when it would be a good time to give gifts, and we will vote at the next team meeting.

JUST BREATHE!

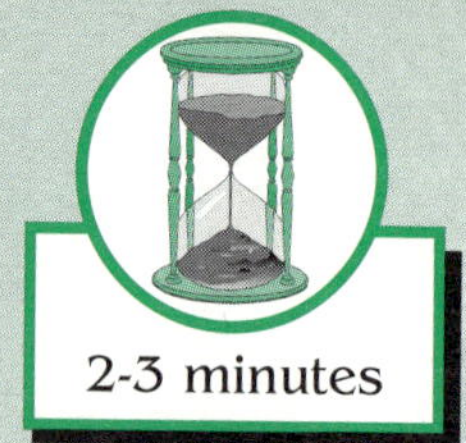

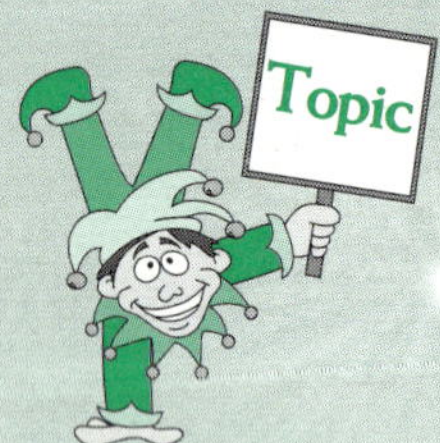

Simple exercise. Use to refocus the team and provide stress relief.

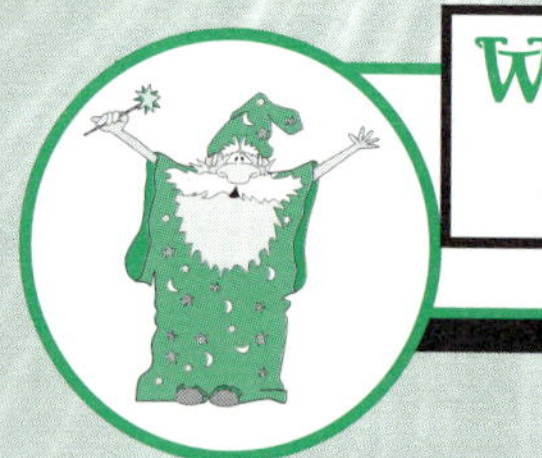

Wizard List

No supplies needed, magic wand (optional)

Preparation

None.

Implementation

1. Explain that you would like to demonstrate a simple technique to relieve tension. We can assume most people are struggling to deal with stress and would welcome a new technique or a refresher if this is familiar.
2. Demonstrate abdominal breathing.
   a. Close your eyes to relax more.
   b. Begin to breathe deeply.
   c. Breathe in through your nose. Your stomach goes in and gets flatter as you exhale.
   d. Breathe out through your mouth. Your stomach goes out and extends as you inhale.
3. Ask the team members to try one or two deep breaths.
4. Suggest that they close their eyes and take ten slow, deep abdominal breaths.
5. Ask for feedback about how they feel now compared to before the exercise.

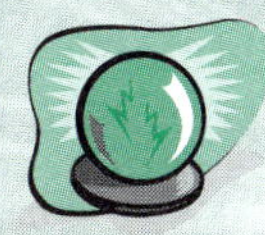

Debriefing

Some people will say they are more relaxed or calm. Others will report feeling light-headed. If no one says this, mention it. Most of us are used to shallow breathing. Explain that more oxygen to the brain promotes better problem solving.

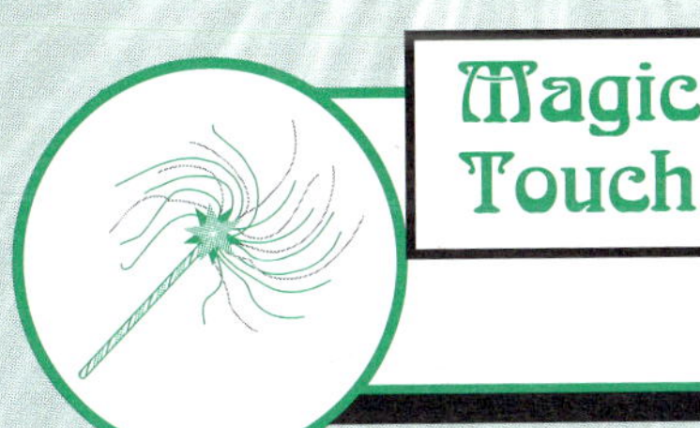

Magic Touch

Add some magic to this simple exercise. Use your magic wand to direct the timing of the breathing pattern.

SHARING SUCCESS

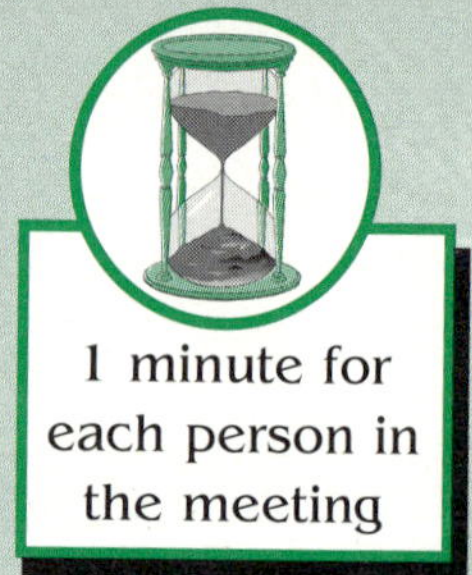

1 minute for each person in the meeting

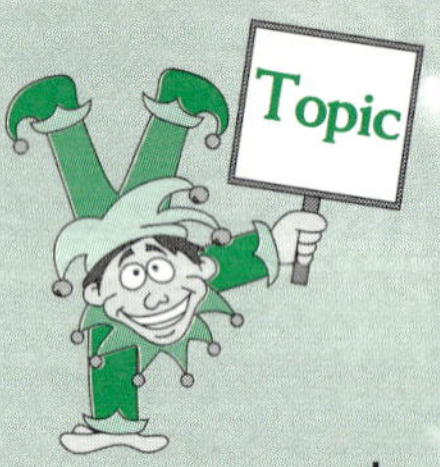

Direction. Use this to refocus on teamwork.

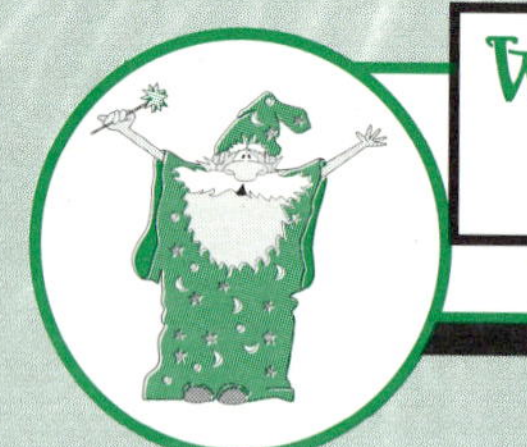

Wizard List

No supplies needed

Preparation

None.

Implementation

1. Ask members to think about a goal they have set in their lives that they have met.
2. Give each person one minute to talk about his or her goal.

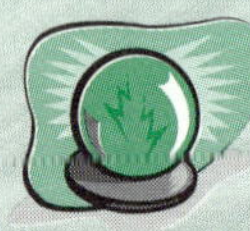

Debriefing

Ask for feedback about the exercise. Explain that sharing our successes creates a positive atmosphere for starting a meeting where success is the goal.

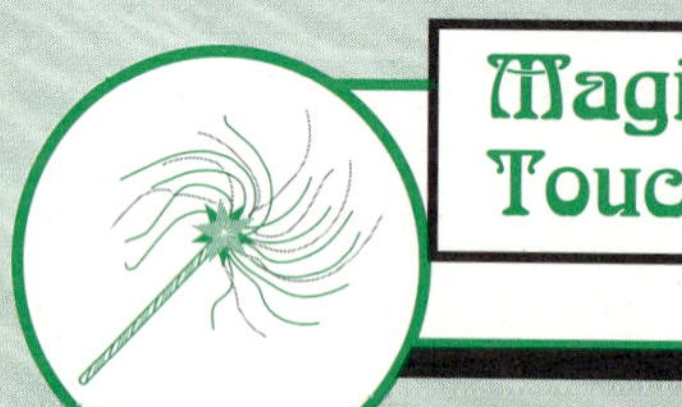

Magic Touch

State: "If you don't know where you are going, anywhere will do."

A CAPITAL IDEA!

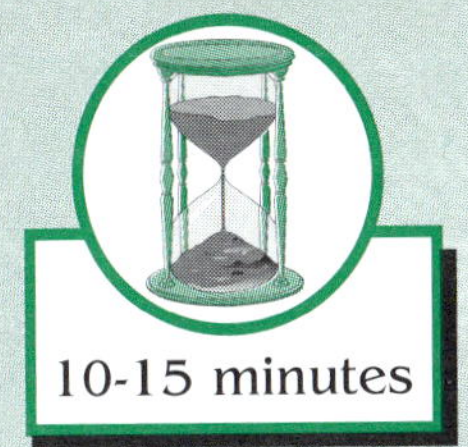

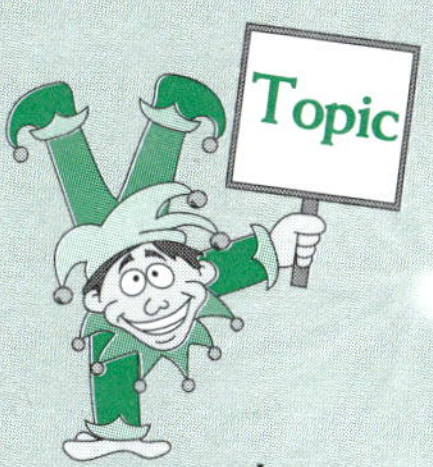

Use to refocus attention and to stress the importance of teamwork.

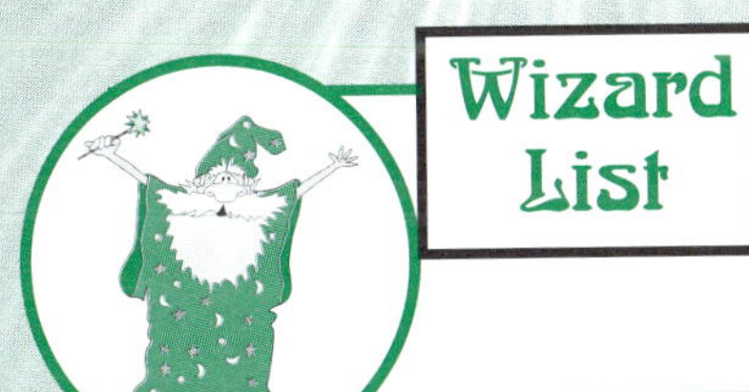

Wizard List

"A Capital Quiz" questionnaire, "A Capital Quiz" answer key, whistle, pens or pencils, small prizes (optional)

Preparation

1. Copy "A Capital Quiz" questionnaire for each team member.
2. Use the "A Capital Quiz" answer key to prepare a transparency, or enlarge the answer key and place it on a flip chart.
3. Provide pens or pencils for each team member. (If possible, select decorated pencils and make these your giveaway prize.)
4. Obtain small prizes such as small erasers or decorated pencils for each team member (optional).

Implementation

1. Explain that you are going to ask each team member to try this "A Capital Quiz" with one other person. Ask the group to divide into pairs.
2. Distribute "A Capital Quiz" and pens or pencils. Blow the whistle to start. Mention there might be prizes involved! Allow 2 to 3 minutes.
3. Blow the whistle and ask the group to combine efforts with another group. Allow 2 more minutes. Blow the whistle to stop the exercise.

4. Display the "A Capital Quiz" answer key, and allow team members to check their own papers.
5. Distribute prizes, if the pencils distributed were not the giveaway.

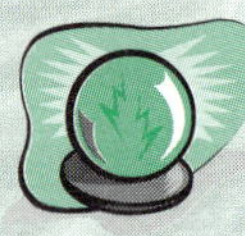

Debriefing

Ask for initial reactions to the quiz. ("Oh, no! I really am being asked about those capitals.") Consider how difficult this might be for someone from a different country who did not learn these as a child in school. Ask members to contrast working alone to working with another team member. What happend when additional brain power was added to the task? Relate this to the benefit of working in teams.

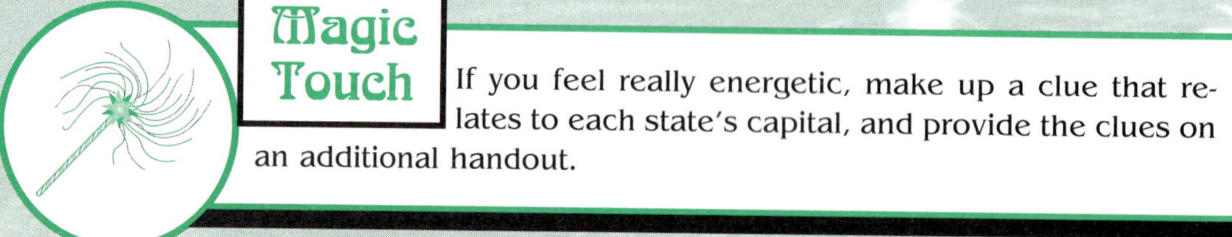

Magic Touch If you feel really energetic, make up a clue that relates to each state's capital, and provide the clues on an additional handout.

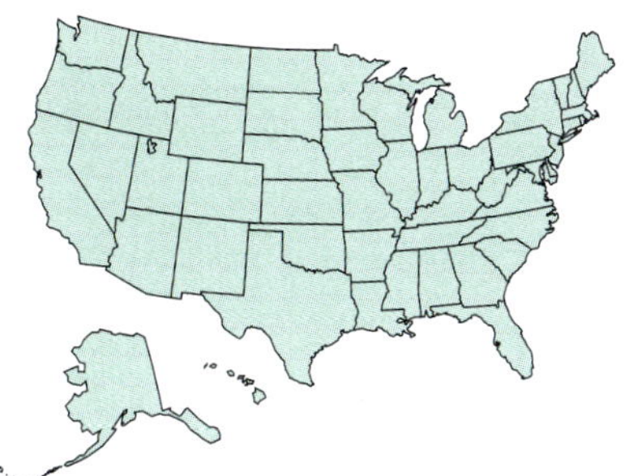

A CAPITAL QUIZ

Questionnaire

STATE	CAPITAL
1. Alabama	________
2. Alaska	________
3. Arizona	________
4. Arkansas	________
5. California	________
6. Colorado	________
7. Connecticut	________
8. Delaware	________
9. Florida	________
10. Georgia	________
11. Hawaii	________
12. Idaho	________
13. Illinois	________
14. Indiana	________
15. Iowa	________
16. Kansas	________
17. Kentucky	________
18. Louisana	________
19. Maine	________
20. Maryland	________
21. Massachusetts	________
22. Michigan	________
23. Minnesota	________
24. Mississippi	________
25. Missouri	________

STATE	CAPITAL
26. Montana	________
27. Nebraska	________
28. Nevada	________
29. New Hampshire	________
30. New Jersey	________
31. New Mexico	________
32. New York	________
33. North Carolina	________
34. North Dakota	________
35. Ohio	________
36. Oklahoma	________
37. Oregon	________
38. Pennsylvania	________
39. Rhode Island	________
40. South Carolina	________
41. South Dakota	________
42. Tennessee	________
43. Texas	________
44. Utah	________
45. Vermont	________
46. Virginia	________
47. Washington	________
48. West Virginia	________
49. Wisconsin	________
50. Wyoming	________

A CAPITAL QUIZ

Answer Key

	STATE	CAPITAL
1.	Alabama	Montgomery
2.	Alaska	Juneau
3.	Arizona	Phoenix
4.	Arkansas	Little Rock
5.	California	Sacramento
6.	Colorado	Denver
7.	Connecticut	Hartford
8.	Delaware	Dover
9.	Florida	Tallahassee
10.	Georgia	Atlanta
11.	Hawaii	Honolulu
12.	Idaho	Boise
13.	Illinois	Springfield
14.	Indiana	Indianapolis
15.	Iowa	Des Moines
16.	Kansas	Topeka
17.	Kentucky	Frankfort
18.	Louisana	Baton Rouge
19.	Maine	Augusta
20.	Maryland	Annapolis
21.	Massachusetts	Boston
22.	Michigan	Lansing
23.	Minnesota	St. Paul
24.	Mississippi	Jackson
25.	Missouri	Jefferson City

	STATE	CAPITAL
26.	Montana	Helena
27.	Nebraska	Lincoln
28.	Nevada	Carson City
29.	New Hampshire	Concord
30.	New Jersey	Trenton
31.	New Mexico	Santa Fe
32.	New York	Albany
33.	North Carolina	Raleigh
34.	North Dakota	Bismarck
35.	Ohio	Columbus
36.	Oklahoma	Oklahoma City
37.	Oregon	Salem
38.	Pennsylvania	Harrisburg
39.	Rhode Island	Providence
40.	South Carolina	Columbia
41.	South Dakota	Pierre
42.	Tennessee	Nashville
43.	Texas	Austin
44.	Utah	Salt Lake City
45.	Vermont	Montpelier
46.	Virginia	Richmond
47.	Washington	Olympia
48.	West Virginia	Charleston
49.	Wisconsin	Madison
50.	Wyoming	Cheyenne

TINY BUBBLES?

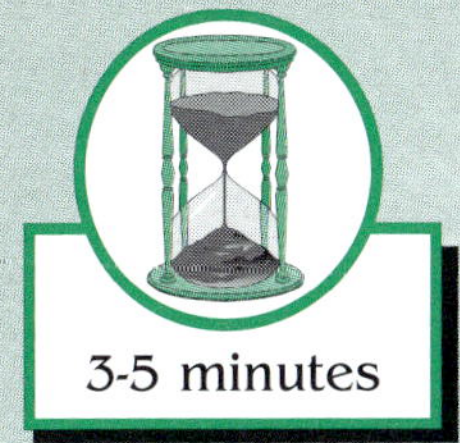

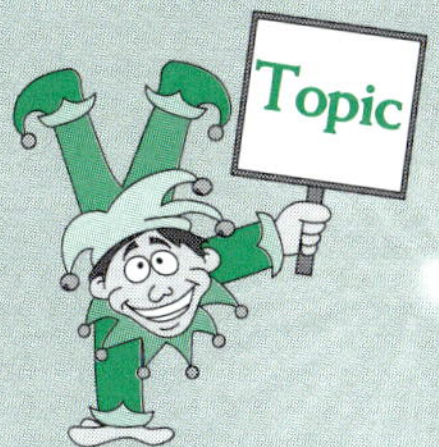

Competition. Use this to start a meeting or when an impasse occurs.

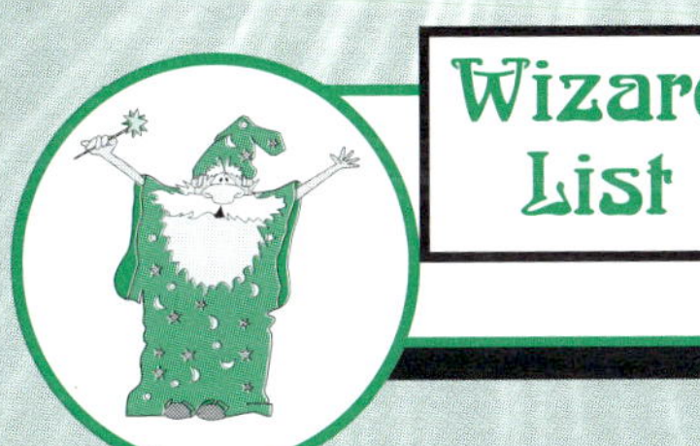

Wizard List

Individually wrapped pieces of bubble gum, several packages of bubble gum, "I Tried" award

Preparation

1. Provide a piece of bubble gum for each team member.
2. Provide packages of bubble gum for prizes.
3. Copy the "I Tried" award.

Implementation

1. Explain to the group that you are going to issue a challenge to them today.
2. Distribute one individually wrapped piece of bubble gum to each team member.
3. Explain that everyone has 30 seconds to see who can make the biggest bubble.
4. Watch carefully so you can give prizes (packages of gum) to the biggest, smallest, first blown bubble, and the "I Tried" award if someone could not blow a bubble.

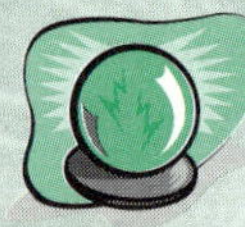

Debriefing

Ask if they liked the activity and tell them a little competition is healthy and there are many ways to win prizes in life!

Magic Touch

Carry bubble gum in your magical team tool kit and share it just for tension relief, as needed! If the group is large, break it into small groups and ask each group to send a representative.

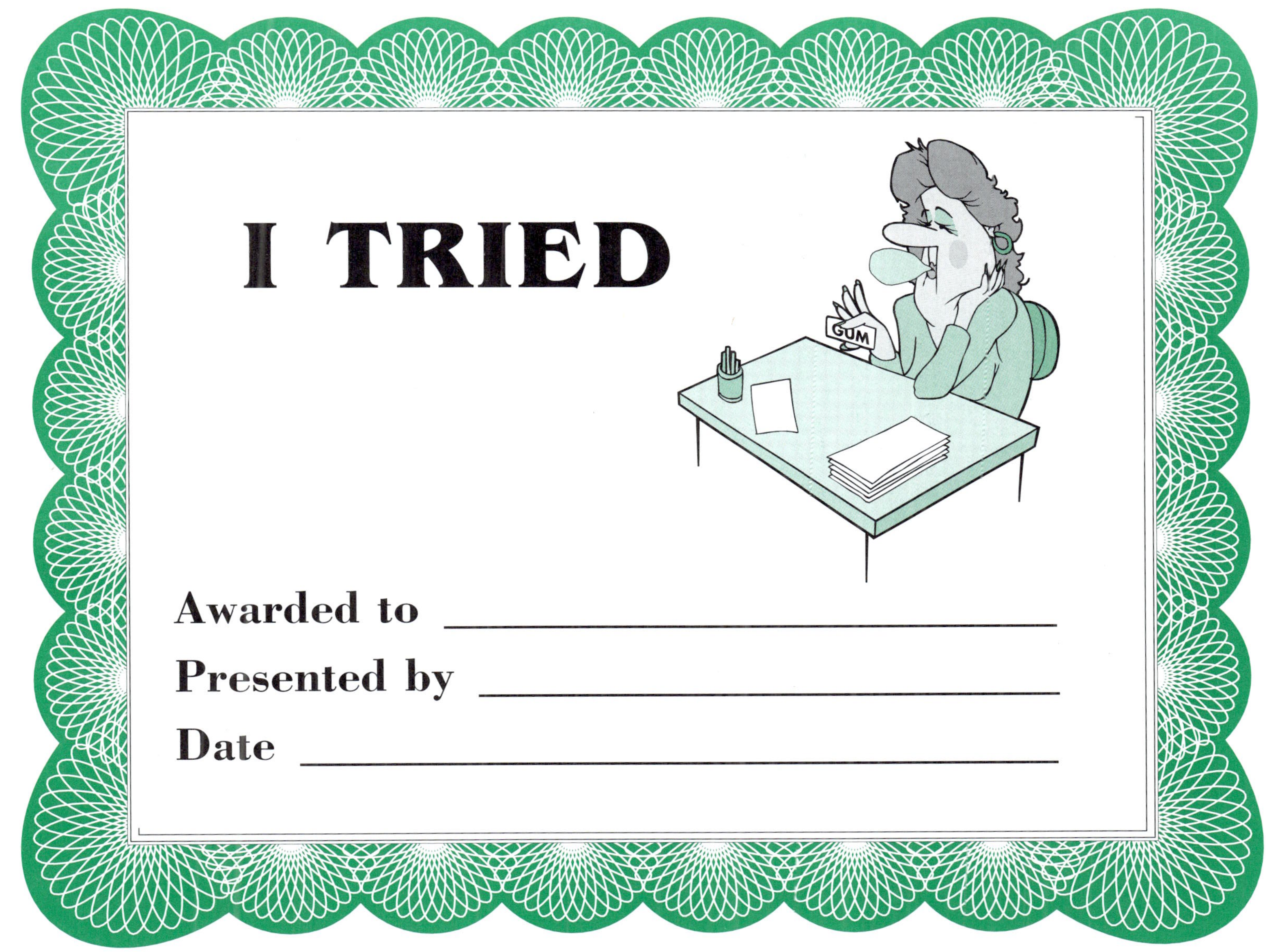

I TRIED

Awarded to ________________

Presented by ________________

Date ________________

DOWN MEMORY LANE

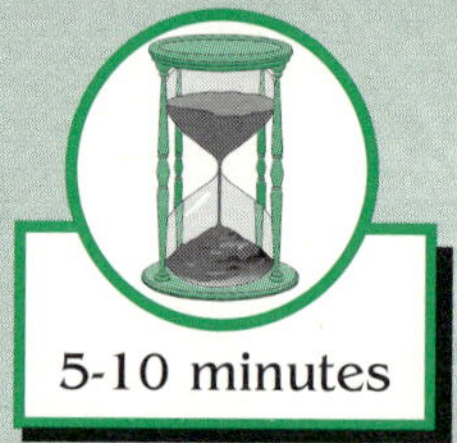

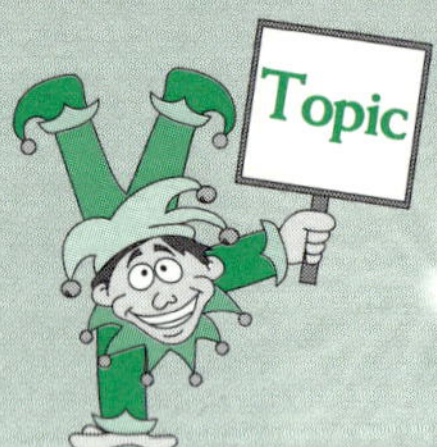

Memory tester. Use when there is an impasse to refocus on team work.

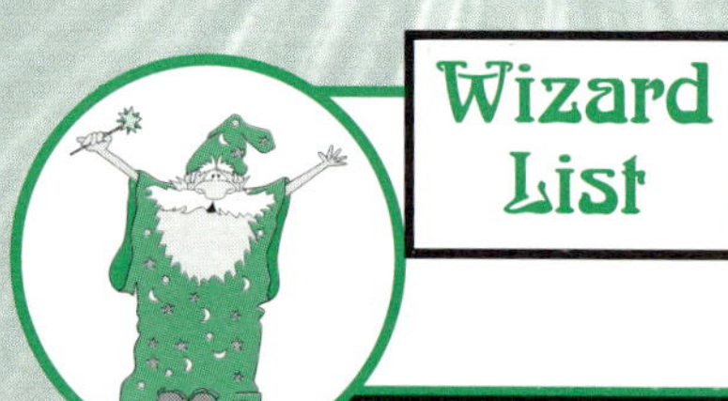

Wizard List

"Memorable Items," paper, pens or pencils, whistle, tray

Preparation

1. Review the "Memorable Item" suggestion list.
2. Select and collect 12 items (all from one category) from the suggestion list, or decide on one of your own.
3. Obtain a serving tray and place the 12 items selected on the tray.
4. Cover the tray with a cloth until ready to begin.

Implementation

1. Ask the team members how good a memory they think they have. (This should evoke some laughter if any of the team members have reached the tender middle years!)
2. Ask the team members if they'd like a test.
3. Distribute paper and pencil or pen to each team member.
4. Explain to the team members that they will be shown a tray of objects for 1 minute. After this, the tray will be covered, and they will have 2 minutes to write down as many items as they can from memory! Announce that you will blow the whistle when the observation time is complete, when they can start writing, and again when time is up.

5. Complete the exercise and ask each team member to count the number of items they have recorded.
6. Remove the cloth from the tray to display the items. Ask members to check their list for accuracy.
7. Announce the winners, give decorated pencils to the winners, and tell the team members they all get prizes for participating. Give out the memo pads to everyone and suggest they use the pads to make lists in case their memory fails them!

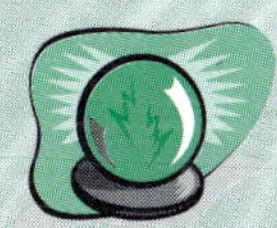

Debriefing

Explain that sometimes we need to test our power of observation to remind us that we can miss even obvious things in the problem-solving journey. This is another illustration of how much more efficient we can be as a team rather than working as individuals.

Magic Touch

To engage team members in the fun and preparation, ask one member to be responsible for bringing 12 items and to keep them a secret! Variation: Choose a theme that represents one or several team members' interests that you know or have learned from working together.

MEMORABLE ITEMS

Suggestion List

FROM THE OFFICE:

- stapler
- staple remover
- tape
- nail clippers
- pencil
- pen
- pad of paper
- hole punch
- box of paper clips
- coffee cup
- highlighter

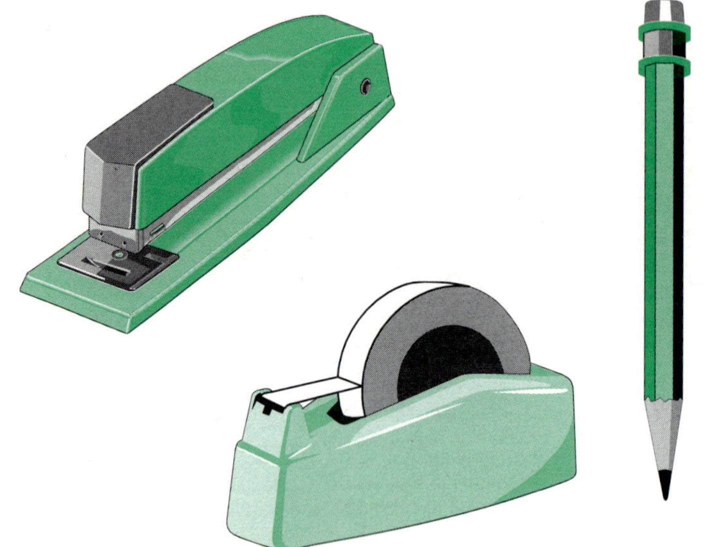

FROM THE KITCHEN:

- measuring cup
- can opener
- wire whisk
- measuring spoons
- spice jar
- spatula
- large spoon
- large fork
- matches
- candle
- trivet
- wine bottle opener
- small strainer

FOR SPORTS FANS:

- golf ball
- whiffle ball
- golf tee
- golf ball marker
- golf glove
- golf towel
- score card
- basketball
- jump rope
- hand weight
- bottle of sports drink
- ball cap

COST-EFFECTIVE, NONINVASIVE, NO-SIDE-EFFECTS STRESS RELIEF!

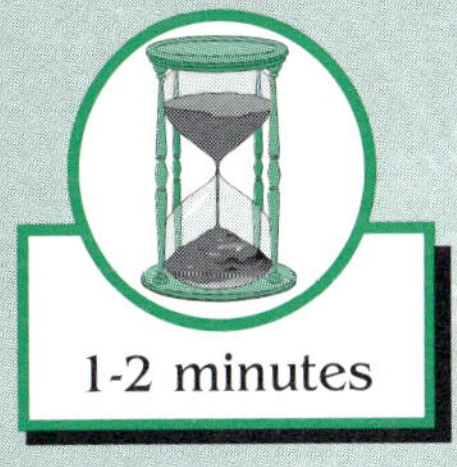

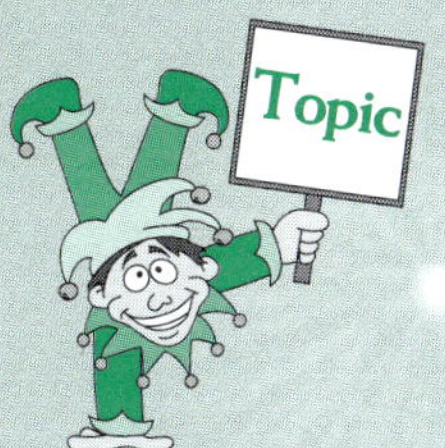

Use for stress relief and fun.

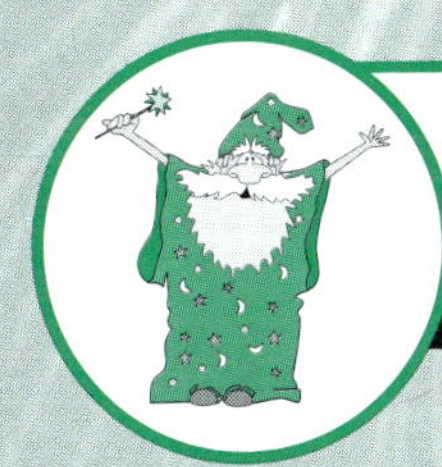

Wizard List Bottle of bubbles, one for each participant (optional)

Preparation

1. Purchase a bottle of bubbles.
2. Purchase a bottle of bubbles for each participant (optional).

Implementation

1. Ask if the group is interested in a cost-effective, noninvasive, no-side-effects technique to manage stress.
2. Blow bubbles. Invite participation by either passing the bottle around or providing each team member with a personal bottle of bubbles to keep!

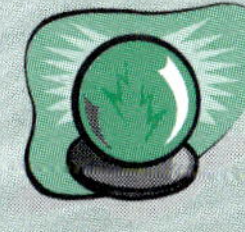

Debriefing

Provide a light discussion on simple things that relieve stress and help us make it through the day.

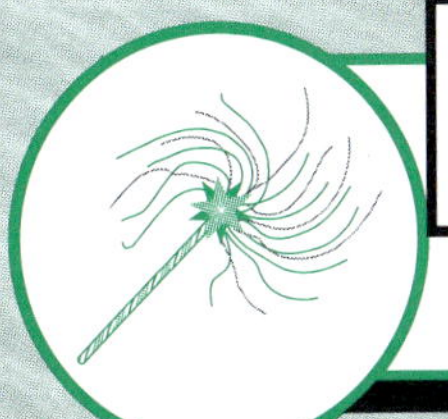

Magic Touch Providing each participant with a small bottle of bubbles is a good take-along reminder that we need to be aware of simple stress relievers.

WANT TO FIND AN EXPERT?

Look in the Mirror

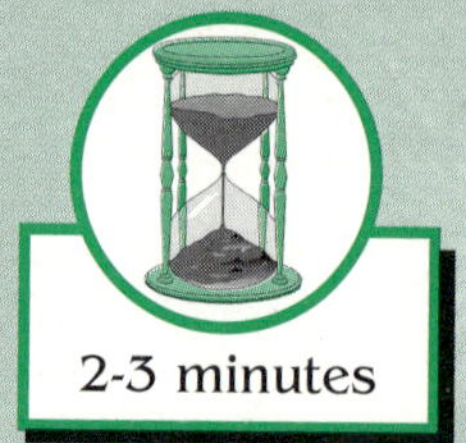

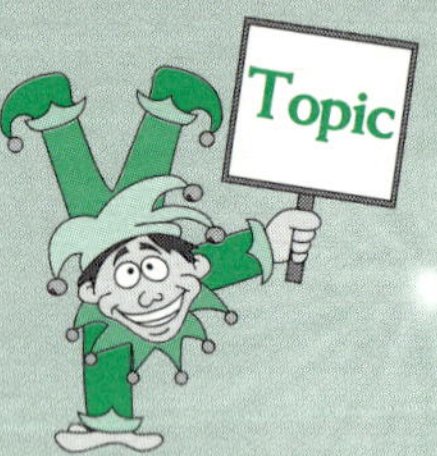

The value of experience. Use for a group impasse.

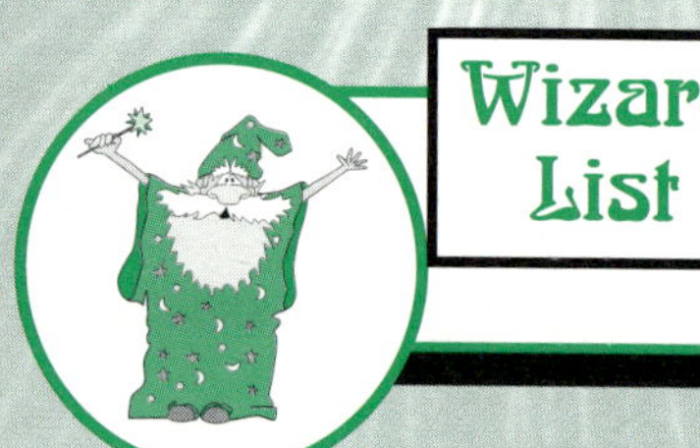

Wizard List Calculator, small note paper, small prize, pens or pencils

Preparation

1. Provide note-sized paper and a pen or pencil for each team member.
2. Provide a small prize.

Implementation

1. Explain that the team members together bring many years of experience to the work of the team, and that, just for fun, you are going to add the total number of years of work experience for the group.
2. Distribute paper and pens or pencils to each participant, and ask them to record a guess.
3. Have participants each tell how many years of experience they have, and ask a team member to add them on the calculator or on paper.
4. Ask who guessed correctly or was the closest, and award the prize.

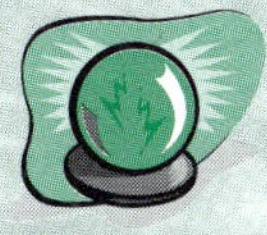

Debriefing

Discuss the value of experience and what it means to a team.

Magic Touch

This activity will probably get a good laugh. Write the number somewhere where the team will see it and refer to it occasionally. No excuses now . . . *We are the experts!*

FOOD FOR THOUGHT

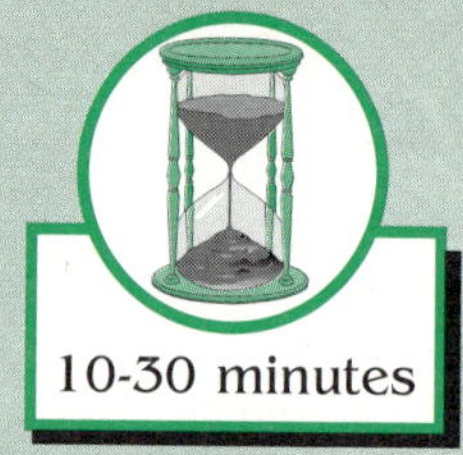

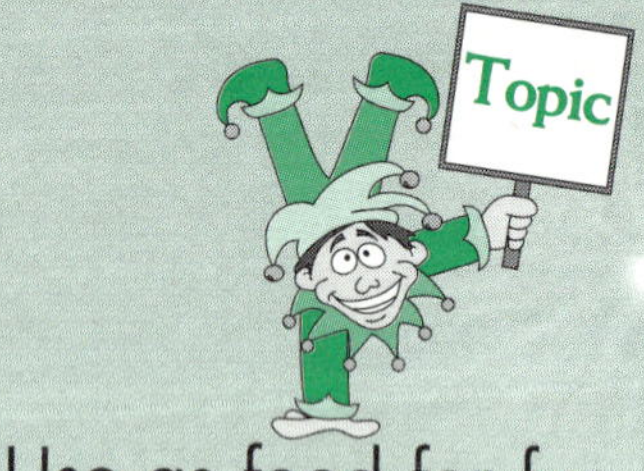

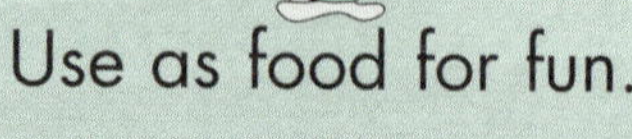

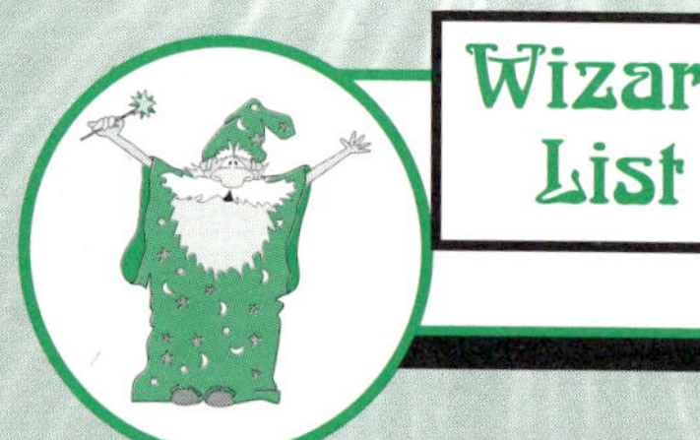

Wizard List

"The Portable Feast," "Pizza," "The Submarine," "The Brainy Brunch," or "A Sundae Party"

Preparation

1. Choose a festive meal or snack. Try to match the food served to an appropriate tie-in.
2. Notify the team that food will be served, or to "Come hungry."
3. Select and post a "Food for Thought" sign. Suggested tie-ins:
   - "The Portable Feast for Thinkers on the Move"—Box lunch with decorative paper tablecloth
   - "Pizza—The Food for Power Thinkers"—Pizza
   - "The Submarine—The Sandwich for Deep Thinkers"—Six-foot-long submarine sandwich
   - "The Brainy Brunch"—Bagels and cream cheese
   - "A Sundae Party for Any Day of the Week"—Ice cream and toppings

Implementation

1. Serve the food.
2. Have fun!

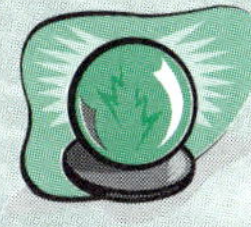

Debriefing

Explain why you chose to serve food at this time: to energize, to reward a task completed, to perk up the team during a difficult step in the process.

Magic Touch

Print your "Food for Thought" sign in color, place it in an inexpensive, plastic stand-up frame, and display it on the food table.

Adapted from: Balzer, Julia W. Humor adds the creative touch to CQI teams. *Journal of Nursing Care Quality.* 8(4):13-19, 1994.

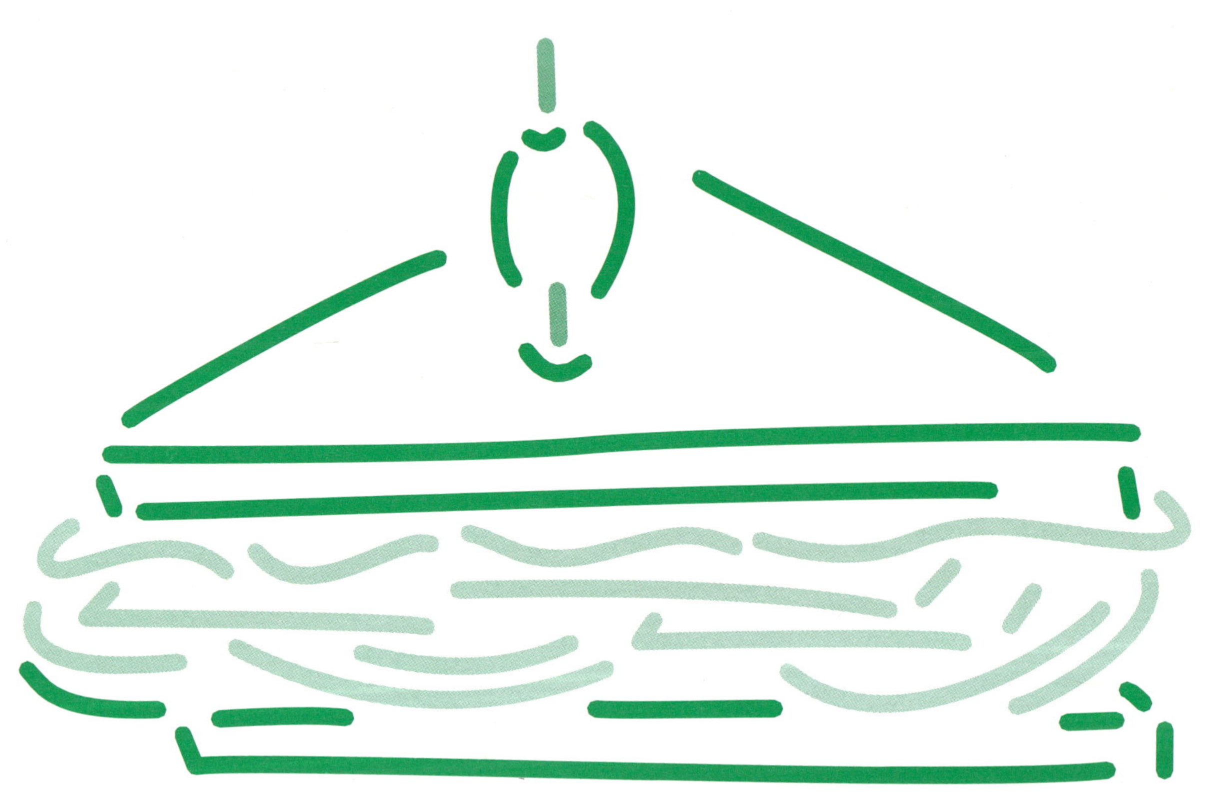

THE PORTABLE FEAST
for Thinkers on the Move

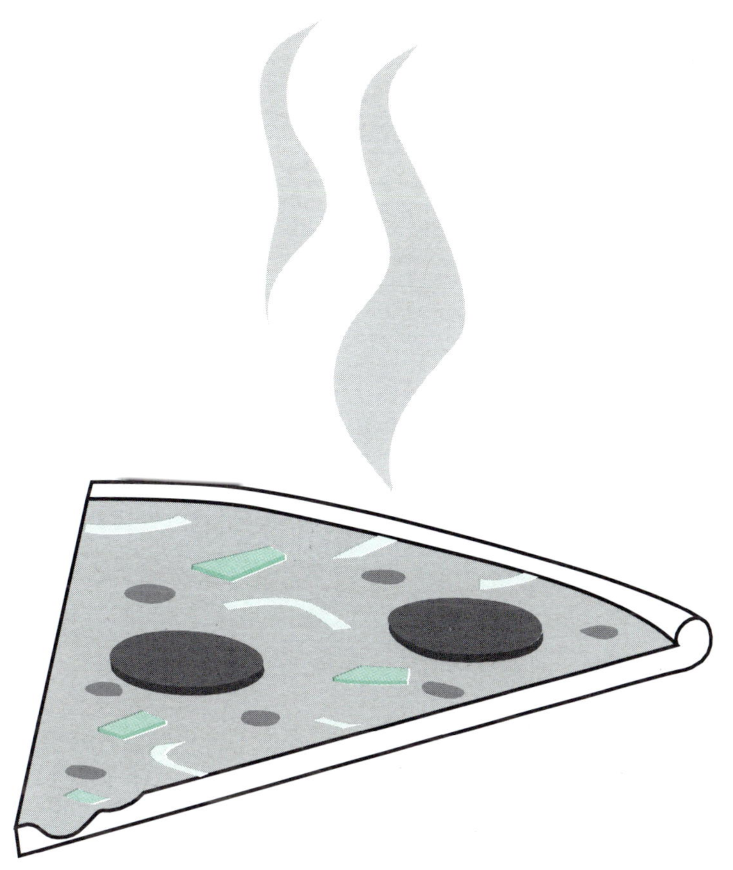

PIZZA

The Food for Power Thinkers

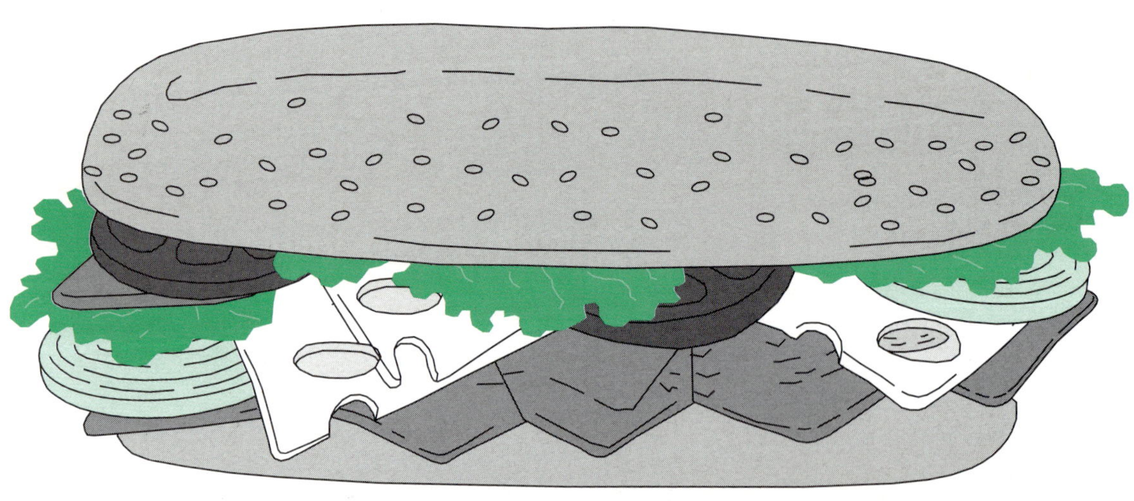

THE SUBMARINE

The Sandwich for Deep Thinkers

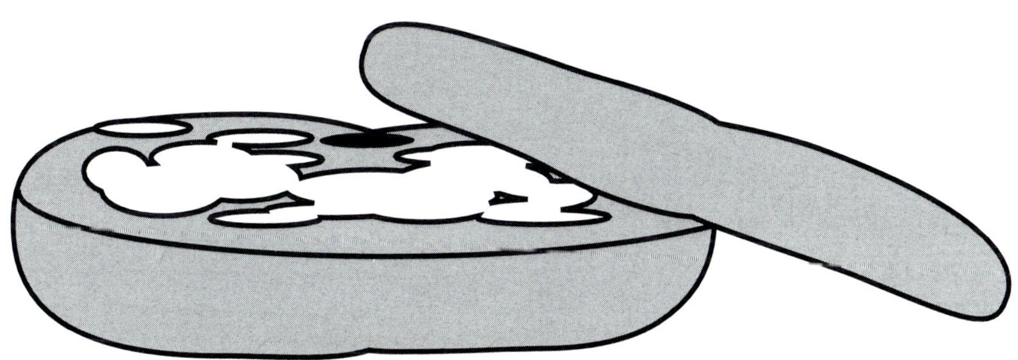

THE BRAINY BRUNCH

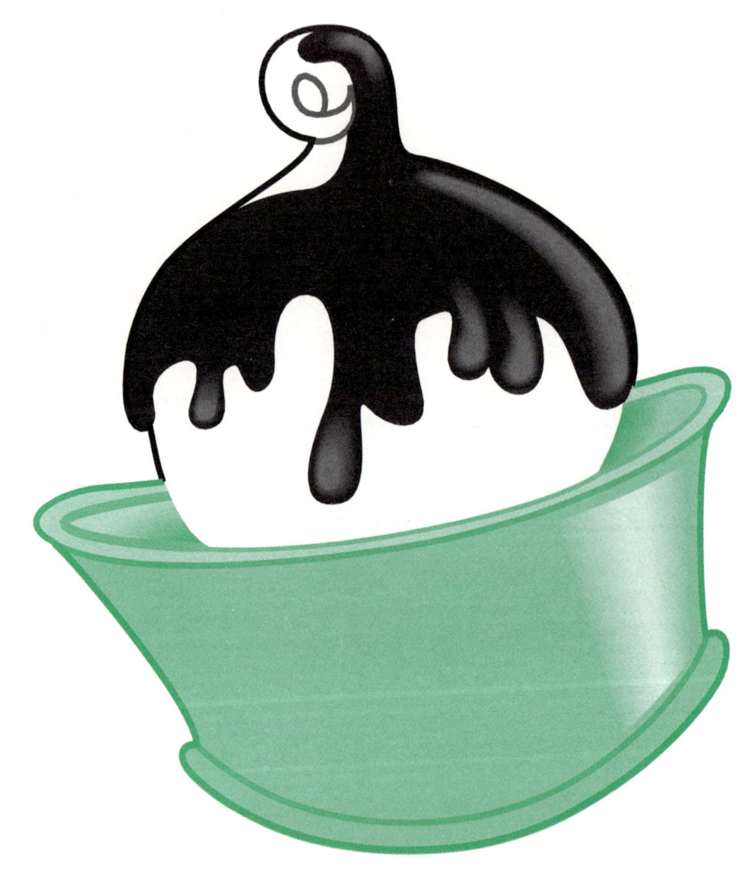

A SUNDAE PARTY
for Any Day of the Week

GROUP RESUME

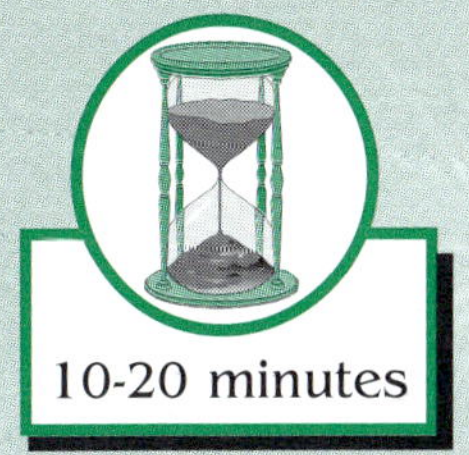

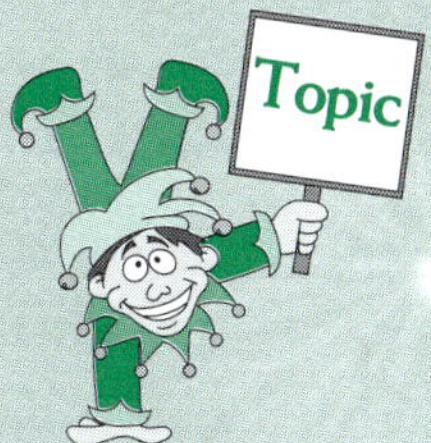

Combined experience. Use this to learn more about team members.

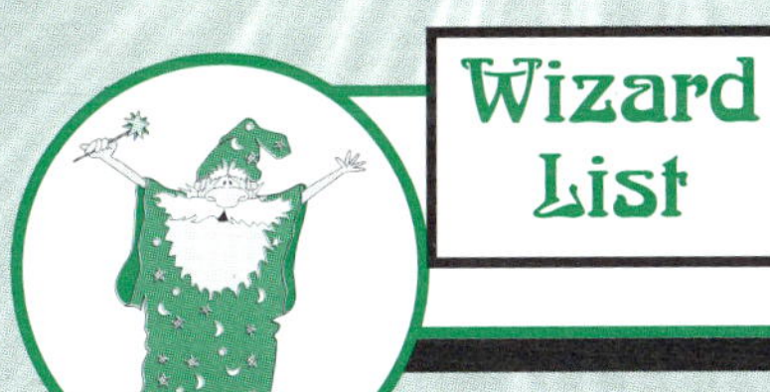

Wizard List

Flip chart, markers, masking tape

Preparation

1. Provide one piece of flip chart paper for every four team members.
2. Provide markers.
3. Bring masking tape.

Implementation

1. Explain that the team members bring rich experiences to the problem-solving process and that sometimes we are unaware of one another's expertise. Explain that the team is going to construct one group resume.
2. Ask for volunteers to write resume categories on the sheets of flip chart paper.
3. Ask the group to generate categories for a resume.
4. Pass the flip chart paper to each member. Have each member write personal information (not in great detail) under each category and then tape the paper to the walls.
5. Review the credentials and experience.

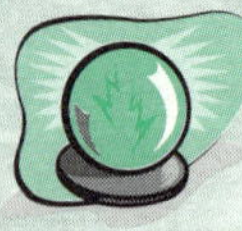

Debriefing

Ask for team members' conclusions, thoughts about the experience, and so forth. Explain that we can work with people a long time and never know the variety of their work experiences and education.

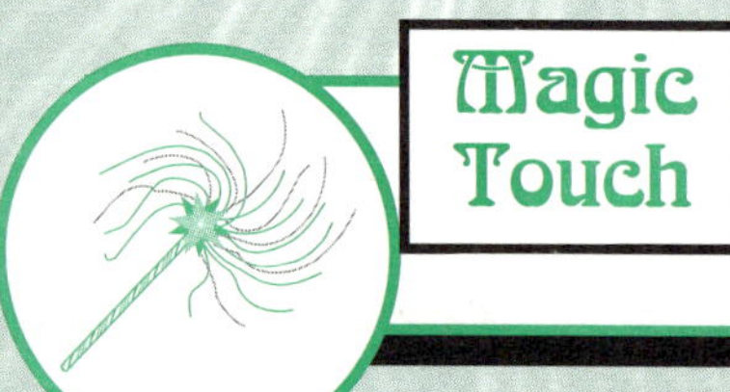

Magic Touch

Reflecting on combined experience provides a sense of quality and gives the team, and its morale, a boost.

PLAY BALL!

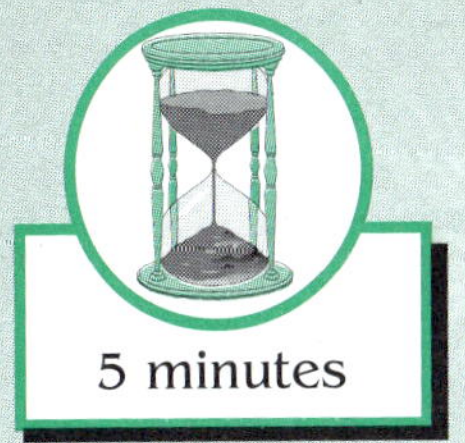

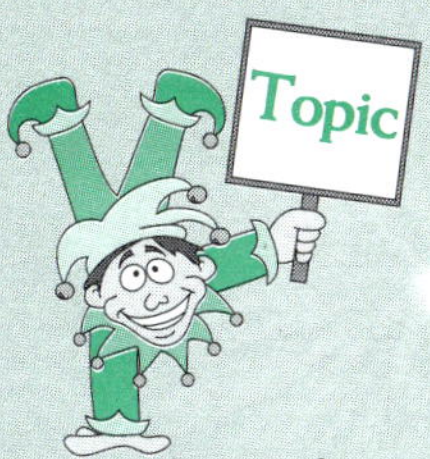

Personal facts. Use for fun or an icebreaker.

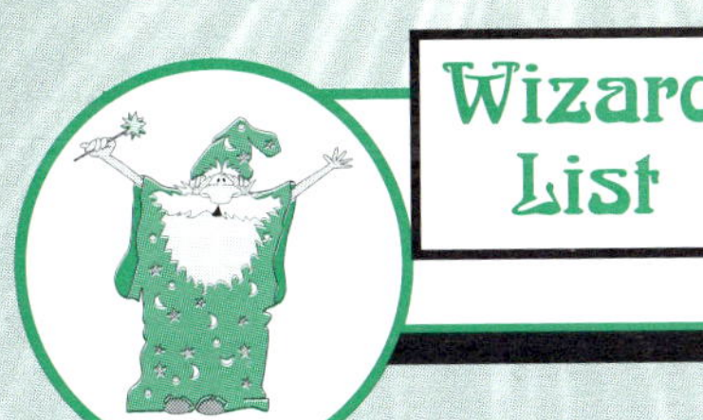

Small, soft ball; whistle; watch with a second hand

Preparation

1. Bring a small, soft ball to the meeting.
2. Bring a whistle and watch with a second hand.

Implementation

1. Announce you are going to warm up the meeting today with a ball game.
2. Explain that each team member is to toss the ball randomly to people on the team. Whoever has the ball in hand must share one fact about his or her life. Give an example from your own life to get the ball rolling.
3. Choose a time limit for playing the game, and announce it to the team.
4. Explain that the sound of the whistle will start and finish the game. Toss the ball to a team member, blow the whistle, and let the game begin!

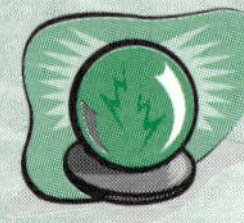

Debriefing

Ask for feedback, and build on this to demonstrate that a little fun and a bit more information about team members make a good warmup for the meeting. Try this activity in the middle of a team meeting if the well of ideas seems dry and a break is needed.

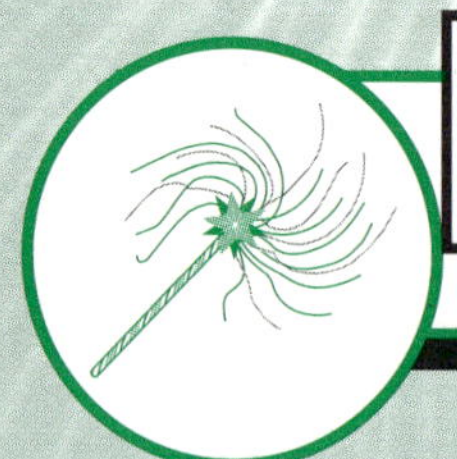

Magic Touch

Check your hat collection for a baseball cap. Wear it and add some zip to the exercise.

TELL ME A STORY

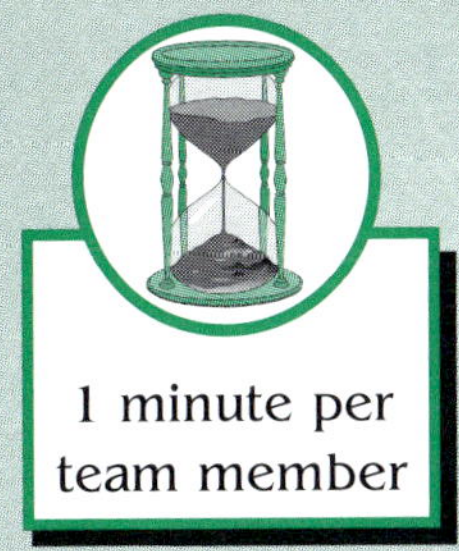

1 minute per team member

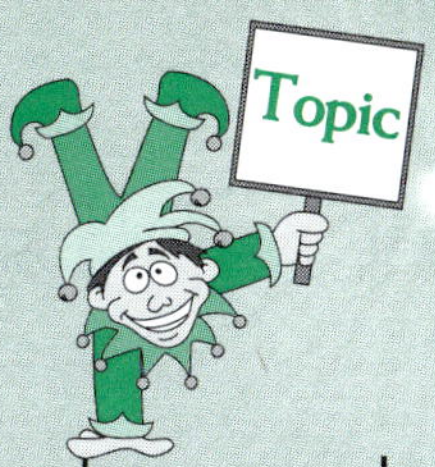

Use to get to know more about group members who have been working together.

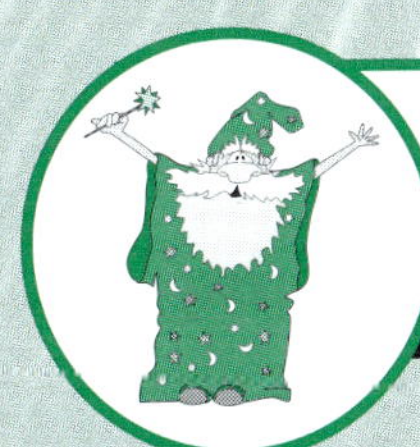

Wizard List

"Tell Me a Story" topics

Preparation

1. Review "Tell Me a Story" topics and select one.

Implementation

1. Suggest that we all have stories to tell, but don't always realize it.
2. State the selected topic and allow 1 minute each for each team member to tell a story.
3. Thank the team members for sharing their stories.

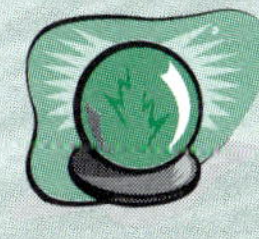

Debriefing

Ask questions to probe for additional information or to make a specific point, but be careful not to make the exercise too long.

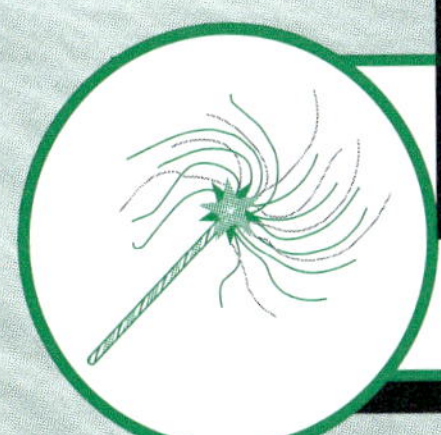

Magic Touch

Telling stories is a fun, safe way to get to know the people with whom you work. It builds trust and speeds the process of learning to work together.

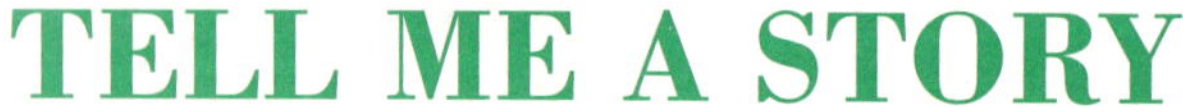

TELL ME A STORY

Topics

1. Can you remember a mentor you have had in your life? What did you learn from the mentor?
2. Recall a favorite movie. Why did you like it?
3. Tell about a memorable person with whom you have worked.
4. Tell about a time you tried to cook something and weren't successful.
5. Tell a story about a trip you would never want to take again.
6. Tell about a holiday or birthday you would like to experience again.
7. Tell about a time you learned something from a child.
8. Tell a story about a favorite pet.
9. Tell about a time when your first impression was wrong.
10. Tell about the time you had a terrible haircut.

Add your own suggestions:

11. ______________________________

____

12. ______________________________

____

13. ______________________________

TELL THE TRUTH

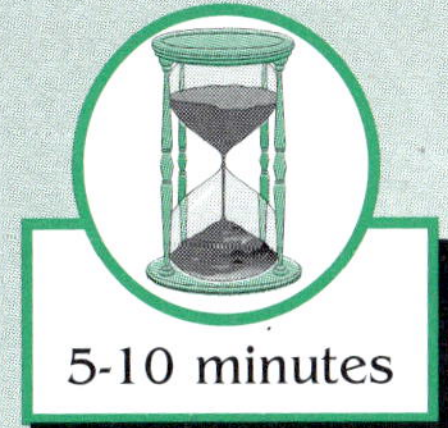

Feedback. Use this to test the climate.

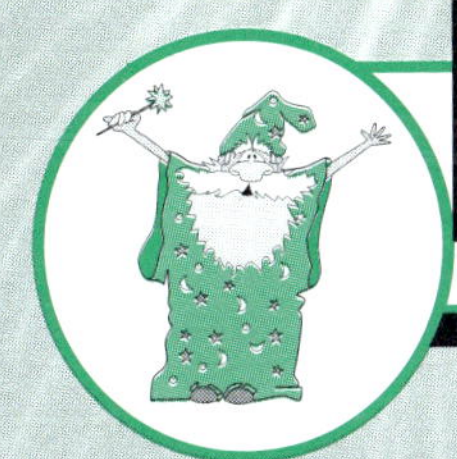

Wizard List "Tell the Truth," pens or pencils

Preparation

1. Copy "Tell the Truth" for each team member.
2. Provide pens or pencils for each team member.

Implementation

1. Explain to the team that you are going to do a quick pretest and posttest of the team's climate.
2. Distribute "Tell the Truth."
3. Ask each member to fill in the dialogue for the first cartoon now and to fill out the caption for the second cartoon at the end of the meeting. Names are optional.

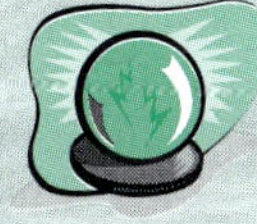

Debriefing

Tell them you will collect them at the end of the meeting for informal feedback.

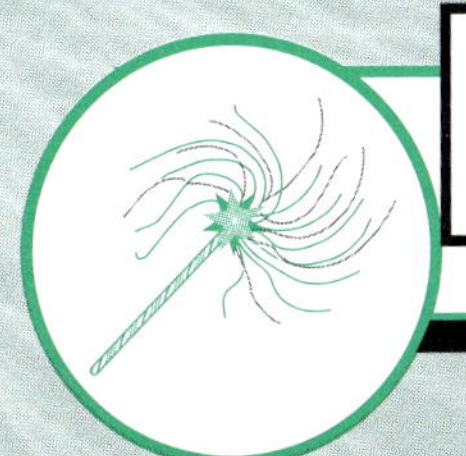

Magic Touch Honest feedback is important to continued success. Never underestimate its worth.

TELL THE TRUTH

Roses are red.
Violets are blue.
What do these cartoons
Say to you?

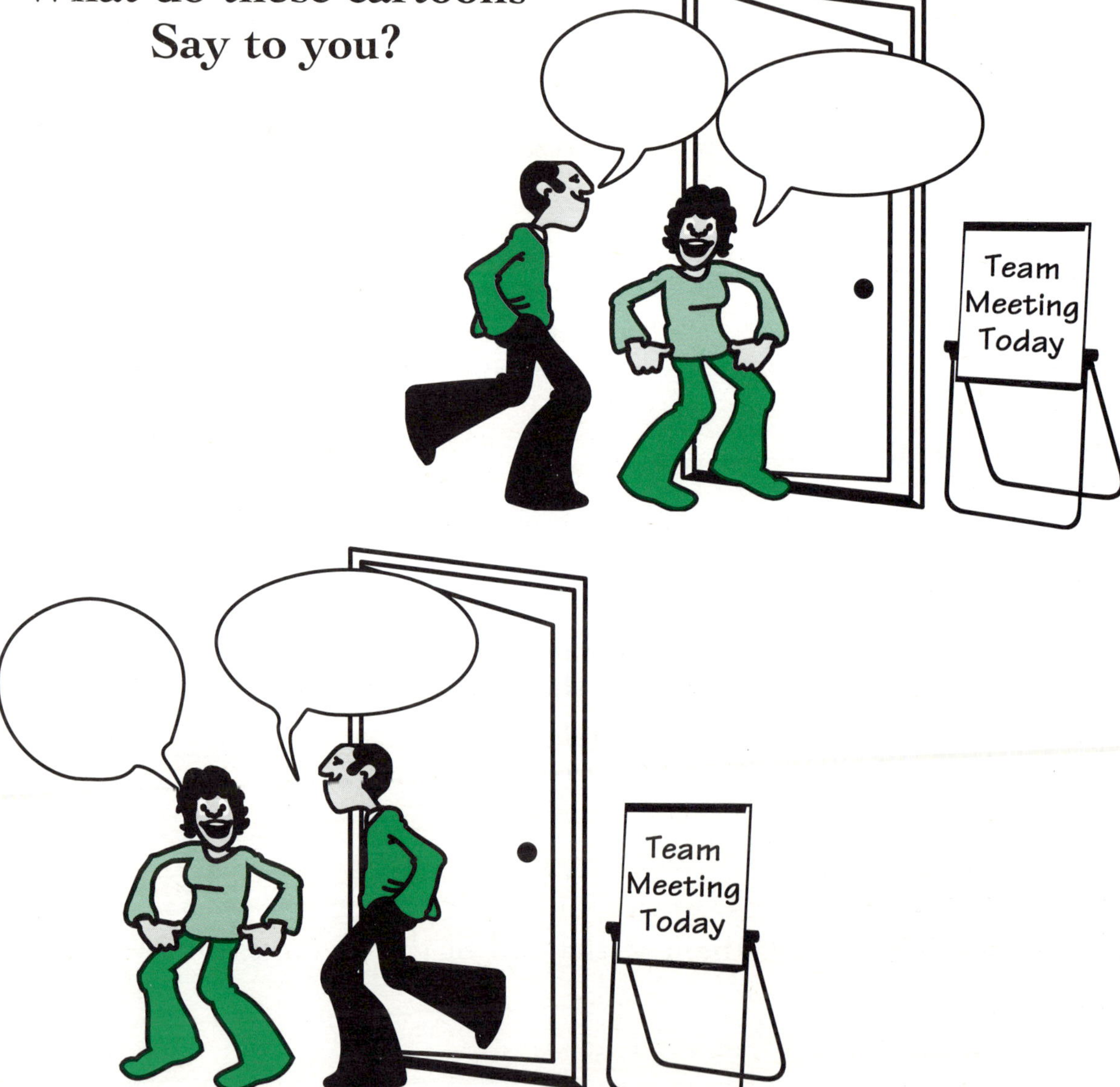

Name (optional)

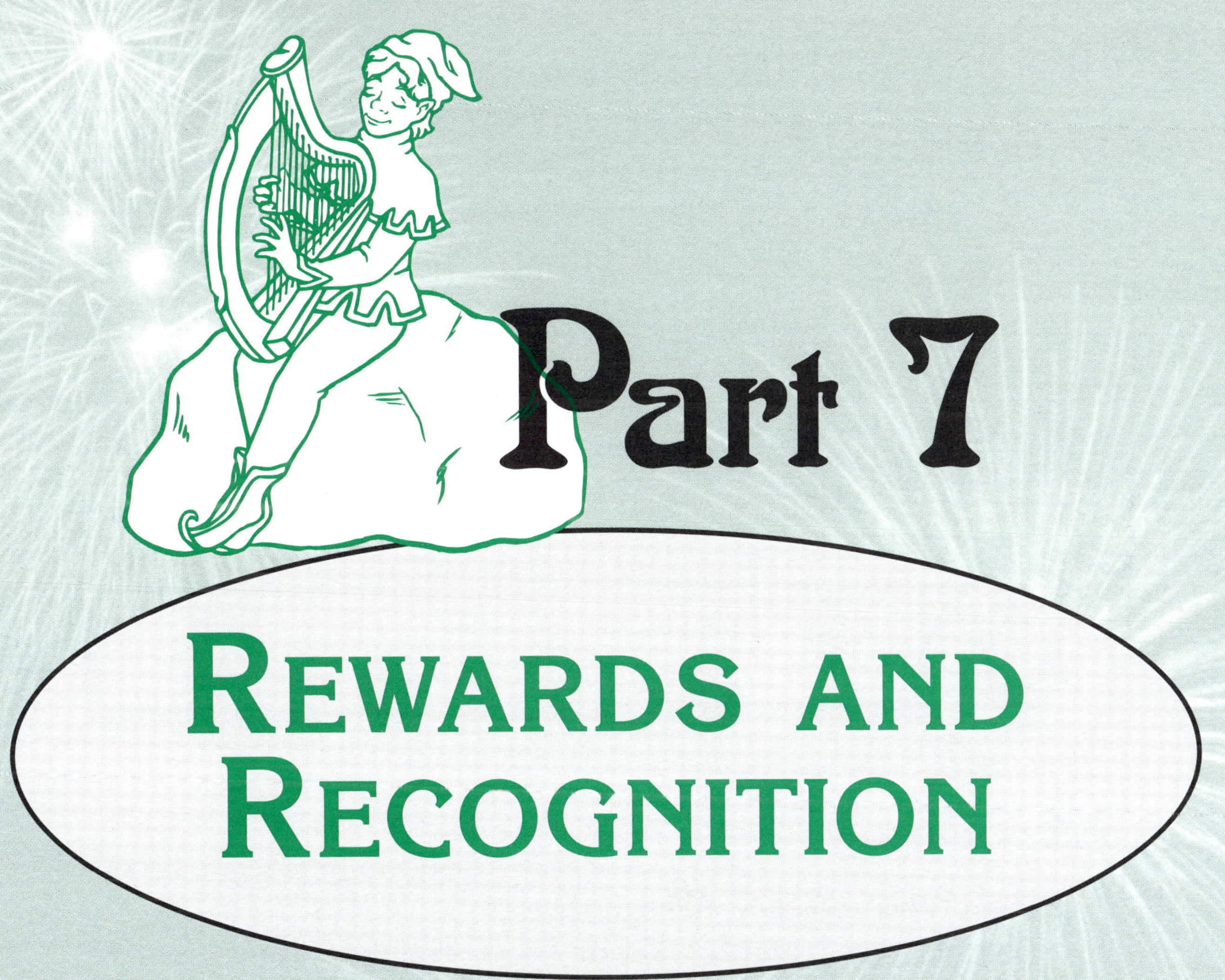

Part 7

Rewards and Recognition

We know that behavior that is rewarded is reinforced. We choose to recognize progress and success, knowing that different forms of recognition are appreciated. Personality style and cultural differences influence what kind of recognition is positive. Here are some activities that have been used successfully to reward individuals, teams, and departments.

Make it a point to ask colleagues in health care and other businesses about their rewards and recognition strategies. Add to the collection and try some of your own . . . psst . . . pass it on!

WHEN SOMETHING IS GOING RIGHT!

Reward and recognition. Use when the team or a team member deserves some recognition.

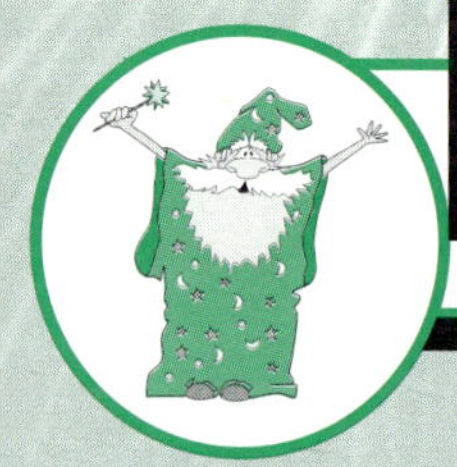

Wizard List "Rewards and Recognition"

Preparation

1. Review "Rewards and Recognition."
2. Select an item from this list or let it stimulate other creative ideas.

Implementation

1. Watch for opportunities that deem reward recognition.
2. Make sure the award/recognition is appropriate.
3. Present the reward in a timely manner.

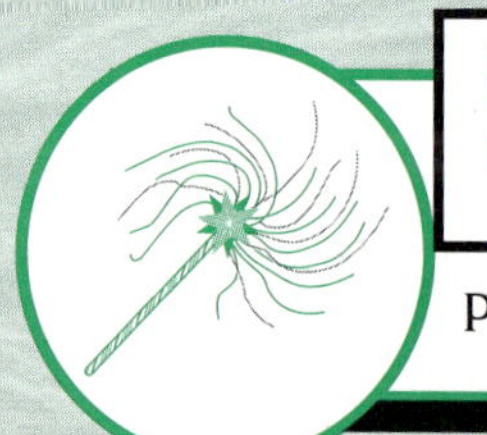

Magic Touch Enough can never be said for positive reinforcement. Use it wisely. A sense of fairness is very important to positive motivation.

REWARDS AND RECOGNITION

Suggestions

Gourmet coffee at meetings
A poem of appreciation shared with a team
Cookies and an appreciation note left at the beginning of a team meeting
A giant "Great Job" memo (Drawn on yellow poster board)
A certificate of appreciation
A basket of candy bars ("Your efforts are worth one-hundred grand"—use the candy bars with this name)
Doughnuts for a staff meeting
Notes of appreciation via E-mail, voice mail, or interoffice mail
An article in the organization's newsletter about an accomplishment
Minutes typed by someone else as a respite
Shared articles about the value of teams and teamwork
A happy song left on voice mail—get a bunch involved and ham it up!
Hugs and Kisses (candy) and a note of appreciation
Praise of an employee shared with that employee's boss
Extra breaks or a long lunch for the team
A card from the group for someone who is having a difficult time
Unsigned notes of praise placed on desks, copier, coffee pot
Flowers placed at someone's work station
A worry stone with a reassuring card
A shared cartoon
An unsolicited letter of recommendation

Add your own!

From a course on rewards and recognition at Athens Regional Medical Center, Athens, Ga.

GO FOR THE GOALS

A Rewarding Experience

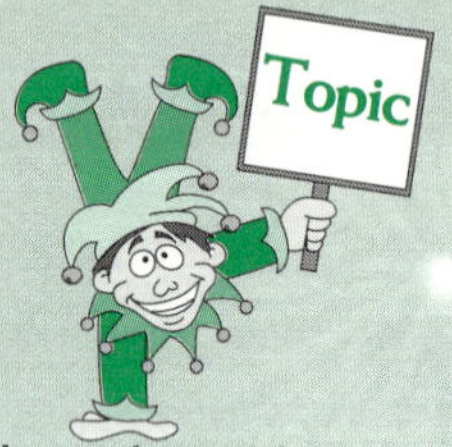

Team recognition. Use to reward behavior, a major goal or breakthrough, or when the team completes its mission.

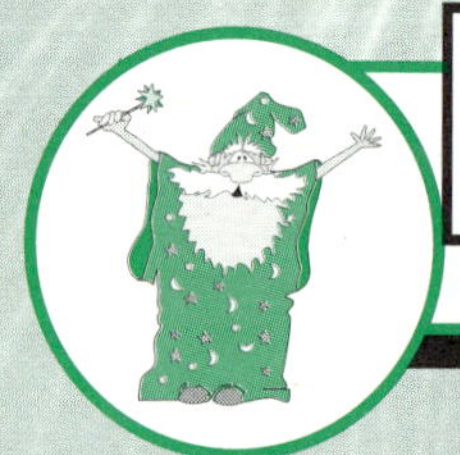

Wizard List

"A Rewarding Experience," gold spray paint, old car parts, glue gun, small pieces of wood

Preparation

1. Review "A Rewarding Experience."
2. Select an idea or use one of your own.
3. Spray paint the selected reward item in gold and glue it to a wood mounting.
4. Make a reward for each participant.

Implementation

1. Announce the award ceremony.
2. Present the awards. (This is the best part.)

Magic Touch

To customize the awards further, have a small brass plate engraved or use a label maker to add the title of the award. Make this a team celebration complete with food and a banner. Use a computer program to make a banner. Involve as many people as possible in getting parts, doing the work, and so forth. It takes a while to make the awards, but it's fun and makes a great impact (former scout leaders or homeroom mothers will love to do this).

By: Jaye Lynn Hall, RN

A REWARDING EXPERIENCE

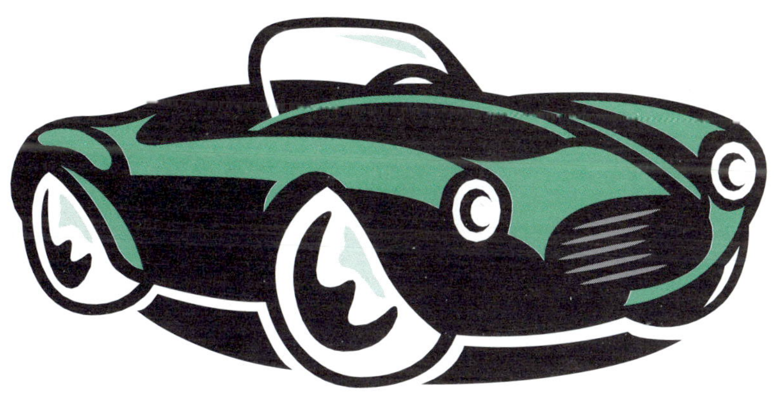

"It takes all my parts to keep me running!"

The Spark Plug Award, for the person who fires us up!

The Turn Signal Award, for the person who keeps us going in the right direction

The Radio Knob Award, for the person who adds music to our life

The Fuel Filter Award, for the person who keeps the negativity out

The Rearview Mirror Award, for the person who carries our history

The Key Award, for the person who gets us started

The Windshield Wiper Award, for the person who clears our vision

You are limited only by your imagination. Let yours go wild. Here is one I can add. How about you?

The Door Handle Award, for the person who helps us handle our disagreements

When They Were Good, They Were Very, Very Good . . .

Special thank-yous. Use to reward or commiserate in the rough spots.

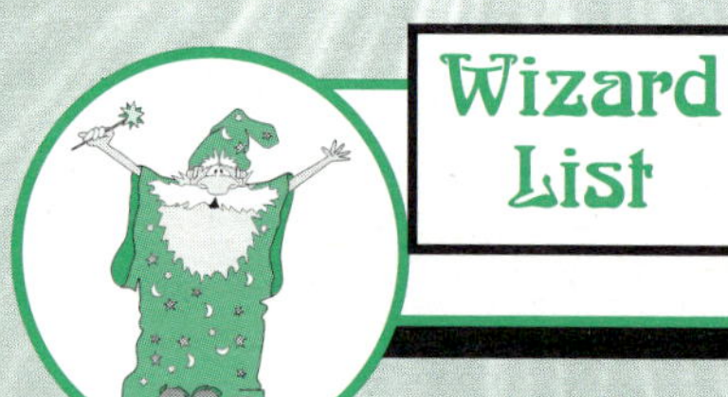

Wizard List

Certificates, "Collecting Coupons"

Preparation

1. Copy an award or coupon and personalize it for the team or individual.
2. Negotiate for possible rewards, such as a free meal.
3. Obtain permission for breaks and time off with the appropriate supervisor.

Implementation

Directions for certificates:

1. Affix one or more fireball candies to the "Whoooee!" certificate.
2. Modify rewards and coupons to fit your needs. (See "Collecting Coupons" page 355.)

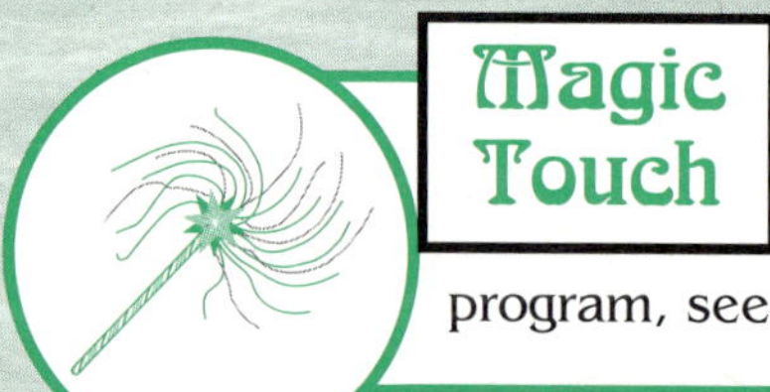

Magic Touch

Distribute with wild abandon; we all need a lift! For an example of an ongoing, hospital-wide recognition program, see "Caring Hands," page 356.

Adapted from: Camilla Bracewell, BS, MA, and Beth Warner

To: ____________________

Whoooee!
What a FIREBALL Presentation Award

Your presentation of the data was *spectacular.* Your delivery was *awesome.* You set the team on fire! **GREAT JOB!**

From : ____________________

Date: ____________________

SPECIAL THANKS!!
SPECIAL THANKS!!

To: ______________________ Date: ______________

Team Name: ______________________

Special thanks for all your help, but especially for your high level of participation in the team.

Your professionalism, dedication, and commitment to high-quality patient care help make this a great place to work.

COLLECTING COUPONS

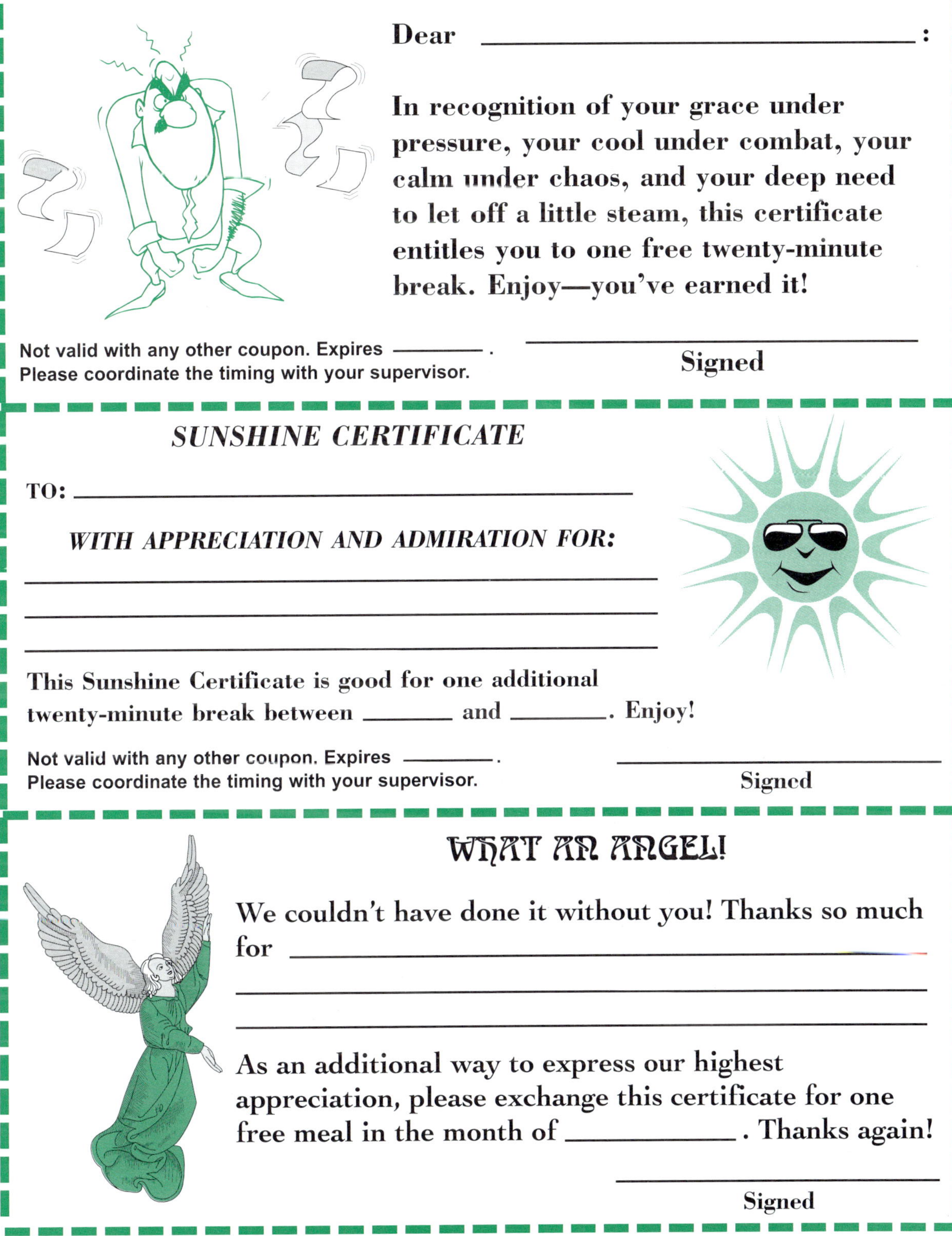

Dear ______________________________:

In recognition of your grace under pressure, your cool under combat, your calm under chaos, and your deep need to let off a little steam, this certificate entitles you to one free twenty-minute break. Enjoy—you've earned it!

Not valid with any other coupon. Expires ________.
Please coordinate the timing with your supervisor.

____
Signed

SUNSHINE CERTIFICATE

TO: ______________________________

WITH APPRECIATION AND ADMIRATION FOR:

____

____

____

This Sunshine Certificate is good for one additional twenty-minute break between ______ and ______. Enjoy!

Not valid with any other coupon. Expires ________.
Please coordinate the timing with your supervisor.

____
Signed

WHAT AN ANGEL!

We couldn't have done it without you! Thanks so much for ______________________________

____

____

As an additional way to express our highest appreciation, please exchange this certificate for one free meal in the month of ____________. Thanks again!

____
Signed

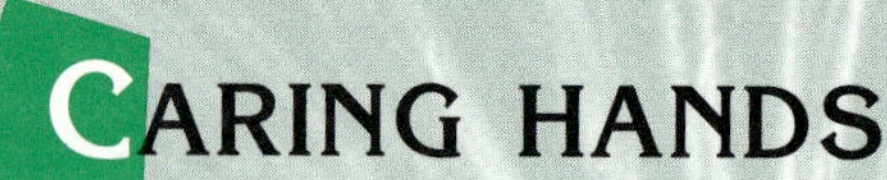

CARING HANDS

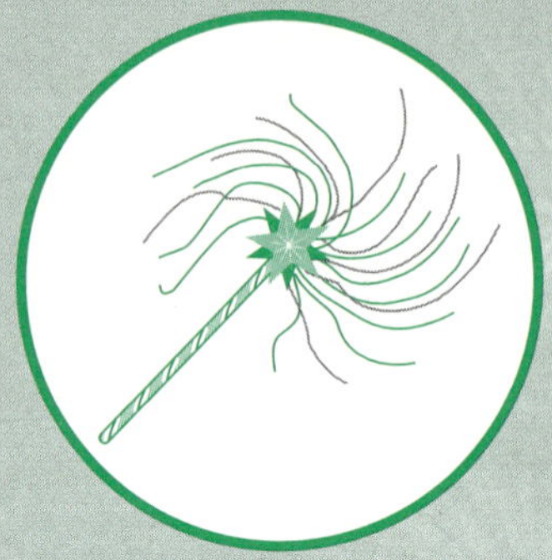

An Example of a Hospital-Wide Reward Program

At Tallahassee Memorial Regional Medical Center in Tallahassee, Florida, Duncan Moore, President and CEO, introduced a staff recognition program based on the story of the *CARING HANDS*. The annual employee recognition gala focuses on these recipients. Following are the story and guidelines for implementation of the program, which were generously shared with permission.

THE CARING HANDS STORY

There is a mission hospital located in the mountains of a very poor country in South America. The country is largely populated by native Indians who live in small, primitive villages and who speak no English. Medical care is limited to a few mission hospitals in various mountain villages.

An international organization reviewing the health care of this country's natives found, to their amazement, that natives would walk for days to get to one particular mission hospital located in one of the country's more inaccessible mountain ranges.

On asking why they came to this particular hospital when they could have gone to one much closer to their village, the natives would answer, "At this hospital, the hands are different."

The study team found that in spite of cultural differences, language barriers, and the great distance over rough terrain, this particular mission hospital had gained the reputation that above all else they truly cared for the natives in everything they did. Thus, the native explanation, "the hands are different."

Likewise, we want people to come to Tallahassee Memorial Regional Medical Center because "the hands are different." In achieving this, we will succeed as few others have.

By: Duncan Moore

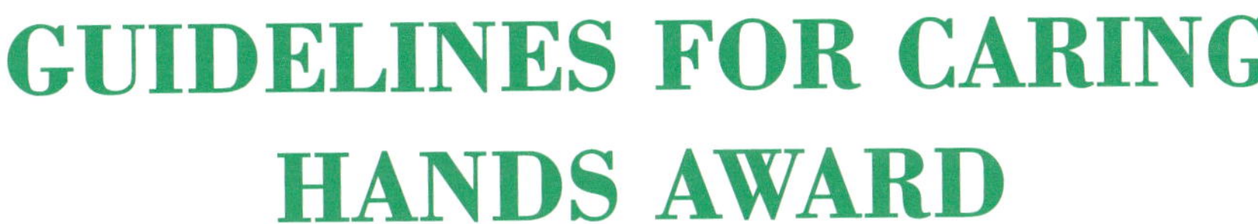

GUIDELINES FOR CARING HANDS AWARD

CRITERIA FOR WINNING A CARING HANDS AWARD

- Nominations to recognize an employee for the award can come from any employee or supervisor.
- We are searching for award-winning activities and caring colleagues.
- Employees can be nominated in any one of the following categories:
  1. Perform an extraordinary singular act that brings credit to the medical center.
  2. Conduct themselves day-in and day-out in such a manner that they are examples for staff to emulate and reinforce the mission and values of the medical center.
  3. Take the time to be different by their attentiveness to their jobs, guest relations, and caring.

CARING HANDS AWARD NOMINATION SHEET

Name of employee to be considered: ______________________

Where they work: ______________________

Who is nominating this employee: ______________________

Date of nomination: ______________________

Reason for nomination: ______________________

Printed with permission from Tallahassee Memorial Regional Medical Center, Tallahassee, Fla.

SEE YOUR NAME IN PRINT

An Invitation to Join the Fun!

How would you like to see your name in print and share your ideas to help others build teams? Yes, we need you! How about sharing your ideas for future editions?

Have you initiated a team activity, exercise, or icebreaker to get the team started, to help establish trust, to teach team dynamics, to facilitate the process, to teach quality improvement tools? Do you have creative or humorous examples of the flow chart, cause-and-effect diagram, or Pareto you could share? What team names do you use?

Please use the form on the following page. Feel free to copy the form and submit as many ideas as you would like! And please supply the following information.

Name: ______________________________

Address: ______________________________

City: ______________ State: ____________ Zip: ____________

Work phone: ____________ Fax: ____________ E-mail: ____________

Home phone: ____________ (authors never sleep)

I can call you for details if you just want to write a brief idea.

Please send your ideas to:

Julia Balzer Riley, RN, MN
P.O. Box 53
Cumming, GA 30128-0053
Toll-free: 800-368-7675
Telephone: 770-844-0584
Fax: 770-844-0280
E-mail: jbriley@mindspring.com

(Suggested Activity Title)

(Suggested Activity Subtitle, if applicable)

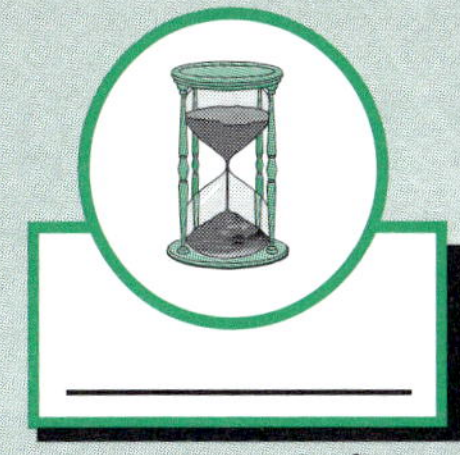

Length of time

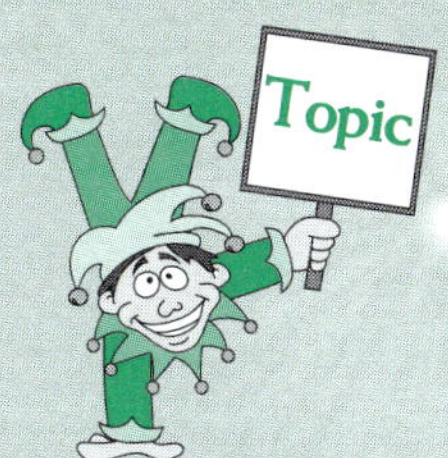

Topic:

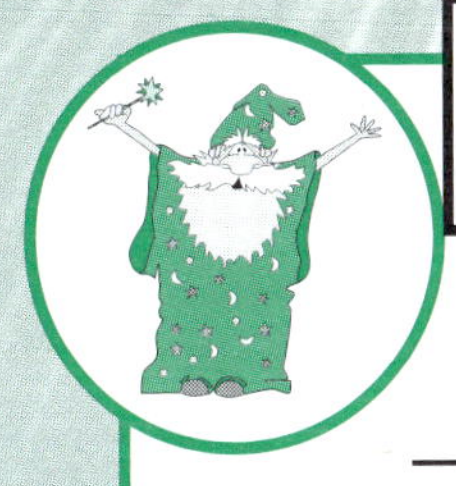

Wizard List (Tools required to implement activity)

Preparation

Implementation

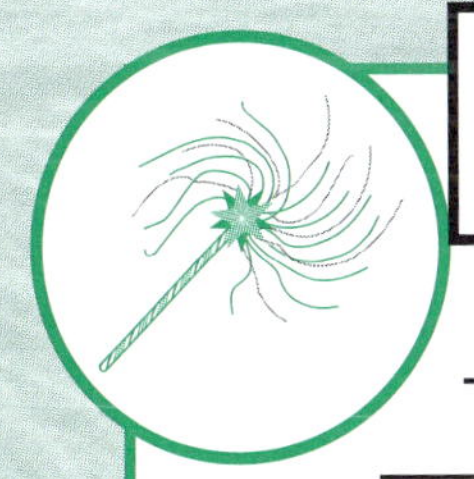

Magic Touch

By:
(Source or author of activity)

RESOURCE LIST

Life-long Learning

Balzer JW: Humor adds the creative touch to CQI teams, *Journal of Nursing Care Quality* 8(4)13-19, July 1994.

Balzer JW: Humor—a missing ingredient in collaborative practice, *Holistic Nursing Practice* 7(4)28-35, 1993.

Balzer Riley, J: *Communications in nursing,* St Louis, 1996, Mosby.

Basso B, Klosek J: *This job should be fun,* Holbrook, MA, 1991, Bob Adams.

Fisher R, Uly W: *Getting to yes: negotiating without giving in,* New York, Penguin.

Garland R: *Making work fun,* San Diego, 1991, Shamrock Press.

Hamilton JM, Kieter ME: *Survival skills for the new nurse,* Philadelphia, 1986, JB Lippincott.

Harrington-Mackin D: *The team building tool kit: tips, tactics, and rules for effective workplace teams,* New York, 1994, AMACOM.

Katz J, Green E: *Managing quality: a guide to system-wide performance management in health care,* St Louis, 1997, Mosby.

Kroeger O, Thuesen JM: *Type talk: the 16 personality types that determine how we live, love, and work,* New York, 1988, Delta.

Lundy JL: *Teams: together each achieves more success,* Chicago, 1992, The Dartnell Corporation.

Martin D: *Team think: using the sports connection to develop, motivate, and manage a winning business team,* New York, 1993, Dutton.

McGee-Cooper A, Trammel D, Lau B: *You don't have to go home from work exhausted,* Dallas, 1990, Bowen & Rogers.

Michalko M: *Thinkpad: a brainstorming card deck,* Berkeley, CA, 1994, Ten Speed Press.

Price Waterhouse Change Integration Team: *Better change: best practices for transforming your organization,* Burr Ridge, IL, 1995, Irwin.

Raben R, Hiyaguha C: *Boldy live as you've never lived before (Unauthorized and unexpected life lessons from Star Trek),* New York, 1995, Morrow.

Schroeder P: *Improving quality and performance: concepts, programs, and techniques,* St Louis, 1994, Mosby.

Schwarz RM: *The skilled facilitator: practical wisdom for developing effective groups,* San Francisco, 1994, Jossey-Bass.

von Oech R: *A kick in the seat of the pants,* New York, 1986, Warner.

von Oech R: *A whack on the side of the head: how to unlock your mind for innovation,* New York, 1986, Warner Books.

von Oech R: *Creative whack pack,* Stamford, CT, 1992, U.S. Games. (An illustrated card deck of ideas to stimulate creative thinking.)

Humor and Health is a newsletter with two purposes: to stimulate a humorous life perspective and to provide information on current developments in humor in medicine, psychology, psychiatry, communication, and human resource development.

Humor and Health, P.O. Box 16814, Jackson, MS 39236-6814.

Conferences, books, and grants for humor projects are available through The Humor Project, Sagamore Institute, 110 Spring Street, Saratoga Springs, NY 12866, (518) 587-8770.